55 Most Common
Medicinal
Herbs

Second Edition

55 Most Common
Medicinal Herbs
Second Edition

The Complete
Natural Medicine Guide

Heather Boon, BScPhm, PhD, and
Michael Smith, BPharm, MRPharmS, ND

Robert
ROSE

For complete cataloguing information, see page 399.

Acknowledgments
We would like to thank the following people for their help in preparing this edition of the book: Bob Hilderley (senior editor) for his patience and guidance through the revision process; Sarah Penney (student, Canadian College of Naturopathic Medicine); Vickie Chang (student, Leslie Dan Faculty of Pharmacy, University of Toronto); and Yuan Zhou (student, Leslie Dan Faculty of Pharmacy, University of Toronto). Without these people's hard work and diligence, the revision of our book would never have been possible.

Disclaimer
This book is a general guide only and should never be a substitute for the skill, knowledge, and experience of a qualified medical professional dealing with the facts, circumstances, and symptoms of a particular case.

The nutritional, medical, and health information presented in this book is based on the research, training, and professional experience of the authors, and is true and complete to the best of their knowledge. However, this book is intended only as an informative guide for those wishing to know more about health, nutrition, and medicine; it is not intended to replace or countermand the advice given by the reader's personal physician. Because each person and situation is unique, the authors and the publisher urge the reader to check with a qualified health-care professional before using any product or procedure where there is a question as to its appropriateness. A physician should be consulted before beginning any exercise program. The authors and the publisher are not responsible for any adverse effects or consequences resulting from the use of the information in this book. It is the responsibility of the reader to consult a physician or other qualified health-care professional regarding his or her personal care.

Editor: Bob Hilderley, Senior Editor, Health
Copy editor: Sheila Wawanash
Design and production: Daniella Zanchetta/PageWave Graphics
Illustrations: Kveta/Three in a Box

We acknowledge the financial support of the Government of Canada through the Book Publishing Industry Development Program (BPIDP) for our publishing activities.

Published by Robert Rose Inc.
120 Eglinton Avenue East, Suite 800, Toronto, Ontario, Canada M4P 1E2
Tel: (416) 322-6552 Fax: (416) 322-6936

Printed and bound in Canada

1 2 3 4 5 6 7 8 9 CPL 17 16 15 14 13 12 11 10 09

To my parents, Shirley and Glenn Boon,
who encouraged me to pursue my academic dreams,
and to my husband, Dr. Albert H.C. Wong, who challenged me
in lively debates regarding the art and science of healing.

– Heather Boon

To my parents, Anne and Jack Smith, for their love, support,
and frequent and much-needed counsel.

– Michael Smith

Contents

PART 2

The Botanical Pharmacy

Foreword

EVERYONE INVOLVED IN the delivery of health care is now aware of the increased interest in complementary and alternative medicine (CAM), especially herbal, or botanical, medicine. According to several recent North American surveys, a growing number of people are using some form of complementary or alternative medicine. In Canada, approximately 70% of the population reports regularly using a natural health product, such as an herb, vitamin, or mineral, but only about 20% of Canadians reported seeing a complementary health-care provider, indicating a high level of self-medication.

Botanical, or herbal, medicine is becoming big business for pharmacists. Almost all retail pharmacies now sell herbal products, and a large proportion of pharmacists report receiving questions about herbs and other natural health products from patients, as well as other members of the health-care team. Although some see botanical medicine as a new "niche" for pharmacy, the debate about whether botanical medicine belongs in pharmacies or in health food stores is becoming heated. The opponents of the sale of botanical products in pharmacies emphasize the fact that most pharmacists have little or no training in this field. Opponents also perpetuate the notion that herbs have not been "scientifically" tested in human studies for their medicinal action and safety. Educating pharmacy students with respect to herbal medicine is increasing, however, and the majority of North American jurisdictions now include some explicit reference to natural health products in standards of practice or guidance documents for pharmacists.

Patients are looking for authoritative information about medicinal herbs — including their effectiveness, safety, and standard dosages — that they can rely on for self-medication and that they can bring to the attention of their physicians or pharmacists. While questions about echinacea and ginseng could once be ignored as a passing trend, health-care professionals are now expected to be knowledgeable about many common herbs. This book is written for the patient and the health-care professional looking for current and authoritative scientific information so as to improve understanding of the medical properties of common herbs and to promote communication between patients and health-care providers.

Initially, this project was planned as a correspondence course with the objective of training pharmacists about botanical medicine. After much deliberation, it was decided that the best approach would be to prepare a series of monographs reviewing the herbal medicines most often seen by pharmacists in

> *This book is written for the patient and the health-care professional looking for current and authoritative scientific information so as to improve understanding of the medical properties of common herbs and to promote communication between patients and health-care providers.*

clinical practice. A very special team had to be created to make sure this project was a success. As one of the primary sites of training in CAM in Canada, the Canadian College of Naturopathic Medicine (CCNM) agreed to manage the day-to-day running of the program. To ensure that the information was correct and balanced, an advisory board of experts was established to review all the material. The majority of the monographs were also submitted to the Canadian Council on Continuing Education in Pharmacy

(CCCEP) for its approval. The project was completed in the summer of 1998 and culminated in the publication of the reference book *The Botanical Pharmacy*, addressed specifically to pharmacists and botanical medicine professionals, in 1999. In 2003, the information was updated to include research conducted in the interim, revised to increase the accessibility of the information for the common reader, and published as *The Complete Natural Medicine Guide to the 50 Most Common Medicinal Herbs*. To prepare this second edition, a complete, systematic review of the scientific literature was conducted for each of the 50 herbs and 5 additional herbs — ashwagandha, bitter orange, hoodia, oregano, and red clover — and a new section on the use of these herbs in managing common health conditions was added as a quick guide for the patient and consumer.

One of the cornerstones of pharmaceutical and medical care is helping patients and customers to make informed decisions about their health care. Likewise, patients owe it to themselves to learn as much as possible about any preventative or therapeutic treatment they may be considering. As patients' options expand to include botanical medicine, or medicinal herbs, as an acceptable form of health care, pharmacists and physicians are being asked to wade through large amounts of information — sometimes reliable, sometimes not — to help patients make the most informed choices possible. When patients choose to make use of botanical products, it is important for pharmacists and physicians to provide monitoring and report adverse effects, as well as herb-drug or herb-herb interactions, when necessary. This role requires pharmacists or physicians who have good working knowledge of botanical medicine and who can apply problem-

solving skills to "fill in the gaps" of our current knowledge of these products.

The authors hope that this book will provide health-care professionals with a foundation of knowledge from which they can with confidence counsel patients about the use of botanical products. For patients and consumers, while this book will not answer all your questions about medicinal herbs, we hope that it will be a useful resource for understanding the safe use of these herbs and for posing informed questions to your pharmacists or physicians. Your good health is what we all want to ensure.

Introduction

Information Sources

In reading this book, it is important to realize not only what medicinal herbs are but also what they are not. Herbal medicine is a complex subject, both a science and an art. No book could cover all the subtle nuances of this fascinating therapy. We have intentionally concentrated on the published scientific material but attempted to incorporate empirical or historical information wherever possible. While many conventional practitioners are not familiar with the traditional elements of herbalism, this empirical knowledge plays a pivotal role in the practice of botanical medicine.

To obtain this information, we conducted extensive searches of Medline, EMBASE, and the Complementary and Alternative Medicine Index. Given that much of the information available on the subject is published in a language other than English — notably, German — a selection of articles was translated for this project.

Legislation

We also consulted the laws governing the manufacture and the sale of herbal medicines in Canada and the United States. Here is a summary of those regulations, designed to ensure safety in using medicinal herbs as drugs and as food.

Canada

In Canada, all botanical medicines are regulated by the federal government as part of a category called natural health products (NHPs). Prior to 2004, all herbs legally for sale in Canada were regulated as either foods or drugs (with drug identification numbers, or DINs) as stipulated by the Food and Drugs Act. The manufacturer of any herb marketed as a food could not print any medicinal claims on the label of the product. In addition, food labeling regulations did not provide for the inclusion of cautions, adverse effects, or other warnings.

Natural Health Products

In response to public demand, the federal Minister of Health created a new Office of Natural Health Products (ONHP) as part of Health Canada in March 1999. The mission of the new office, now known as the Natural Health Products Directorate (NHPD), was to "ensure that all Canadians have ready access to natural health products [including herbs] that are safe, effective and of high quality, while respecting freedom of choice and philosophical and cultural diversity." On January 1, 2004, new regulations governing the manufacture, packaging, labeling, storage, importation, distribution, and sale of natural health products (including herbs) in Canada came into force. The new regulations are part of the current Food and Drugs Act but are specific to NHPs, effectively identifying them as a category distinct from foods and drugs. Requirements apply to all persons who sell NHPs, namely manufacturers, distributors, importers, packagers, and labelers. A transition period of up to 6 years for certain elements of the regulations will allow those affected sufficient time to come into compliance with the new regulations. Detailed information about the regulations is available on the NHPD website at www.hc-sc.gc.ca/dhp-mps/prodnatur/index-eng.php.

> *We have intentionally concentrated on the published scientific material but attempted to incorporate empirical or historical information wherever possible. While many conventional practitioners are not familiar with the traditional elements of herbalism, this empirical knowledge plays a pivotal role in the practice of botanical medicine.*

The definition of a natural health product has two components: a functional and a substance component. The functional component is related to the intended function of a substance and states that NHPs include those substances that are manufactured, sold, or represented for use in

- Diagnosis, treatment, mitigation or prevention of a disease, disorder, or abnormal physical state or its symptoms in humans;
- Restoring or correcting organic functions in humans; or
- Maintaining or promoting health or otherwise modifying organic functions in humans.

The substance component of the NHP definition provides for an "inclusion" list that outlines the medical ingredients that can be contained within NHPs and an "exclusion" list that specifically identifies those substances that are not considered NHPs.

For herbal medicines, the inclusion list specifically identifies that the following will be classified as NHPs:

- Plant or plant material, alga, fungus, or non-human animal material;
- Extract or isolate of this material, the primary molecular structure of which is the same as that which it had prior to its extraction or isolation, as natural health products.

In addition, the NHPD and the Food Directorate provide a list of herbs that are considered NHPs, regardless of their dosage form. These specific herbs are not allowed to be sold as foods because of their known physiologic or pharmaceutical properties and lack of food purpose. This list is available on the NHPD website.

Under the new regulations, all NHPs sold in Canada require product licenses. The intent of requiring pre-market approval is to provide a mechanism for assessing and managing the benefits and risks associated with the use of NHPs. The regulations set out the requirements — including the quantity of the medical ingredients, the purpose for which the NHP is intended to be sold, and supporting safety and efficacy data — for submitting an application for a product license.

Site licenses are also required for all buildings where NHPs are manufactured, packaged, or labeled prior to sale. In addition, importers and distributors require a site license for all locations where NHPs are stored and handled prior to sale. One of the key prerequisites for obtaining a site license is the adoption and maintenance of good manufacturing practices (GMPs). Details about the good manufacturing practice standards for natural health products, developed in consultation with stakeholders, is available on the NHPD website. This document provides standards for control of materials, process control, a self-inspection program, a contractor inspection program, recall procedures, quality control, assessment of stability, record keeping, sterilization procedures, testing of samples, and reporting recalls. In recognition of the diversity in capacity among industry stakeholders, the GMPs are results- and outcomes-based — they do not dictate the processes used to achieve the results.

NHP Labels

The new regulations focus on ensuring that NHP labels will assist consumers in selecting products that meet their particular needs and expectations, and in understanding the merits and limitations of the products they choose. Among other things, all NHP labels are required to contain the following information:

- Brand name
- Product number (issued with the product license, preceded by the designation NHP or, in French, PSN)
- Dosage form
- Net amount of the NHP in terms of weight, measure, or number

- Name and address of the product license holder
- Proper name and, if any, the common name of each medicinal ingredient
- Strength or potency of the medicinal ingredients (by proper name)
- Qualitative list of all non-medicinal ingredients
- Recommended use or purpose
- Recommended route of administration
- Recommended dose and, if any, the duration of use
- Risk information relating to the NHP, including any cautions, warnings, contraindications, or known adverse reactions associated with the use of that NHP
- Recommended storage conditions, if any
- Lot number
- Expiration date
- Description of the source material from which the medicinal ingredients are derived or obtained (e.g., root of the plant)
- Key information, as designated by the regulations, must be provided in both French and English. Any other language(s) may used in addition.

The new regulations focus on ensuring that NHP labels will assist consumers in selecting products that meet their particular needs and expectations, and in understanding the merits and limitations of the products they choose.

Standards of Evidence

A standards of evidence framework has been developed in conjunction with the new regulations. The aim of this framework is to ensure that product claims are supported by appropriate evidence, which can include both scientific and traditional evidence, depending on the type of claim being made. All claims must be pre-approved by the NHPD before the product is granted a license.

The Licensed Natural Health Products Database (LNHPD), available on the NHPD website, provides a list of all natural health products currently licensed in Canada. By 2010, all natural health products legally sold in Canada are expected to have product licenses.

The United States

In the United States, herbal products are regulated as dietary supplements as defined by the Dietary Supplement Health and Education Act (DSHEA) of 1994. This definition also encompasses nutritional supplements, such as vitamins, minerals, amino acids, and botanical medicines. Companies marketing "dietary supplements" cannot make specific therapeutic claims regarding their products (i.e., about using them to diagnose, prevent, mitigate, treat, or cure a specific disease). However, they may make "statements of nutritional support" or "structure and function claims" (statements explaining how the product may affect the structure of function of the body) and "general health claims" (claims about the effects on "well-being" achieved by consuming the supplement). Under the DSHEA regulations, manufacturing companies may also indicate to customers possible areas of concern, such as potential side effects and contraindications.

Manufacturers are required to ensure that they can substantiate any claim made and that any statements made about their products are truthful and not misleading, but they are not required to seek pre-approval from the Food and Drug Administration (FDA). In all cases where the claims have not been approved by the FDA, the following disclaimer must be placed on the label: "This statement has not been evaluated by the Food and Drug Administration. This product is not intended to diagnose, treat, cure or prevent any disease."

In response to concerns about product quality, US regulatory authorities are implementing good manufacturing practices for herbal products.

Botanical Dosage Forms

Herbal medicines are prepared in a variety of forms, including teas, liquids, solids, and standardized extracts.

Herbal Teas: Decoctions and Infusions

A time-honored method of taking herbal medicines is in the form of a tea. There are primarily two kinds: decoctions and infusions. A decoction is normally reserved for fibrous plant material, such as stems, bark, roots, and rhizomes, and is made by boiling the plant material until it is reduced to a specific volume. Steeping the more delicate plant parts (flowers, leaves) in either hot or cold water makes an infusion. The temperature of the water will influence the constituent extracted.

The use of these dosage forms is often limited by poor palatability and the fact that only water-soluble constituents are extracted.

Liquid Dosage Forms: Tincture and Fluid (Liquid) Extracts

A tincture is made by macerating or percolating the plant material in a mixture of water and alcohol. The components extracted are determined by the ratio of alcohol to water used in the solvent. While the percentage of alcohol can be as high as 90%, it is more commonly in the range of 25% to 60%. The strength of the tincture is usually given as the ratio of solid herbal product used compared to the total volume of the solution. The most common range is between 1:3 and 1:5 (plant: total solution).

A fluid (liquid) extract is also a hydroalcoholic product, but in these products, one unit of the preparation is equivalent to one unit of the original plant product (i.e., they are more concentrated than tinctures). While this increased potency definitely has its advantages, questions have been raised about the way in which some commercial products are manufactured. Many of the commercially available fluid extracts are made by simply evaporating the solvent from a tincture and then reconstituting the residue to the appropriate volume. This method can cause degradation of the more unstable constituents.

> *Manufacturers are required to ensure that they can substantiate any claim made and that any statements made about their products are truthful and not misleading, but they are not required to seek pre-approval from the Food and Drug Administration (FDA).*

Unfortunately, in practice, the terms "tincture" and "fluid extract" are often used interchangeably. In addition, it is uncommon for liquid dosage forms to indicate either alcohol content or strength on the label. Tincture and fluid (liquid) extracts are usually ingested in a little water. Using warm water causes most of the alcohol present to evaporate, thus reducing its undesirable effects. These dosage forms have the advantage of containing both alcohol and aqueous soluble components and of allowing prescribers to combine herbs. As with herbal teas, poor palatability is often a problem.

A glycerite is a tincture-like product in which glycerin is used as a solvent. These preparations appear to be particularly useful in the management of pediatric conditions or where alcohol is strictly contraindicated.

Solid Dosage Forms

Herbal medicines are available in a range of solid doses, including capsules, tablets, freeze-dried products, and lozenges. While capsules usually simply contain the dried herbs, tablets are often made from concentrates. Concerns have been raised regarding the small quantity of herbs often contained in these dosage forms.

Standardized Extract

A standardized extract is a product in which a specific concentration of a particular constituent or group of constituents is guaranteed. While all the original constituents may still be present, they are often not in the proportions found in the original herb. While this approach is attractive to the conventional medical model, it depends on the existence, extraction, and identification of a discrete single active constituent or group of constituents. The effect of this approach on the synergy reputed by herbalists to exist between components has yet to be clarified.

To assure quality, some preparations may be standardized to a "marker" component guaranteeing that the correct plant was harvested and used. This marker agent need not necessarily be the active constituent.

> *A standardized extract is a product in which a specific concentration of a particular constituent or group of constituents is guaranteed.*

Dosage Considerations

Botanical medicine is not practiced in a homogeneous manner. Different groups follow distinct philosophies that favor specific dosage systems. Suggested dose regimens may come from herbal traditions (Chinese, Ayurvedic), established European pharmacopoeias, or clinical and pharmacological evaluation. This situation presents the practitioner and consumer with a dilemma regarding a standard dosing regimen for any given herb. As a general rule, doses used by practitioners trained in North America are usually lower than those used by their European counterparts. For this project, the authors have attempted to include a variety of dosage regimens commonly seen in North America.

Safety Issues

A misconception often shared by practitioners and the public alike is that complementary therapies are completely safe. Unfortunately, this is not the case. Adverse effects from a number of complementary therapies, including botanical medicine, have been noted. The dangers of complementary medicine can be classified as falling into one of four categories.

Sins of Omission

Sins of omission are those in which the patient deteriorates because the CAM practitioner does not recognize the seriousness of the condition and does not refer the patient to appropriate medical care. The quality of education and the professional character of complementary health-care providers play a role in determining both their safety and competence. While many "professional" associations of Canadian herbal practitioners do exist, none have the authority to regulate the practice. With the exception of the practice of naturopathic medicine in Ontario, Manitoba, Saskatchewan, and British Columbia, no federal or provincial regulations exist for the practice of herbal medicine. This results in little uniformity between herbal practitioners. Cases in which a patient self-medicates inappropriately would also fall in this category.

Intrinsic Procedural Risks

Intrinsic procedural risks are those arising as a direct result of the administration of the therapy. Examples of adverse reactions that result directly from the use of a specific herbal product, including allergic responses, have been reported. Complications and ill effects have also been noted due to misidentification of the herbal content, intentional or unintentional adulteration of the product with heavy metals or pharmaceuticals, and suspected interactions with conventional medication.

> *A misconception often shared by practitioners and the public alike is that complementary therapies are completely safe. Unfortunately, this is not the case.*

Situational Amplifications

Situational amplifications occur in cases where CAM therapy aggravates an existing condition. The use of some herbs, especially as part of a "detoxifying" protocol, may exacerbate a patient's condition at the onset of treatment. Critical and objective evidence on the use of herbal medicines in certain populations, such as children, the elderly, or pregnant women, is lacking. Most information in this area comes from anecdotal and historical sources, the importance of which has yet to be investigated.

Worthless Procedures

The final category is the delivery of worthless procedures for financial or other gains on part of the practitioner. Unfortunately, as the popularity of "natural" medicine increases, so does the opportunity for misrepresentation of its use. This is especially a concern when effective treatment, either conventional or unconventional, exists for the condition.

Caveat Emptor

One aim of this book is to protect patients from these dangers by providing the most current and accurate information available on the 55 common herbs reviewed, including clearly identifying any false or dubious claims, adverse effects, cautions or contraindications, and drug interactions. Although herbal medicines have been shown to be effective for preventing and treating health problems, we are not advocating any single herb or herbal procedure, nor are we suggesting that medicinal herbs can replace other conventional drug treatments for serious illness. We strongly recommend that you consult with your doctor, medical or naturopathic, and your pharmacist before taking any medicinal herb for any health condition. Irrespective of the amount of evidence for a particular herbal medicine, many conditions can only be treated safely and effectively after consultation with an appropriately trained health-care professional.

Book Format

This book has two sections: Medicinal Herbs for Common Health Conditions and The Botanical Pharmacy. The first section will assist you in quickly identifying the herbs used in managing 55 specific common health conditions, from acne to yeast infections. For most health conditions, several herbs are briefly listed, which can then be explored in detail in the second section of this book, where the relevant research or scientific literature for the medical action of each of 55 herbs is reviewed.

> *We strongly recommend that you consult with your doctor, medical or naturopathic, and your pharmacist before taking any medicinal herb for any health condition.*

Like the book as a whole, the information for each herb reviewed in the Botanical Pharmacy section increases in level of complexity, with a thumbnail sketch providing a concise summary of the entire review, the introduction a presentation of basic botanical information, and the section titled "Relevant Research" a summary of published scientific studies and empirical evidence.

Scholars of botanical medicine and clinicians can pursue this research further at the IN-CAM website (www.incamresearch.ca), where the medical literature on each herb is fully documented. Reviews of new research studies and clinical trials will be posted on this site from time to time.

The book thus unfolds from section to section, gaining in complexity, and offers ongoing access to the best information available.

Selected References

Baseline Natural Health Products Survey Among Consumers, March 2005 (http://www.hc-sc.gc.ca/dhp-mps/pubs/natur/eng_cons_survey-eng.php); accessed Sept 24, 2008.

Boon H, Hirschkorn K, Griener G, Cali M. The ethics of dietary supplements and natural health products in pharmacy practice: A systematic documentary analysis. International Journal of Pharmacy Practice 2008; in press.

Charrois T, Hill R, Vu D, et al. Community pharmacist survey of natural health product adverse events and drug interactions. Annals of Pharmacotherapy 2007;41:1124–29.

Chevallier A. The Encyclopedia of Medicinal Plants. Westmount, Quebec: Readers Digest, 1996.

Dietary Supplement Health and Education Act of 1994. U.S. Food and Drug Administration Center for Food Safety and Applied Nutrition, 1995 (http://www.cfsan.fda.gov/~dms/dietsupp.html); accessed May 2, 2006.

Dvorkin L, Gardiner P. Regulation of dietary supplements in the United States of America. Clinical Research and Regulatory Affairs 2003;20(3):313–25.

Ernst E. Interactions between herbal medicinal products and synthetic drugs. International Journal of Risk & Safety in Medicine 2000;13(2–3):77–79.

Ernst E. Possible interactions between synthetic and herbal medicinal products Part 1: A systematic review of the indirect evidence. Perfusion 2000;1:4–15.

Farrell J, Reis N, Boon H. Pharmacists and natural health products: a systematic analysis of legal responsibilities in Canada. Pharmacy Practice 2008;6(1):33–42.

Johnson T, Boon H, Jurgens T, et al. Canadian pharmacy students' knowledge of herbal medicine. American Journal of Pharmacy Education 2008;72(4):article 75.

Kwan D, Boon H, Hirschkorn K, Welsh S, Jurgens T. Consumers' influence on pharmacists' professional responsibilities with respect to natural health products. BMC Complementary and Alternative Medicine 2008;8(40).

Kwan D, Hirschkorn K, Boon H. U.S. and Canadian pharmacists' attitudes, knowledge, and professional practice behaviors toward dietary supplements: a systematic review. BMC Complementary and Alternative Medicine 2006;6(31).

Natural Health Products Directorate. Licensed Natural Health Products Datatbase (http://www.hc-sc.gc.ca/dhp-mps/prodnatur/applications/licen-prod/lnhpd-bdpsnh-eng.php); accessed Sept 24, 2008.

Natural Health Products Directorate. Site Licensing (http://www.hc-sc.gc.ca/dhp-mps/prodnatur/applications/licen-site-exploit/index-eng.php); accessed Sept 24, 2008.

Natural Health Products Directorate of Health Canada. Natural Health Products (http://www.hc-sc.gc.ca/dhp-mps/prodnatur/index-eng.php); accessed Sept 24 2008.

Natural Health Products Directorate Health Products and Food Branch Health Canada. Product Licensing (http://www.hc-sc.gc.ca/dhp-mps/prodnatur/applications/licen-prod/index-eng.php); accessed Sept 24, 2008.

Park J. Use of alternative health care. Health Reports (Statistics Canada) 2005;16(2):39–42.

Williamson E. Drug interactions between herbal and prescription medicines. Drug Safety 2003;26(15):1075–92.

PART 1

Medicinal Herbs for Common Health Conditions

Preface

FOR CENTURIES, HERBAL doctors in many different cultures worldwide have recommended herbs for treating various health conditions. While these remedies carry with them the authority of folk wisdom, only relatively recently have herbs been tested using conventional scientific methods to assess their efficacy in treating illness and promoting good health. *55 Most Common Medicinal Herbs: The Complete Natural Medicine Guide* presents the "Traditional Use" for each herb discussed, which in some cases has been verified in controlled clinical trials, as well as the "Current Medicinal Use" of each herb, which is based on existing scientific research and medical evidence. When you look at all the evidence, both traditional and scientific, a single herb can have many uses.

In this section of the book, the medical background of 55 common health conditions is briefly described and the medicinal herbs used to treat these conditions, traditionally and currently, are summarized and evaluated. Fascinating folklore and facts about these herbs are briefly presented in snippets derived from the second section of the book, where you will find a complete botanical pharmacy if you want to know more about any herb listed in the first section.

The general aim of this book is to help you make informed choices about herbal medicines, not to make recommendations or present prescriptions. Be sure to consult a qualified health-care professional for more information on the use of these herbs for specific health conditions.

Acne (Acne vulgaris)

Medical Background

Contrary to the old wives' tale, acne is not made worse by having too much sex or not washing a dirty face. Acne is a relatively common inflammatory condition that results in the development of pimples or pustules from blocked or inflamed hair follicles. These can present as whiteheads (flesh-colored or whitish closed bumps on the skin), blackheads (with dark centers), acne pimples, or blemishes.

Because changes in hormone levels can trigger these symptoms, acne most often affects teenagers during puberty and women during pregnancy or during their menstrual

> *Contrary to the old wives' tale, acne is not made worse by having too much sex or not washing a dirty face.*

cycle. Other triggers include some oil-based cosmetics or cleansing agents, clothing that prevents evaporation of skin moisture, humid conditions, sweating, and severe or prolonged stress. Although the scientific evidence that acne is affected by diet is currently inconclusive, some dietary changes (such as decreasing consumption of chocolate, restricting fatty foods, and avoiding fast foods) have been reported to be helpful. Since the sun has natural anti-inflammatory effects, acne may improve during the summer.

Common Medicinal Herbs

Herbal medicines are often used by practitioners in combination with other herbs and other types of treatment. The following herbs have been used in the management of acne:

🌿 Chaste Tree

For acne related to hormone changes, chaste tree has been used traditionally.

Dandelion and Burdock

Herbal medicines used to support the liver and aid digestion, such as dandelion and burdock, are also sometimes recommended in cases of acne and other skin conditions.

Tea Tree Oil

There is evidence from one clinical trial that 5% tea tree oil gel helps to treat acne and has fewer adverse effects than conventional benzoyl peroxide medication.

Cautions

If you are taking other medications or supplements, talk to a health-care professional before starting any herbal medicines. If you are unsure whether you have acne, consult a qualified health-care professional. If the acne does not respond to 6 weeks of herbal treatment, seek medical advice. Topical or oral antibiotics are used to treat more severe or widespread acne.

Allergies and Hay Fever
(Allergic Rhinitis)

Allergies and hay fever are characterized by irritation of the mucous membranes of the eyes, nose, throat, and lungs and are caused by the immune system overreacting to airborne environmental allergens. Symptoms of allergies include itching of the eyes, nose, and throat, bouts of sneezing, runny nose, swollen eyelids, headache, wheezing, nasal congestion, irritability, and malaise. The allergens that trigger allergies may also worsen symptoms of asthma.

Allergies can affect people of all ages and may begin as early as 2 years of age. Allergies may be caused by seasonal allergens, such as pollen and fungal spores, or perennial allergens, such as dust, pet dander, and cigarette smoke.

Most treatments for allergies and hay fever focus on increasing the patient's comfort level and quality of life. Common treatments include avoiding sources of allergens wherever possible, over-the-counter or prescription antihistamines to mildly suppress the immune system, and immunotherapy, where low amounts of allergens are injected into the body to prime the immune system and thereby prevent an allergic reaction.

Common Medicinal Herbs

Herbal medicines are often used by practitioners in combination with other herbs and other types of treatment. The following herbs have been used in the management of allergies and hay fever:

Ma Huang

Ma huang, also known as ephedra, may provide symptomatic relief for congestion associated with allergies but is not available in all jurisdictions because of safety concerns.

Ma huang constricts the blood vessels, resulting in a decrease in mucus production. Decongestants containing ma huang are available in Canada.

Nettle Leaf

There is evidence from one clinical trial that two 300 mg capsules of nettle leaf taken at the onset of hay fever symptoms was more effective at reducing the symptoms than a placebo.

> *While nettle has enjoyed a long medicinal history in many different models of traditional herbalism, it is considered by many members of the public to be a noxious weed.*

Caution

If you are taking other medications or supplements, talk to a health-care professional before starting any herbal medicines. If you are unsure whether you have allergies or hay fever, consult a qualified health-care professional.

Anxiety

Medical Background

Anxiety is the most prevalent of all psychiatric disorders. In general, anxiety is a normal emotion that can encourage preparation and appropriate caution required for daily activities. When anxiety becomes severe, however, it can be debilitating and reduce quality of life.

Anxiety is characterized by physical and emotional feelings of distress and unease that can arise from a variety of triggers. The causes of anxiety are often unclear. In some cases, the mere suggestion or anticipation of an event can cause the onset of anxiety.

Anxiety disorders are classified into different categories based on the type of symptoms. Categories include generalized anxiety disorder, anxiety disorder due to a general medical condition, substance-induced anxiety disorder, obsessive-compulsive disorder, panic attacks and panic disorder, phobic (fear-based) disorders, and stress disorders. Anxiety must be diagnosed and managed by a trained health-care professional, such as a physician or psychiatrist. Treatments may vary based on the type of anxiety but usually include some combination of psychotherapy and sedative or antidepressant drugs.

Common Medicinal Herbs

Herbal medicines are often used by practitioners in combination with other types of treatment. The following herbs have been used in the management of anxiety:

❧ Bitter Orange

Several animal studies have suggested that this herb decreases anxiety. Clinical trials are needed to investigate this application in humans.

❧ Chamomile (German)

Compounds found in chamomile have been shown to have a sedative, mildly hypnotic effect in humans and mice. For this reason, chamomile tea is often recommended to treat mild anxiety and insomnia. Clinical trials are needed to confirm its effectiveness for treating anxiety.

❧ Kava

Kava products have traditionally been used to treat nervous conditions, and there is evidence from clinical trials that, compared to a placebo, 100 mg capsules of kava, standardized to 70 mg kavalactones and taken three times daily, can significantly improve anxiety symptoms. Concerns about a possible association between kava use and liver toxicity have limited the availability of kava in many countries.

> *Kava plays an important role in many of the social and religious customs of the indigenous peoples of Polynesia. A kava beverage is used during funeral and marriage ceremonies, as well as to honor guests and visiting dignitaries.*

❧ Lemon Balm

There is evidence from one clinical study that taking one tablet containing 80 mg of lemon balm and 160 mg of valerian daily before bed was as effective at promoting sleep as the sedative triazolam. The use of lemon balm for anxiety is supported by animal studies.

❧ Passionflower

Positive results have been seen in several studies using passionflower extract or a combination product containing passionflower to treat anxiety. These findings are supported by animal studies.

🌿 *Scullcap*

While not yet supported by scientific trials, scullcap is traditionally used to treat symptoms of nervous tension and exhaustion.

🌿 *Valerian*

Valerian has historically been used as a sedative, and this is supported by animal studies. However, human trials have reported mixed results on its efficacy as a sleep aid. Further research is needed before firm conclusions can be drawn.

Caution

If you are taking other medications or supplements, talk to a health-care professional before starting any herbal medicines. If you are unsure whether you have an anxiety disorder, consult a qualified health-care professional. Anxiety is a serious health concern, and self-treatment is not recommended.

Arthritis (Osteoarthritis)

Osteoarthritis is the most common joint disorder, most often presenting in older adults and seniors. Men and women are equally affected. Arthritis is characterized by inflammation of the joints, causing pain, swelling, and stiffness. In the case of osteoarthritis, these symptoms are caused by joint changes and a loss of joint cartilage. Osteoarthritis is a localized joint inflammation, usually of the hands, resulting from small changes in the cartilage. It must be diagnosed and managed by a trained health-care professional, such as a physician or orthopedic specialist.

Osteoarthritis usually presents with joint pain, joint stiffness, reduced range of motion, friction in joints, joint deformity, and joint enlargement with bony swellings. Symptoms are worsened by weight bearing, overuse of the joint, trauma, lack of physical activity, repetitive movements, and obesity. If left untreated, and often even with treatment, osteoarthritis can result in severe joint destruction and deformity. Most treatments for arthritis aim to relieve pain, increase joint flexibility, and stop the inflammatory processes. Treatment plans often include non-steroidal anti-inflammatory drugs (NSAIDS), steroids, muscle relaxants, rest, and physical therapy.

Common Medicinal Herbs

Herbal medicines are often used by practitioners in combination with other herbs, dietary modifications, and other types of treatment. The following herbs have been used in the management of arthritis:

🌿 *Capsicum*

There is clinical evidence that topically applied capsicum creams and ointments are effective in treating the pain associated with osteoarthritis.

🌿 *Devil's Claw*

Two systematic reviews have concluded that devil's claw taken daily can improve pain, range of motion, and the time needed to recover from stiffness associated with osteoarthritis.

> *After devil's claw was introduced to European herbal medicine, it became so popular that, by 1976, it was estimated that 30,000 arthritic patients in the United Kingdom alone were using it.*

🌿 *Ginger*

Traditionally used in Asia for its anti-inflammatory properties, ginger has been found in case and clinical studies to be effective at reducing the pain and swelling associated with arthritis.

🌿 *Meadowsweet*

Meadowsweet has a long history of use for treating arthritic pain in traditional medicine. It was the first plant from which acetylsalicylic acid (aspirin) was synthesized. While this herb does contain constituents with demonstrated painkilling properties, scientific research is needed to confirm this traditional use.

🌿 *Nettle*

Nettle also has a long history of use for treating arthritic pain in traditional medicine. While not conclusive, test tube and clinical studies suggest that nettle's anti-inflammatory properties may be effective at reducing the pain and disability associated with arthritis. Further research is needed before firm conclusions can be drawn.

🌿 *Willow*

One clinical trial suggests that willow extract may decrease pain associated with osteoarthritis.

Caution

If you are taking other medications or supplements, talk to a health-care professional before starting any herbal medicines. If you are unsure whether you have arthritis, consult a qualified health-care professional.

Arthritis (Rheumatoid)

Medical Background

Rheumatoid conditions are a general category of autoimmune conditions that mainly affect the joints. The most common rheumatic condition is rheumatoid arthritis. In this condition, the supporting structures of joints are attacked by the immune system, causing weakness and degradation.

The onset of rheumatoid arthritis usually occurs between 30 and 50 years of age, although symptoms can start at any age. It affects about 1% of the population and occurs twice as often in women as in men. Pain in rheumatoid arthritis is initially caused by inflammation and later becomes a result of mechanical stress. Over time, the joints are progressively destroyed.

Symptoms are hard to detect at first but include stiffness in the morning that worsens with time, fatigue, possibly low fever, and overall feelings of weakness. Joints eventually become swollen, painful, and stiff. A characteristic feature of rheumatoid arthritis is a pattern of swelling that is symmetrical (the same on each side of the body). Most commonly, joints in the fingers and toes, wrists and ankles, shoulders, elbows, and hips are involved. Deformity at these joints may develop.

Conventional medical treatments include diet and rest, medication that helps prevent joint destruction, medication that relieves the joint pain, and physical support, such as splints, for the joints.

Common Medicinal Herbs

Herbal medicines are often used by practitioners in combination with diet and lifestyle modifications, as well as other types of treatment. The following herbs have been used in the management of rheumatic conditions:

🌿 *Capsicum*

There is some clinical evidence that topically applied capsicum creams and ointments may be effective in treating the pain associated with rheumatoid arthritis.

> *Capsicum is one of the oldest and most widely used medicinal and culinary herbs in the world. Approximately 25% of the world's population uses capsicum on a daily basis.*

🌺 Cat's Claw

A clinical trial has shown a modest benefit to joint pain and swelling when patients with rheumatoid arthritis who were already taking conventional medication started taking an extract of cat's claw. Further research is needed to confirm these results.

🌺 Evening Primrose

There is limited evidence that evening primrose is effective at relieving some of the symptoms of rheumatoid arthritis. Further research is needed before firm conclusions can be drawn.

🌺 Meadowsweet

Meadowsweet is commonly used as an anti-inflammatory and may help mediate symptoms of rheumatoid arthritis. Research on using meadowsweet to treat rheumatoid arthritis is needed to assess its effectiveness.

🌺 Turmeric

Several clinical studies indicate that turmeric is effective at treating rheumatoid arthritis, including joint swelling, walking speed, and morning stiffness.

Caution

If you are taking other medications or supplements, talk to a health-care professional before starting any herbal medicines. It is important to be assessed by a health-care professional to confirm the presence of rheumatoid arthritis. If you are already taking medication for rheumatoid arthritis, consult a health-care professional before taking any herbs.

Asthma

Medical Background

Asthma is characterized by inflammation of the airway, caused by a range of stimuli that trigger partially or completely reversible constriction of the bronchioles. Asthma must be diagnosed and managed by a trained health-care professional. Asthma symptoms include wheezing, shortness of breath, and a feeling of tightness in the chest, especially at night or in the early morning. Patients may have intermittent or persistent symptoms that range from mild to severe. Worsening of symptoms can be triggered by allergens from the environment, infections, cold or dry air, air pollution, exercise, excitement, and anxiety. Smoking can make asthma symptoms worse, but there is no evidence that air cleaners or purifiers help.

Asthma affects 4% to 7% of the world's population and is on the increase in the industrialized world. It is more common in children and in people who live in urban environments. It is the most common cause of hospitalization for children and accounts for a large proportion of absenteeism from elementary school. Untreated asthma can cause sleep problems, impair physical activity, and affect learning. If mild symptoms are not addressed, they can potentially escalate into serious and sometimes life-threatening asthma episodes.

Most treatment for asthma focuses on preventing symptoms. Individualized treatment plans usually include long-term agents for reducing and preventing symptoms, as well as agents that provide quick relief in the event of a serious worsening of asthma symptoms.

Common Medicinal Herbs

Herbal medicines are often used by practitioners in combination with other herbs, dietary modifications, and other types of treatments. The following herbs have been used in the management of asthma:

🌺 Cat's claw

Cat's claw has traditionally been used in the management of asthma, probably because of its anti-inflammatory properties. To date, however, no clinical trials have assessed how well it works. Cat's claw should not be used as a substitute for asthma medications prescribed by a physician.

✽ Ginkgo

Several small clinical studies suggest that ginkgo may have beneficial effects for individuals diagnosed with asthma; however, additional research is needed to confirm these preliminary findings.

✽ Lobelia

Lobelia is traditionally used to treat a wide range of respiratory conditions, including asthma. Clinical trials are needed to investigate its effectiveness for asthma.

✽ Ma Huang

Ma huang has a long history of use for treating respiratory conditions, including asthma, in traditional Chinese medicine and contains substances with known bronchodilating effects. It is not recommended for self-medication, but it may be suggested and monitored by a qualified health-care professional.

> *Ma huang – or, more correctly, its constituent ephedrine – was probably the first traditional Chinese herbal product to receive acceptance in the West.*

Caution

If you are taking other medications or supplements, talk to a health-care professional before starting any herbal medicines. If you are unsure whether you have asthma, consult a qualified health-care professional. Asthma is a serious health concern, and self-treatment is not recommended.

Back Pain

Medical Background

Low back pain may present in a variety of ways: sharp or dull, constant or intermittent, shallow or deep, mild to severe. Most often, low back pain is caused by a sedentary lifestyle, which over time causes weakening of supportive back muscles. Poor posture, inadequate shoes or mattresses, exercising improperly or while tired, physical labor, muscle or ligament trauma, being overweight, smoking, and sudden bursts of activity in an otherwise sedentary lifestyle are also common triggers. Less often, low back pain may signal the presence of an underlying illness, such as arthritis, spine injuries, spinal tuberculosis, cancer, or diseases of the kidneys, pancreas, liver, bladder, uterus, or prostate. Symptoms may be worsened by excessive bed rest.

Low back pain affects up to 80% of individuals at some time in their lives and is second only to the common cold as the leading cause of missed work days among adults aged 18 to 45. The prevalence of low back pain increases with age, affecting up to 50% of seniors at any given time. Left untreated, serious episodes of low back pain may increase in frequency and severity.

Most treatment for low back pain focuses on decreasing pain and increasing ability to perform daily activities. Individualized treatment plans usually include long-term protocols, such as exercise, massage, and chiropractic, for reducing and preventing symptoms, as well as agents that provide quick relief in the event of a serious worsening of symptoms. These agents include ice, heat therapy, topical and oral pain relievers, and acupuncture.

Common Medicinal Herbs

Individual herbal medicines are often used by practitioners in combination with manual therapies, such as chiropractic and massage, and other types of treatment. The following herbs have been used in the management of low back pain:

🌿 Devil's Claw

Two systematic reviews concluded that devil's claw appears to reduce low back pain significantly better than a placebo.

🌿 Willow

Several clinical trials suggest that willow may be effective at treating the symptoms of chronic low back pain.

> *Salicylic acid was first extracted from the flowering buds of meadowsweet, or spiraea, as it was once known. The term "aspirin" (acetylsalicylic acid) means "from spiraea."*

🌿 Meadowsweet

Meadowsweet has a long history of use for treating pain in traditional medicine. It was the first plant from which acetylsalicylic acid (aspirin) was synthesized. While this herb does contain constituents with demonstrated painkilling properties, scientific research is needed to confirm this traditional use.

Caution

If you are taking other medications or supplements, talk to a health-care professional before starting any herbal medicines. If your low back pain does not improve after 1 week of herbal treatment, seek the advice of a qualified health-care professional.

Bladder Infection
(Cystitis)

Medical Background

Bladder infections are usually characterized by urgent and painful urination, frequent urination, pain above the pubic bone, or cloudy or bloody urine. Infections are primarily caused by *E. coli* gram-negative bacteria. Symptoms may be mild to severe, depending on the individual, and in some cases an infection may occur even though there are no symptoms. Bladder infections should be diagnosed and managed by a trained health-care professional, such as a physician.

In general, more women than men are affected by bladder infections because of their shorter urethra length and the close proximity of the urethra to the anus and vagina, which can both be sources of bacteria. Other factors that increase the risk of bladder infections include pregnancy; sexual intercourse; use of spermicides; use of a diaphragm; diabetes; urinary stones or obstructions; enlarged prostate; structural or functional abnormalities of the urinary tract, including use of a catheter; and a history of bladder infections or infections of the urinary tract in general. If left untreated, a bladder infection may progress up the ureters to the kidneys, resulting in a kidney infection, which can be very serious.

Treatment for bladder infections focuses on eliminating the causative bacteria. Antibiotics are typically administered, usually for about 3 days, until symptoms subside, indicating that the bacteria have been successfully eliminated. In more severe cases, antibiotic treatment may be recommended for up to several weeks. Prevention measures are generally directed at women and include drinking lots of water to ensure good urine flow to wash out the bladder, wiping from front to back, urinating soon after sexual intercourse, and wearing loose-fitting, breathable clothing and underwear.

Common Medicinal Herbs

Individual herbal medicines are often used by practitioners in combination with other herbs and other types of treatments. The following herbs have been used in the management of bladder infections:

🌺 Cranberry

The results of two studies suggest that cranberry (180 mL of juice or 800 mg capsules) may be effective at *preventing* bladder infections. Cranberry is not, however, an effective *treatment* for bladder infections and should not be used as a substitute for antibiotics.

🌺 Juniper

This herb has traditionally been used for the treatment of uncomplicated bladder infections. Scientific research is needed to confirm this traditional use.

🌺 Uva-Ursi

Uva-ursi has traditionally been considered one of the most effective herbal antiseptics for uncomplicated bladder infections. Scientific research is needed to confirm this traditional use.

> *Uva-ursi produces small, leathery, oblong leaves and small, pale pink flowers. Bears are thought to like the sour red berries, which gave rise to the popular name "bearberry."*

Caution

If you are taking other medications or supplements, talk to a health-care professional before starting any herbal medicines. If you are unsure whether you have a bladder infection, consult a qualified health-care professional, who will typically provide antibiotics if you have an infection.

Blood Pressure (High)

Medical Background

High blood pressure, also known as hypertension, is characterized by either a systolic blood pressure above 140 mm Hg or a diastolic blood pressure above 90 mm Hg. Systole occurs when the left ventricle of the heart is contracting to push blood throughout the body, and diastole occurs when the left ventricle is relaxed. The blood pressure numbers reflect the pressure in the arteries at these different times.

High blood pressure does not usually produce any symptoms unless it is prolonged or becomes very severe, at which time it damages organs, such as the eyes, kidneys, heart, lungs, and brain. It also damages the arteries and increases the risk of death. Less severe symptoms of prolonged high blood pressure include nausea, vomiting, headache, trouble breathing, and general malaise. High blood pressure is a serious illness that should be diagnosed by a trained health-care professional, such as a physician.

High blood pressure affects about a third of all North Americans over the age of 20 and affects black people more than Caucasians. Approximately 30% of individuals with high blood pressure do not know they have it. And among those who do know they have high blood pressure, 40% are not receiving treatment — likely because it can be difficult to continue a treatment plan when one is not experiencing very many symptoms.

Treatment for high blood pressure tends to focus on lifestyle changes, such as diet and exercise, in addition to pharmaceutical treatments. Lifestyle recommendations often include reduction of salt and alcohol consumption, weight loss, and home monitoring of changes in blood pressure. One problem with pharmaceutical treatments is that the drugs may have side effects.

Common Medicinal Herbs

Individual herbal medicines are often used by practitioners in combination with other herbs, stress management, lifestyle changes, and other types of treatment. The following herbs have been used in the management of high blood pressure:

Ashwagandha

Several animal studies suggest ashwagandha may lower blood pressure. However, more research is needed to confirm these preliminary findings.

Garlic

The results of clinical studies have been conflicting; thus, there is insufficient evidence to routinely recommend garlic for the management of blood pressure.

> In ancient Britain, the hard wood and berries of hawthorn were thought to have magical powers. Many Christians believe that the crown of thorns worn by Jesus was made of hawthorn.

Hawthorn

Hawthorn is traditionally used as a general heart tonic, but there are only a couple of small scientific studies, with conflicting results. It is unlikely that hawthorn will help severe forms of high blood pressure. Further research is needed to confirm whether it may be beneficial for people with mild hypertension.

Caution

If you are taking other medications or supplements, talk to a health-care professional before starting any herbal medicines. If you are unsure whether you have high blood pressure, consult a qualified health-care professional. Untreated high blood pressure can have serious long-term health consequences.

Boils and Skin Ulcers

Medical Background

Boils and skin ulcers are characterized by the appearance of large, pimple-like nodules that are inflamed, painful, and filled with pus. They occur most often on the face, neck, breasts, or buttocks and are caused by an infection with a bacterial organism called *Staphylococcus aureus*. This is a bacterium that can easily become antibiotic resistant and cause serious health problems, so prompt medical treatment by a trained health-care professional, such as a physician, is advised. Occasionally, multiple boils may join together, creating something called a carbuncle. Patients with a carbuncle may experience additional symptoms, including fever and general weakness.

Boils and skin ulcers may affect anyone but are most often seen in those who are overweight, elderly, immunocompromised, or diabetic. Hot, humid climates and crowded or unhygienic living conditions may increase the risk of boils.

Treatment for boils and skin ulcers tends to focus on hot compresses to promote self-drainage and local antibiotics to kill the bacteria. In certain cases, when this protocol is not effective or the patient has a high risk of complications, incision-induced drainage and treatment with oral antibiotics may be required.

Common Medicinal Herbs

Individual herbal medicines are often used by practitioners in combination with other herbs and other types of treatment. The following herbs have been used in the management of boils and skin ulcers:

🌺 *Calendula*

Calendula has traditionally been used to treat a variety of skin conditions. It is often applied as an external cream or gel to treat skin abrasions and sores. Animal studies support this use.

> *Traditionally, the colorful flowers of calendula were thought to lift spirits and encourage cheerfulness. The flowers are edible and are often added to salads or made into teas and cordials.*

🌺 *Echinacea*

Echinacea has traditionally been used in treating sores and ulcerations topically because of its anti-inflammatory activity. Further research is needed to investigate this use.

🌺 *Slippery Elm*

Slippery elm has traditionally been used externally to treat boils and skin ulcers, likely due to its soothing, astringent properties. Further research is required to investigate this use.

Caution

If you are taking other medications or supplements, talk to a health-care professional before starting any herbal medicines. If you are unsure whether you have a boil or skin ulcer or if it is due to an underlying condition, such as diabetes, consult a qualified health-care professional. Untreated boils or skin ulcers can have serious long-term health consequences.

Breastfeeding Complications

Medical Background

Breastfeeding benefits both the infant and the mother in many ways. It provides important nutrients for a newborn and gives infants immune complexes to help them defend against infections, as well as providing protection against various health conditions, such as diabetes and allergies. Breastfeeding benefits the mother by offering protection against osteoporosis and some cancers, and helps her return to her pre-birth condition more quickly.

Complications for the mother can include excessive breast enlargement, tender nipples, and inflamed milk ducts. Mastitis is a common condition in which a section of the lactating breast is blocked from emptying properly. Symptoms of mastitis appear as a flushed, tender, section of the breast, which could eventually lead to infection. Complications for the infant are mainly related to malnutrition. If the infant is not getting enough breast milk, symptoms of malnutrition can develop, including a drop in weight, constant fussiness, and dehydration. The infant could have difficulties getting breast milk because of mechanical problems latching on or because the mother is not producing enough milk.

Common medical treatments for breastfeeding difficulties include stimulation of breast milk, counseling on breastfeeding, or a switch to a breast pump or formula. Many drugs and herbs taken by the mother can be detected in breast milk, so it is important to consult a health-care professional before any medication or herbs are taken.

Common Medicinal Herbs

Herbal medicines are often used by practitioners in combination with other herbs, dietary modifications, and other types of treatment. The following herb has been used in the management of breastfeeding difficulties:

🌺 *Chaste Tree*

Two studies have reported that chaste tree stimulates milk production in lactating mothers. Further research is needed to investigate these preliminary findings and to establish whether chaste tree is safe for use by women who are breastfeeding.

> *Wives of Roman legionnaires spread the aromatic leaves of the chaste tree on their beds while their husbands were at war. It was included in monks' diets (hence the common name "monk's pepper"), planted liberally in the grounds of many Catholic monasteries, and worn in the clothing to promote celibacy.*

Caution

If you are taking other medications or supplements, talk to a health-care professional before starting any herbal medicines. It is important to consult a health-care professional before taking any kind of medication or herbal product when breastfeeding.

Burns (Minor)

Medical Background

More than two million Americans suffer from burns every year, with children and the elderly being most affected. Almost all (80%) minor burns occur in the home, while sunburn is the most common minor burn that occurs outside the home. Burns can be caused by contact with high heat, hot water, and electricity, as well as exposure to chemicals or to UV radiation.

The severity of the burn depends on the duration of contact with the heat source. Burns can be classified as superficial, superficial partial thickness, deep partial thickness, and full thickness. These terms replace the old classification system of first, second, or third degree burns. Minor superficial burns are the only ones that may be safely treated at home. All other burns should be immediately treated by a trained health-care professional, such as a physician.

Superficial burns are small, superficial, and shallow, usually caused by a brief contact with a heat source. They do not extend down past the top layer of skin. Symptoms include pain, swelling, and redness, rarely with blistering. Sunburns usually fall in this category.

Superficial partial thickness burns result from more prolonged exposure to a heat source that still only affects the skin surface. Symptoms include pain, temperature sensitivity, weeping blisters, and redness that whitens (blanches) with pressure.

Deep partial thickness burns extend down below the skin's surface, affecting a layer called the dermis as well. These burns may be a result of scalding, flash ignition, and flames. Symptoms include intense pain in some areas with loss of sensation in others, large blisters, and a patchy red and white appearance indicating a loss of blood vessels.

Full thickness burns completely burn away all the layers of skin, resulting in a dry, leathery surface that lacks sensation. These types of burns penetrate deeply, sometimes affecting muscle and bone in addition to skin.

Treatment for minor burns tends to focus on relieving the pain, protecting the burn, and minimizing the chance of infection and scarring. Cool running water, cold compresses, topical steroid and antibiotic creams, wound dressings, and oral over-the-counter pain medications are usually recommended.

Common Medicinal Herbs

Individual herbal medicines are often used by practitioners in combination with other herbs and other types of treatment. The following herbs have been used in the management of minor burns:

Aloe Vera

The results of several clinical studies suggest that aloe vera may be effective at treating minor burns by increasing the rate of healing. Further research is needed to confirm these findings and to determine the exact dosage form (ointment, cream, or gel) that is most effective.

There are many legends about the powers of aloe vera, including that it was the secret of Cleopatra's beauty – which may account for its use in a variety of health and beauty aids – and that it was applied to the body of Jesus Christ after his crucifixion.

Calendula

Calendula has a history of traditional use as a treatment for minor scalds, likely due to its anti-inflammatory effects. Though more detailed human research is needed to confirm this use clinically, animal research is promising, showing that calendula supports skin regeneration.

Echinacea

Echinacea has been used traditionally to treat skin ailments, such as burns, topically because of its anti-inflammatory activity. Further research is needed to investigate this use.

Caution

If you are taking other medications or supplements, talk to a health-care professional before starting any herbal medicines. If you are unsure of how serious your burn is, consult a qualified health-care professional. Untreated severe burns can have serious long-term health consequences.

Cancer

Medical Background

Approximately 40% of women and 45% of men will develop some form of cancer during their lives. Cancer is a very serious illness that can affect any part of the body. Because of this, there is no single set of symptoms that characterize cancer. Cancer usually starts out as a small mass of disorganized cells that steadily grows until it produces symptoms in the local area. Symptoms usually arise because the mass of the cancer starts to push on an organ, blood vessel, or nerve and somehow impede function or cause pain. Symptoms depend primarily on the location of the cancer. Some general warning signs include, but are not limited to, sudden weight loss, unexplained fatigue, night sweats, sudden appetite loss, persistent pain or discomfort, blood in the urine or stool, and recurring nausea or vomiting. Cancer can only be diagnosed by a trained health-care professional, such as a physician or oncologist.

Treatment for cancer tends to focus on eliminating all cancer cells. This is done through chemotherapy, radiation, hormonal or immunotherapy, and surgery. Depending on the type of treatment, side effects can include vomiting, nausea, mouth sores, fatigue, lethargy, weight loss, and hair loss. A cancer is considered cured if the patient does not have any cancer cells for a period of 5 to 10 years, depending on the type of cancer.

Common Medicinal Herbs

Individual herbal medicines are often used by practitioners in combination with other herbs and other types of treatment. Though not curative, the following herbs have been used in the management of cancer:

Astragalus (adjunctive)

The results of several clinical and animal studies suggest that astragalus may have immune-stimulating effects, including in cases where patients are being treated for cancer. Scientific research is needed to investigate these preliminary findings.

Garlic (preventative)

The results from high-quality epidemiological studies suggest that garlic may have a preventative effect against several types of cancer, including colon cancer. Test tube and animal studies support this finding. Further research is needed to confirm these results.

❧ *Red Clover (preventative)*

This herb has traditionally been used to prevent breast cancer, although several clinical trials have shown no benefit to markers that may indicate breast cancer development. Further studies are needed.

Caution

If you are taking other medications or supplements, talk to a health-care professional before starting any herbal medicines. If you suspect you have cancer, immediately consult a qualified health-care professional. While herbal medicines can be taken with conventional cancer medication and radiation therapy, this should only be done under the care of a qualified health-care professional. Untreated cancer can have serious long-term health consequences.

> *During the past 100 years, more than 1,300 scientific papers have reported on the chemical constituents, mechanisms of action, and clinical applications of garlic, making it one of the most extensively researched medicinal plants.*

Canker Sores

Medical Background

Canker sores are characterized by a shallow ulcer on a mucosal surface of the mouth, including the inside surface of the lips or cheeks, the floor of the mouth, the ceiling of the mouth, the throat, or the tongue. The sores may persist from 4 to 14 days and resolve spontaneously without leaving a scar. They are rounded and small, between about 0.5 to 2.0 centimeters, although larger sores are occasionally seen. Colorwise, they may be gray to grayish yellow, surrounded by an inflamed red border. Canker sores are usually very painful, and the pain is generally worsened with eating, drinking, swallowing, talking, and brushing the teeth. Some patients experience a burning sensation a few days before the canker sore appears, and many patients suffer recurring episodes.

Canker sores are very common, affecting 25% of Americans, most often individuals in their 20s and 30s. The exact cause of canker sores remains unknown, but there seems to be a familial link. Stress, local trauma, immune and nutritional deficiencies, hormonal changes, smoking cessation, and the consumption of chocolate, coffee, peanuts, eggs, cereals, almonds, strawberries, cheese, or tomatoes are also thought to be contributing factors.

There is no known cure for canker sores, and treatment tends to focus on controlling pain, promoting healing, and preventing recurrence. Depending on the suspected cause of the sores, immune and nutritional deficiencies are addressed through diet or dietary supplements and offending foods are avoided. Ice, mouth rinses, and oral pain-relieving products are often recommended to provide temporary pain relief. In certain cases, pain medications may also be recommended.

Common Medicinal Herbs

Individual herbal medicines are often used by practitioners in combination with other herbs, dietary modifications, and other types of treatment. The following herbs have been used in the management of canker sores:

❧ *Kava*

Topical application of kava has traditionally been used to ease the pain of canker sores. Scientific research is needed to confirm this use.

❧ *Licorice*

While preliminary, the results of one clinical study in which participants used a mouthwash containing licorice suggest that licorice may help to reduce the pain of canker sores and prevent their occurrence.

> *Licorice is arguably the most common herbal medicine because it is frequently added to natural health products as a flavoring agent.*

❋ *St. John's Wort*

A small clinical trial reported that a mouthwash made from hypericum (found in St. John's wort) helped heal recurrent mouth sores. Additional research is needed to confirm this preliminary finding.

Caution

If you are taking other medications or supplements, talk to a health-care professional before starting any herbal medicines. Any mouth sore that lasts for more than 10 days should be examined by a qualified health-care professional.

Cholesterol (High)

Medical Background

High cholesterol, also known as hyperlipidemia, is characterized by above-normal blood levels of low-density lipoprotein (LDL, or bad cholesterol) and below-normal blood levels of high-density lipoprotein (HDL, or good cholesterol), as determined by a blood test. The ratio between the two is of particular importance. High cholesterol has no symptoms until levels are extremely elevated, when heart disease, enlarged liver and spleen, and pancreatic inflammation may occur. Excess cholesterol is sometimes stored in the skin and tendons, creating bumps known as xanthomas. High cholesterol can only be diagnosed by a trained health-care professional, such as a physician.

High cholesterol affects men and women equally. More men are affected than women until women enter menopause, when their blood cholesterol levels tend to rise. Genetics also play a significant role; having a close family member with high cholesterol is an important risk factor. Eating a diet high in fat and cholesterol, smoking, being overweight, consuming alcohol, and being inactive are also risk factors. High cholesterol may also develop as a symptom of liver disease and thyroid dysfunction.

Treatment of high cholesterol tends to focus on reducing exposure to risk factors through diet and lifestyle changes. Depending on the severity of the problem, lipid-reducing drugs may also be prescribed.

Common Medicinal Herbs

Individual herbal medicines are often used by practitioners in combination with other herbs, diet modification, and other types of treatment. The following herbs have been used in the management of high cholesterol:

❋ *Alfalfa*

The results of several animal studies and one small human study suggest that alfalfa may help to prevent and lower high cholesterol. Further scientific research is needed to confirm these preliminary findings.

> *Alfalfa was first described in literature by Pliny (AD 23–79) as being introduced to Greece by Darius, King of Persia (550–486 BC).*

❋ *Ashwagandha*

Several animal studies suggest that ashwagandha may lower cholesterol levels. However, more research is needed to confirm these preliminary findings.

❋ *Elder*

Preliminary human studies show mixed results from using elderberry juice to lower cholesterol. Additional clinical trials are needed.

🌿 *Garlic*

Several clinical trials show mixed results on garlic's ability to lower cholesterol, and proper doses are difficult to determine. Findings on this use are inconclusive, and further clinical trials are needed.

🌿 *Milk Thistle*

Two small clinical trials suggest that milk thistle may help reduce cholesterol levels. Additional studies are needed to confirm these preliminary results.

🌿 *Turmeric*

Several small studies report that turmeric may lower serum cholesterol levels. Randomized, double-blind, controlled studies are needed to confirm these preliminary findings.

Caution

If you are taking other medications or supplements, talk to a health-care professional before starting any herbal medicines. If you suspect you have high cholesterol, consult a qualified health-care professional. Untreated high cholesterol can have serious long-term health consequences.

Cold Sores

Medical Background

Cold sores, also known as fever blisters, are characterized by the appearance of one or more painful, weeping blisters that burst, leaving a sore that persists for about 1 week, at which point it scabs over and falls off without leaving a scar. Cold sores typically appear on the lips but can also occur in the mouth, eyes, lungs, brain, esophagus, and genitals. They are caused by infection with a virus called *Herpes simplex*, which remains present in the body for life and goes through periods of activation and latency.

Cold sores are extremely common, with 98 million episodes reported every year in the United States. By the age of 40, 84% of American adults have antibodies to *Herpes simplex* in their blood, indicating that they have been exposed to the virus. The virus can survive outside the body for several hours, meaning that some infections may be caused by indirect exposure to the virus, transmitted through contact with surfaces.

Occasionally, in the days leading up to the cold sore, there is a burning or tingling sensation at the site. Additional symptoms may include swelling, fever, and aches and pains. Cold sores are usually triggered during periods of decreased immune function, such as illness, stress, excessive sun exposure, menstruation, and exposure to certain medications. Extreme temperatures, dental procedures, and trauma may also play a role. The virus that causes cold sores is highly infectious and can be easily transmitted to different sites on the body and to other people. During onset of a cold sore, precautions should be taken to avoid transmission by avoiding kissing and sexual intercourse, sharing glasses or lip products, and touching the sore.

Treatment for cold sores tends to focus on pain relief, preventing transmission to other sites of the body and to others, and preventing secondary bacterial infections. These goals are achieved through icing the sores, applying over-the-counter antibiotic creams, and cleansing the area with soap and water.

Common Medicinal Herbs

Individual herbal medicines are often used by practitioners in combination with other herbs and other types of treatment. The following herbs have been used in the treatment of cold sores:

🌿 *Lemon Balm*

The results of one clinical study suggest that lemon balm may be effective at decreasing the frequency of cold sore outbreaks.

Like most members of the mint family, lemon balm, or melissa, is aromatic, producing a characteristic lemony scent when bruised or crushed. The name "melissa" derives from the Greek for "bee," referring to the attraction the plant holds for bees.

🌺 Licorice

This herb has traditionally been used topically to treat cold sores because of its anti-inflammatory and immune-boosting properties. One clinical trial reported beneficial effects, but more studies are needed to confirm these findings.

🌺 Tea Tree Oil

The results of one small clinical study suggest that 6% tea tree oil gel may be effective at increasing the rate of healing of cold sores. Further research is needed to confirm these preliminary findings.

Caution

If you are taking other medications or supplements, talk to a health-care professional before starting any herbal medicines. If you are unsure whether you have a cold sore, consult a qualified health-care professional.

Colic

Medical Background

Colic affects approximately 25% of infants. It most often begins at 1 month of age and clears up on its own sometime between 4 and 6 months. Colic is characterized by episodes of prolonged crying and fussiness for no discernible reason. Additional symptoms include gas and abdominal bloating. Although the cause is unknown, colic does not affect the baby's growth, development, or appetite. However, concerned parents should always consult a trained health-care professional, such as a physician or pediatrician, to ensure that the symptoms are not due to an underlying illness.

Treatment of colic tends to focus on keeping the baby as comfortable as possible through rocking, patting, playing soft music, and tight swaddling.

Common Medicinal Herbs

Individual herbal medicines are often used by practitioners in combination with other herbs, dietary modifications, and other types of treatment. The following herb has been used in the treatment of colic:

🌺 Chamomile

Chamomile has a history of traditional use as a treatment for colic, likely due to its relaxing effects. Scientific research studies are needed to investigate this traditional use.

Chamomile helped Peter Rabbit get over a particularly indulgent trip to Farmer McGregor's vegetable garden. It takes a brave skeptic to argue with evidence like that.

Caution

If your child is taking other medications or supplements, talk to a health-care professional before starting any herbal medicines. If you suspect that your infant has colic, consult a qualified health-care professional.

Common Cold (Upper Respiratory Tract Infection)

Medical Background

The common cold is associated with many symptoms that affect respiration, often including a cough or laborious breathing because of phlegm obstructing the airways. These acute upper respiratory infections are caused by respiratory viruses, which may cause accompanying symptoms, such as a sore throat or runny nose.

The common cold can affect people of all ages and is experienced most frequently during the spring and fall. It is mainly spread by person-to-person contact, and after entry into the body, the virus can take up to 3 days to start showing symptoms. The first sign is often a sore throat. This is followed by sneezing and excess mucus production in the nose, which usually starts out a clear color but becomes cloudy after a few days. Temperature usually remains normal during a common cold, and symptoms should decrease and disappear within 10 days. There are no vaccines for the common cold, and susceptibility is not influenced by health, environmental temperature, or nutrition.

Treatments for the common cold are mainly used to support the immune system and treat individual symptoms. For specific symptom treatments, see the sections titled "Coughs" and "Sore Throat."

Common Medicinal Herbs

Herbal medicines are often used by practitioners in combination with other herbs and/or other types of treatment. The following herbs have been used in the management of respiratory conditions:

Echinacea

Although this is a popular herb for preventing and treating cold symptoms and upper respiratory tract infections, clinical studies have shown conflicting evidence. Generally, the research suggests that echinacea will not help *prevent* cold symptoms, but some forms of echinacea may be beneficial in reducing the severity and duration of symptoms if taken within the first 48 hours of the onset of symptoms. Further research is needed to confirm the effects of this herb.

Echinacea species were used extensively as medicinal herbs by native North American tribes, reportedly to treat a variety of ailments, including mouth sores, toothaches, colds, sore throats, burns, and snake bites.

Elder

Elder flowers have traditionally been used to treat respiratory conditions, including colds, flus, and bronchitis. Two clinical trials with a combination product containing elder as a main ingredient lend support for this indication, but additional trials with elder as a single agent are needed.

Garlic

One clinical trial suggests that garlic may be helpful in preventing the common cold. Additional research is needed to confirm this finding.

Ginseng (Asian and American/Canadian)

Several clinical trials suggest that ginseng, both Asian and North American, may be helpful in preventing the common cold.

Goldenseal

Goldenseal is traditionally used to treat symptoms of the common cold, such as upper respiratory tract infections. Further scientific research is needed to investigate this traditional use.

Ma Huang

Ma Huang has an active ingredient called ephedrine, which dilates the bronchioles to facilitate breathing and decreases mucus production. Products containing ephedrine for treating respiratory symptoms are sold in Canada.

🌺 *Oregano*

Oregano has traditionally been used to treat respiratory conditions; however, there are no clinical studies at this time. Scientific research is needed.

Caution

If you are taking other medications or supplements, talk to a health-care professional before starting any herbal medicines. It is important to be assessed by a health-care professional if respiratory conditions do not resolve within 10 to 14 days or if they worsen over time.

Coughs

Medical Background

Coughs are the number one symptom that causes North Americans to seek medical attention. Approximately 20% of all medical visits are due to diseases associated with coughing, and more than one billion dollars is spent annually in North America to treat coughs.

A cough is characterized by a deep inhalation followed quickly by contraction of the chest, abdomen, and diaphragm, resulting in a forceful expulsion of air from the lungs. Under normal circumstances, this coughing reflex is a productive defense mechanism for the body to prevent foreign material from remaining in the lungs or to clear mucus from the lungs. Productive coughs are often seen when a patient has a respiratory infection from a bacterium or virus, causing a buildup of excess mucus in the lungs. Other causes of productive coughs include sinusitis and asthma.

When a cough persists beyond 8 weeks, however, or is unproductive (it is dry, not clearing the lungs of foreign material or mucus), it may be a sign of a more serious underlying problem, such as postnasal drip syndrome, gastroesophageal disease, pharyngeal (voice box) dysfunction, heart disease, or cancer. Coughing may also be a side effect of some medications. The underlying cause of such coughs can only be diagnosed by a trained health-care professional, such as a physician.

The treatment of coughs varies greatly depending on the root cause of the cough. A doctor may prescribe mucus thinners (expectorants) or cough suppressants to improve the patient's comfort while the cause of the cough is being treated. Staying hydrated, using room humidifiers, and taking over-the-counter lozenges may also help alleviate symptoms.

Common Medicinal Herbs

Individual herbal medicines are often used by practitioners in combination with other herbs and/or other types of treatment. The following herbs have been used in the treatment of coughs:

🌺 *Elder*

Elder flowers have a history of traditional use as a treatment for coughs due to colds. Scientific research studies are needed to investigate this traditional use.

> *In rural England, it was considered a grave offense to damage any part of the elder tree, because it was thought to be inhabited by the Elder Mother and intrinsically linked to Mother Earth.*

🌺 *Licorice*

Licorice has a history of traditional use as a treatment for coughs, likely due to its mucus-thinning and cough-suppressing properties. More research is needed to confirm this traditional use.

🌺 *Lobelia*

Lobelia has a history of traditional use as a treatment for coughs, likely due to its mucus-thinning properties and the depressant effect it has on the respiratory system. Scientific research studies are needed to investigate this traditional use.

Thyme
The results of test tube and animal studies provide some scientific support for thyme's traditional use in the treatment of coughs, probably due to its anti-spasmodic effect on the lungs. Further studies are needed to confirm these preliminary findings.

Caution
If you are taking other medications or supplements, talk to a health-care professional before starting any herbal medicines. Any person with a cough that lasts for more than 10 days should be examined by a qualified health-care professional.

Depression

Medical Background
Depression is a persistent feeling of sadness that interrupts normal functioning. This condition can manifest as a loss of interest or enjoyment in activities, drowsiness, decreased sexual interest, and menstrual abnormalities. It is normal to feel sadness after a disappointment or loss of a loved one, but symptoms of depression last for weeks or months instead of days.

Depression can happen at any age but is most common in women and usually develops between the teenage years and the age of 40. The cause is unknown, although some influences may involve genetics, major life stressors, physical conditions, and changes in the balance of brain chemical signals. Some medications and nutritional deficiencies may also cause symptoms of depression.

Conventional medical treatments include prescription medication and counseling, often at the same time. When you are experiencing symptoms of depression, it is important to consult a health-care professional for a proper diagnosis and to determine any factors that may be influencing the condition. Always consult a health-care professional for severe forms of depression, including thoughts of suicide.

Common Medicinal Herbs
Herbal medicines are often used by practitioners in combination with other herbs, dietary modifications, and other types of treatment. The following herbs have been used in the management of depression:

Ginkgo
One small clinical trial suggests that ginkgo may have beneficial effects in those diagnosed with depression; however, additional research is needed to confirm these preliminary findings.

Lemon Balm
Lemon balm has traditionally been used to improve mood and dispel anxiety. Clinical trials are needed to investigate this use.

Scullcap
This herb has traditionally been used to treat conditions of nervous tension and exhaustion. Clinical trials are needed to investigate its application in depression.

St. John's Wort
In clinical trials, St. John's wort has been shown to be effective when treating mild to moderate short-term depression. This herb does not appear to be effective for treating severe depression.

> *St. John's wort has been associated with a colorful mythology involving St. John the Baptist, and a variety of customs use the plant as a talisman to ward off misfortune. It was mentioned in the texts of Hippocrates, Pliny, and Galen as helpful for wound healing and pain.*

Caution

If you are taking other medications or supplements, talk to a health-care professional before starting any herbal medicines. Consult a health-care professional for a proper diagnosis of and a safe treatment plan for depression. In most cases, it is not recommended to attempt self-treatment.

Diabetes

Medical Background

Diabetes is a condition characterized by high levels of sugar in the blood. Symptoms of diabetes include high blood sugar levels, frequent urination, increased thirst, weight loss, nausea, vomiting, and possibly increased appetite.

Type 1 diabetes appears when the immune system destroys cells that produce insulin (a hormone released by the body that stimulates sugar uptake by tissues). Symptoms usually start appearing before the age of 30, and commonly in childhood. Type 1 diabetes is influenced by genetics, and risk factors include family history, ethnicity, and race.

Type 2 diabetes also seems to be associated with family history and is often correlated with weight gain. Symptoms usually start appearing in adulthood but are now occurring earlier in life with increasing rates of childhood obesity. Insulin levels usually start out high in type 2 diabetes, but the blood sugar is also high because the tissues are insulin resistant and not absorbing the sugar. Insulin resistance eventually causes a decrease in insulin production.

The long-term effects of high blood sugar levels can have implications for blood vessels and nerves, cause blindness, increase the chance of liver failure, and increase the chance of infection. Conventional medical treatments include regular monitoring of blood sugar levels, exercise, dietary changes, and oral medications. Insulin injections are also prescribed when needed.

Common Medicinal Herbs

Herbal medicines are often used by practitioners in combination with other herbs, dietary and lifestyle modifications, and other types of treatment. The following herbs have been used in the management of diabetes:

Ashwagandha

One clinical case series and several animal studies suggest that ashwagandha may have beneficial effects for those with diabetes. However, more research is needed to confirm these preliminary findings.

> *The Indian (Ayurvedic) herb ashwagandha is traditionally used for its purported overall effects on health, including helping the body resist physical and psychological stress.*

Elder

Elder has traditionally been used to treat diabetes, and preliminary test tube studies show promising results. Further research is needed.

Evening Primrose

Though preliminary, results from several clinical trials have reported positive results from using evening primrose to treat nerve damage caused by diabetes.

Ginseng (American/Canadian)

This herb has traditionally been used to treat diabetes, but clinical trials of using ginseng to treat high blood sugar levels have shown mixed results. More scientific research is needed to investigate this use.

Milk Thistle

One small clinical trial suggests that adding milk thistle to conventional therapy for patients with type 2 diabetes might improve their glycemic profile. Additional research is needed to confirm this preliminary finding.

Caution

If you are taking other medications or supplements, talk to a health-care professional before starting any herbal medicines. Consult a health-care professional for a proper diagnosis of diabetes and a safe treatment plan.

Diarrhea

Medical Background

Diarrhea is defined as an increase in the daily weight of stools, which can often be equated with an increase in fluidity of the stool. Stool consistency and amount varies greatly with diet and among individuals. The intestine usually absorbs 99% of the water that passes through it, and when this absorption is impaired, more fluid is passed in the stool. This creates the loose, fluid stools commonly known as diarrhea.

Diarrhea is a familiar occurrence in North America, occurring on average once a year per person. It is most often experienced by children under 5 and is rare in the elderly over 65. Serious episodes may require hospitalization and can potentially be fatal because of the drastic decrease in the body's water content. Causes of acute diarrhea in North America are mostly food-borne illnesses and viruses, whereas chronic diarrhea can be caused by drugs, surgery, tumors, medical conditions, or dietary reactions.

Conventional medical treatments for diarrhea include increasing fluid intake to compensate for lost fluid and administering drugs to help stop the diarrhea. It is important to bring prolonged diarrhea to the attention of a health-care professional for proper assessment and treatment. Diarrhea with mucus or blood in it or that is accompanied by dehydration or weight loss should be treated immediately.

Among North American First Nations peoples, slippery elm bark was mixed with water to produce a thick, viscid mucilage used both externally and internally in conditions where the mucous membranes were inflamed and irritated.

Common Medicinal Herbs

Herbal medicines are often used by practitioners in combination with other herbs and other types of treatment. The following herbs have been used in the management of diarrhea:

Chamomile

Chamomile has traditionally been used to treat digestive upset, such as diarrhea, especially when symptoms include spasms and pain. Scientific research is needed to investigate this use.

Goldenseal

Berberine, a compound found in goldenseal, has been found in several clinical trials to improve diarrhea. It is not clear whether all goldenseal products will have this activity.

Red Raspberry

Largely due to its astringent action, red raspberry has traditionally been used to treat diarrhea. Scientific research is needed to investigate this use.

Slippery Elm

Slippery elm has traditionally been used to treat digestive conditions associated with inflammation of the mucous membranes, including diarrhea. Scientific research is needed to investigate this use.

Caution

If you are taking other medications or supplements, talk to a health-care professional before starting any herbal medicines. Consult a health-care professional for treatment of diarrhea if it persists or becomes severe.

Dysmenorrhea
(Painful Menstruation)

Medical Background

Menstruation is the monthly blood loss and shedding of uterine lining experienced by women of childbearing age. This is part of the menstrual cycle and is triggered by hormones. Menstruation lasts 5 to 7 days in most women. Unpleasant symptoms can include severe cramping in the abdomen and lower back, nausea and vomiting, fatigue, and headache. These symptoms are collectively called dysmenorrhea and usually occur just before or during the first 3 days of menstruation.

Dysmenorrhea is most common in adolescents. It usually arises soon after menstrual cycles begin, sometimes persisting into a woman's 20s, and its causes are unknown. If symptoms begin after adolescence, pelvic abnormalities could be the cause. Factors contributing to symptoms could include stress surrounding the menstrual cycle, an abnormally positioned uterus, and lack of exercise.

Common medical treatments include drugs to help manage the pain of cramping, birth control pills to help lessen the severity of monthly symptoms, application of heat to the abdominal region, and regular exercise.

Common Medicinal Herbs

Herbal medicines are often used by practitioners in combination with other herbs, dietary modifications, and other types of treatment. The following herbs have been used in the management of painful menstruation:

🌿 Cat's Claw

Cat's claw has traditionally been used to treat menstrual irregularities. Scientific research is needed to investigate this use.

🌿 Chaste Tree

Several small clinical studies suggest that chaste tree extract might help to relieve menstrual symptoms. Further clinical trials are needed to confirm these preliminary findings.

🌿 Dong Quai

This herb has traditionally been used to treat menstrual symptoms; however, attempts to quantify its effects in clinical trials have been largely unsuccessful.

🌿 Wild Yam

This herb is traditionally used to treat painful menstruation. Scientific research is needed to investigate this use.

> *The Aztecs, Mayans, and other native peoples of North and Central America used wild yam for treating painful menstruation and labor.*

Caution

If you are taking other medications or supplements, talk to a health-care professional before starting any herbal medicines. Consult a health-care professional if menstrual symptoms are severe or do not respond to non-prescription painkillers.

Dyspepsia

Medical Background

Dyspepsia is an uncomfortable or painful feeling in the upper abdomen. It is often explained as a sensation of gassiness, burning, indigestion, or becoming full after a small intake of food. About 25% of the North American population suffers from recurrent symptoms of dyspepsia. This can be caused by many different factors, including problems with the esophagus; underlying conditions, such as diabetes or heart complications; drugs; muscle spasms; or ulcers. It is important to consult a health-care professional for a proper diagnosis of dyspepsia to determine any underlying causes. Conventional medical treatments for dyspepsia include treating any underlying diseases, as well as oral medications to help decrease symptoms.

Common Medicinal Herbs

Herbal medicines are often used by practitioners in combination with other herbs, dietary modifications, and other types of treatment. The following herbs have been used in the management of dyspepsia:

Devil's Claw

While its use is yet to be confirmed with clinical studies, devil's claw, because of its bitter properties, has traditionally been used to treat symptoms of dyspepsia.

Lemon Balm

Oral consumption of lemon balm is traditionally thought to help digestive upset and is mild enough to use in children. Clinical trials are needed to confirm this indication.

Peppermint

Traditionally, peppermint is used as a carminative, relaxing and soothing the digestive tract. Trials have reported mixed results with using peppermint to treat symptoms of indigestion; more detailed research is required.

Turmeric

One small study suggests that turmeric may decrease symptoms of dyspepsia; however, further research is needed to confirm this preliminary finding.

> *Historically, turmeric has also been used for both its flavor (it is a major ingredient in curry powder) and its color (it is used in the preparation of mustard).*

Caution

If you are taking other medications or supplements, talk to a health-care professional before starting any herbal medicines. Consult a health-care professional for proper diagnosis and treatment of dyspepsia.

Eczema (Dermatitis)

Medical Background

Eczema is a condition characterized by red, inflamed, flaking, and itchy areas of skin. Thickening of the skin may eventually occur because of repetitive scratching. This collection of symptoms can be caused by many factors, including immune reactions, drugs, and other conditions. Eczema can be localized on one patch of skin or, in some types, it can be all over the body. It is common in children but can appear at any age.

Atopic dermatitis, caused by the body's immune reactions, is a type of eczema that may be determined by genetics. It is most common in children living in developed countries, affecting 5% of children in North America. Children are usually less sensitive after 5 years of age, although episodes can appear up until 30 years of age. Atopic dermatitis can be acute or chronic and is usually triggered by exposure to certain environmental factors.

Contact dermatitis is another type of eczema, resulting from physical contact with an irritant or allergen. An episode of contact dermatitis may take up to 3 weeks to resolve and may recur after exposure to the trigger.

Conventional medical treatments for eczema include cold compresses, topical or oral drugs to control immune responses or decrease symptoms, and avoidance of known triggers. Moisturizing with oils or creams and soothing the rash with oatmeal baths may also be recommended.

Common Medicinal Herbs

Herbal medicines are often used by practitioners in combination with other herbs, dietary modifications, and other types of treatment. The following herbs have been used in the management of eczema:

🌿 Burdock

Due to its reputation as a detoxifying herb, burdock has traditionally been taken orally for the management of skin conditions. Scientific research is needed to investigate this use.

> *In Western and Chinese herbalism, burdock is used as a detoxifying agent to "cleanse" the blood, removing toxins from the body.*

🌿 Calendula

While they are limited to animal studies, findings indicate that calendula has an anti-inflammatory effect, potentially supporting its traditional use in the treatment of skin conditions. Further scientific research is needed to investigate the use of calendula for treating eczema specifically.

🌿 Echinacea

This herb has traditionally been used to treat a variety of skin abrasions, possibly because of its anti-inflammatory activity. Scientific research is needed to investigate this use.

🌿 Elder

Topical preparations using elder have traditionally been used to treat skin conditions. Scientific research is needed to investigate this use.

🌿 Evening Primrose

Clinical trials have reported conflicting results surrounding the use of evening primrose to decrease symptoms of atopic dermatitis.

Caution

If you are taking other medications or supplements, talk to a health-care professional before starting any herbal medicines. Consult a health-care professional for proper diagnosis and treatment of eczema.

Erectile Dysfunction

Medical Background

Erectile dysfunction is the inability for a male to have or maintain an erection, preventing sexual intercourse. This can happen for many reasons, including psychological reasons, problems with blood flow or nerve impulses, hormonal changes, or drug use. Psychological factors can include anxiety, stress, or mood. Erectile dysfunction can also result from more serious conditions, such as diabetes or deterioration of blood vessels. The prevalence of erectile dysfunction increases with age and may not be experienced with every incidence of attempting sexual intercourse.

Common medical treatments for erectile dysfunction include treatment of any underlying condition, psychological counseling, and prescription medication.

Common Medicinal Herbs

Herbal medicines are often used by practitioners in combination with other herbs and other types of treatment. The following herb has been used in the management of erectile dysfunction:

🌿 Ginkgo

Clinical trials using ginkgo to treat erectile dysfunction have reported mixed results; more detailed studies are required to confirm this indication.

Caution

If you are taking other medications or supplements, talk to a health-care professional before starting any herbal medicines. Consult

Ginkgo is one of the most widely used and well-researched herbal medicines. It has been estimated that the ginkgo tree has existed for more than 200 million years, making it the oldest known tree species on earth. Charles Darwin is reported to have called the ginkgo tree a living fossil.

a health-care professional for a safe and effective treatment plan for treating erectile dysfunction.

Fatigue

Medical Background

Fatigue is a temporary condition involving feelings of drowsiness, decreased alertness, and low levels of concentration during the day. Both physical and mental fatigue are possible. It can be caused by lack of sleep, excessive physical or mental exertion, or the effects of drugs. Individuals particularly at risk of fatigue are not able to maintain a regular sleeping pattern, such as shift workers or individuals who are on call for their jobs. Prolonged episodes of fatigue that interrupt daily living may indicate chronic fatigue syndrome and should be treated by a health-care professional.

Chemicals in the brain induce feelings of drowsiness, and several stimulants used to treat fatigue work against these chemicals. Caffeine (e.g., in soft drinks, tea, and coffee) is the most common stimulant used to combat fatigue. However, excess consumption of caffeine could lead to symptoms of fatigue by impairing sleep.

Conventional medical treatments for fatigue include non-prescription and prescription products. Encouraging good sleep habits may also help to resolve fatigue.

Common Medicinal Herbs

Herbal medicines are often used by practitioners in combination with other herbs and other types of treatment. The following herbs have been used in the management of fatigue:

🌿 Asian and American/Canadian Ginseng

While ginseng has a long record of traditional use in preventing fatigue, clinical trials using the Asian and North American varieties of this herb to treat *physical* fatigue have shown mixed results. Preliminary trials using them to treat *mental* fatigue have reported positive results.

🌿 Siberian Ginseng

While preliminary, findings from small clinical trials using Siberian ginseng to increase physical performance and decrease physical fatigue have reported positive results. Further trials are needed to further investigate this use.

The name "ginseng" means "essence of the earth in the form of a man" and refers to the resemblance of the Asian and American/Canadian ginseng plant root to a human form.

Caution

If you are taking other medications or supplements, talk to a health-care professional before starting any herbal medicines. Consult a health-care professional before taking ginseng if you have any other health conditions or are taking medications.

Gastritis
(Stomach Inflammation)

Medical Background

Gastritis is a gastrointestinal disorder involving inflammation of the stomach lining. It is commonly caused by *H. pylori* bacteria, alcohol consumption, psychological stress, or frequent use of non-steroidal anti-inflammatory drugs (NSAIDs), such as aspirin and ibuprofen. Symptoms of gastritis appear as indigestion, causing discomfort in the upper abdomen, heartburn, bloating, gas, and nausea. Chronic inflammation of the stomach lining can cause tissue death, gastrointestinal bleeding, and decreased secretion of stomach acid.

Common conventional medical treatments for gastritis include symptomatic treatment with drugs to decrease the acidity of stomach secretions and removal of any potential causes.

Common Medicinal Herbs

Herbal medicines are often used by practitioners in combination with other herbs and other types of treatment. The following herbs have been used in the management of gastritis:

Peppermint

Peppermint has traditionally been used to soothe symptoms of indigestion and other digestive conditions. Further research is needed to investigate this use.

> *Although it is native to Europe, peppermint is now an important aromatic and medicinal crop grown throughout North American temperate zones, especially in the states of Indiana, Wisconsin, Oregon, Washington, and Idaho.*

Licorice

This herb has been used traditionally for centuries and in conventional medicine for decades to treat gastrointestinal conditions. Licorice may provide a protective layer for the gastrointestinal tract by increasing mucus production and quality.

Caution

If you are taking other medications or supplements, talk to a health-care professional before starting any herbal medicines. Consult a health-care professional for a proper diagnosis of and a safe and effective treatment plan for gastritis.

Headaches
(Tension and Sinus)

Medical Background

Tension headaches are characterized as pain that is distributed across the head, possibly extending down to the shoulders and neck. This is the most common kind of headache, experienced by 75% of the North American population at some point in their lives. Tension headaches originate from muscle tension in the muscles of the face. This can result from fatigue, stress, anxiety, or other emotions. Tight muscles in areas surrounding the head can also cause tension headaches.

Sinus headaches are also common, characterized by pain in the face where the sinuses are located. Sinus headaches occur when inflammation in the sinuses irritates the sinus walls. This inflammation can result from an infection or blockage of the sinus. People can have rare or chronic sinus headaches.

Common conventional medical treatments for headaches include prescription and non-prescription drugs to help manage the pain. If headaches are recurring or persist, a health-care professional should be consulted.

Common Medicinal Herbs

Herbal medicines are often used by practitioners in combination with other herbs, dietary modifications, and other types of treatment. The following herbs have been used in the management of headaches:

🌸 *Meadowsweet*

This herb has traditionally been used to decrease inflammation and relieve pain, and may benefit patients with headaches. Clinical trials are needed to investigate this use.

🌸 *Willow*

Although there are no clinical studies to support its use in treating headaches, willow has traditionally been used as a painkiller and may benefit patients with headaches.

> *Willow products are considered to be natural painkillers. Since willow does not contain aspirin (acetylsalicylic acid), it should not be used as a substitute for aspirin in thinning the blood.*

Caution

If you are taking other medications or supplements, talk to a health-care professional before starting any herbal medicines. Do not use meadowsweet or willow during pregnancy or while breastfeeding. Consult a health-care professional for a safe and effective protocol for treating chronic or severe headaches.

Hemorrhoids

Medical Background

Hemorrhoids are enlarged blood vessels in the anal region. They can be positioned close to the external opening of the anus or farther inside the body. Hemorrhoids can be swollen and painful, causing irritation, or they can be asymptomatic. If the hemorrhoid is external, it can sometimes be seen as a swollen, purplish protrusion during visual inspection of the anus.

About 5% of the North American population experiences hemorrhoids, most commonly in males and during pregnancy in females. Hemorrhoids can occur in both adults and children, although incidence increases with age. They can be caused by many factors, including pregnancy, heavy lifting, straining, and prolonged diarrhea or constipation. Symptoms include pain around the anus, a small amount of bleeding after a bowel movement, and a feeling of incomplete emptying.

Common conventional medical treatments for hemorrhoids include symptomatic treatments with non-prescription or prescription medication and sitz baths, in which only the buttocks and hips are submersed in warm water.

Common Medicinal Herbs

Herbal medicines are often used by practitioners in combination with other herbs and other types of treatment. The following herbs have been used in the management of hemorrhoids:

🌸 *Horsechestnut*

Horsechestnut seed extract could potentially be used to treat hemorrhoids. Scientific research is needed to investigate this use.

> *While horsechestnut products are not sold widely in North America, they are very popular in Europe, and especially in Germany, where in 1996 horsechestnut was the third-bestselling herbal product, with estimated sales of US$51 million.*

🌺 *Dandelion*

Traditionally, herbs that support liver function, such as dandelion, have been used to treat hemorrhoids. Scientific research is needed to investigate this use.

Caution

If you are taking other medications or supplements, talk to a health-care professional before starting any herbal medicines. Do not use horsechestnut seed extract during pregnancy.

Infections (Minor)

Medical Background

Minor skin bacterial infections occur when small skin wounds are colonized by bacteria. Symptoms of an infection include redness and tenderness and minor swelling in the area. Infections can be avoided by cleaning a wound as soon as it happens and keeping the area as clean as possible. After a day or so, it is important to uncover the wound if it has been tightly bandaged, to prevent colonization of bacteria from trapped moist body heat.

Minor bacterial infections are usually self-limiting and respond to local treatments. Both prescription and non-prescription antibacterial ointments are available. If the infection progresses or does not resolve, oral antibiotics may be recommended.

Common Medicinal Herbs

Herbal medicines are often used by practitioners in combination with other herbs and/or other types of treatment. The following herbs have been used in the management of minor infections:

🌺 *Echinacea*

Topical products containing echinacea could be helpful in treating minor infections because it has anti-inflammatory actions and possibly weak antibacterial properties. Scientific research is needed to investigate this use.

🌺 *Tea Tree Oil*

Tea tree oil has traditionally been used as a topical antiseptic. Scientific research is needed to investigate this use.

> *The indigenous people of Australia have long prized the aromatic leaves of the tea tree, both for religious purposes and for medicinal use as an antiseptic and antifungal agent in treating skin, oral, and vaginal infections.*

Caution

If you are taking other medications or supplements, talk to a health-care professional before starting any herbal medicines. Consult a health-care professional if a minor infection progresses or does not resolve.

Insomnia

Medical Background

Insomnia is defined as having difficulty falling asleep or experiencing sleep that is not restful, regardless of its duration. Problems staying asleep and frequent waking may also be symptoms of insomnia. Lack of sleep can affect emotions, memory, motor skills, concentration, and general awake-time functioning. Insomnia is often correlated with underlying conditions, including depression, diabetes, and arthritis.

Symptoms of insomnia are experienced by half of all North Americans, the highest prevalence being found among individuals 65 years of age or older. Symptoms of insomnia can last anywhere from a few days to years. Factors that can cause insomnia include emotional stress, anxiety, physical conditions that cause discomfort or pain, and mental or mood disorders, such as depression. Lifestyle habits, such as alcohol or caffeine consumption, late-night exercise or stimulation, and late-night meals can also contribute.

Common medical treatments for insomnia include resolution of the underlying condition if one is present, reconstructing a sleeping pattern, and avoiding factors that cause insomnia. Prescription and non-prescription medications to aid in sleep are also available.

Common Medicinal Herbs

Herbal medicines are often used by practitioners in combination with other herbs and other types of treatment. The following herbs have been used in the management of insomnia:

Chamomile

Chamomile contains constituents with a demonstrated sedative effect, which fits with its traditional use in calming nervous tension and treating insomnia. Scientific research is needed to investigate this use.

Hops

This herb has traditionally been used as a mild sedative, often in combination with valerian. Scientific research is needed to investigate this use.

Lemon Balm

This herb has traditionally been used as a mild sedative and can be combined with valerian. Scientific research is needed to investigate this use.

Passionflower

Passionflower has traditionally been used to treat restlessness and sleeping difficulties. Scientific research is needed to investigate this use.

> *The flowers of the passionflower plant are thought to represent the elements of Christ's Passion. For example, the fringe-like crown is said to represent the crown of thorns, while the five anthers represent the five stigmata.*

Scullcap

Scullcap has traditionally been used to treat insomnia. Scientific research is needed to investigate this use.

Valerian

Studies of valerian as a sleep aid have shown mixed results. Additional scientific clinical trials are needed to draw firm conclusions about its effectiveness.

Caution

If you are taking other medications or supplements, talk to a health-care professional before starting any herbal medicines. The herbs listed above may have sedative and hypnotic properties, and should be consumed with caution. Consult a health-care professional if symptoms of insomnia do not resolve or get worse.

Irritable Bowel Syndrome

Medical Background

Irritable bowel syndrome is a gastrointestinal disorder characterized by abdominal cramps, often relieved by defecation, and a frequent change in consistency of the stool or frequency of bowel movements that can manifest as periods of diarrhea or constipation. Symptoms appear in irregular bouts and can also include bloating, gas, and nausea.

Symptoms of irritable bowel syndrome usually appear between adolescence and 30 years of age. The cause is unknown, and no anatomical origin has been found. Factors that trigger bouts of symptoms are thought to be both psychological and physical. Psychological triggers include stress, depression, and anxiety. Physical triggers include a change in bowel mobility and genetic and environmental influences. There are no known risk factors for irritable bowel syndrome, and it occurs more frequently in men than in women.

Common medical treatments for irritable bowel syndrome include dietary therapy (e.g., avoiding foods that may trigger symptoms), drug therapy, and psychological counseling.

Common Medicinal Herbs

Herbal medicines are often used by practitioners in combination with other herbs, dietary modifications, and other types of treatment. The following herbs have been used in the management of irritable bowel syndrome:

Hops

While there is a lack of scientific research, hops has traditionally been used to calm nervous tension associated with irritable bowel syndrome. Scientific research is needed to investigate this use.

> *Hops is an essential plant in the brewing of beer, making it arguably one of the most commonly used herbs.*

Lemon Balm

Due to its soothing qualities, lemon balm has traditionally been used to calm nervous tension associated with irritable bowel syndrome. Scientific research is needed to investigate this use.

Peppermint

Several clinical trials have reported that peppermint, administered mainly as enteric-coated capsules, helped decrease the severity of irritable bowel syndrome symptoms.

Caution

If you are taking other medications or supplements, talk to a health-care professional before starting any herbal medicines. Consult a health-care professional for a safe and effective protocol to decrease symptoms of irritable bowel syndrome.

Liver Conditions

Medical Background

The liver plays a number of important roles in the body, including detoxification, production of bile, and regulation of cholesterol. Damage that impairs these functions can result from several sources, including drugs, infection, or lack of oxygen to the liver. Specific symptoms of liver impairment are most accurately exposed through blood testing but could manifest as fatigue, loss of appetite, nausea, jaundice, and gastrointestinal bleeding. The liver is made out of a tissue that can regenerate, so depending on the nature of damage to the liver, it may be able to repair itself after trauma.

Two main categories of liver conditions are hepatitis and cirrhosis. Hepatitis is a specific type of liver disorder characterized by acute or chronic inflammation of the liver. It can be caused by a virus, drug use, or immune reactions. Some types of hepatitis are reversible. In cirrhosis, chronic injury to the liver causes large amounts of scar tissue, leading to liver dysfunctions. It can be caused by some medical disorders, drugs, chemicals, or infection. Cirrhosis is usually not reversible, and treatment is targeted at supporting the liver.

Common conventional medical treatments for liver conditions include treatment of underlying disorders and complications, administration of therapeutic drugs, and avoidance of damaging substances, such as alcohol and certain drugs and herbs.

Common Medicinal Herbs

Herbal medicines are often used by practitioners in combination with other herbs and/or other types of treatment. The following herbs have been used in the management of liver conditions:

🌺 Dandelion

Dandelion root has traditionally been used to promote bile production and excretion by the liver. While this action is supported by evidence from animal studies, clinical trials are needed to investigate this property.

> *In the British herbal tradition, dandelion root is used for liver and digestive problems and the leaves for their diuretic properties in cases of edema. This latter action is demonstrated eloquently by the French name* pissenlit, *or "urinate in bed."*

🌺 Milk Thistle

Despite the fact that milk thistle has a long historical tradition of use in the prevention and management of liver conditions, several meta-analyses of clinical trials have reported equivocal or non-significant results for using milk thistle to treat hepatitis or cirrhosis. Further research is warranted to allow firm conclusions to be drawn.

🌺 Turmeric

Turmeric has traditionally been used to provide protection for the liver. Clinical trials are needed to investigate this use.

Caution

If you are taking other medications or supplements, talk to a health-care professional before starting any herbal medicines. Because an accurate diagnosis of the problem is essential, if you suspect you have liver problems, consult a health-care professional for a safe and effective treatment protocol.

Memory Loss and Dementia

Medical Background

Because recollection of past events is a part of daily life, impairment of memory can have a drastic impact on our lives. Memory impairment comes in two main forms: difficulty making new memories and difficulty recalling past events. Natural aging or traumatic injuries can result in memory loss, and it may be a symptom of some diseases.

Not everyone experiences memory loss as they age. In those who do experience age-related memory loss, progression is gradual and usually manifests as forgetfulness, especially for names and events. Memory loss due to trauma can result from physical brain injury or prolonged oxygen deprivation. This type of memory loss can be dramatic and irreversible. No specific treatments for memory loss exist in conventional medicine. If an underlying illness is causing the memory loss, the illness is treated.

In dementia, there is a deterioration of other mental functions, including reasoning, knowledge, awareness, thinking, and judgment, in addition to memory loss. Loss of these abilities occurs in stages and generally worsens with time. A natural decline in these functions, mainly memory, may happen with age, but dementia is characterized by more severe changes that impair activities of daily living. Symptoms of dementia could worsen with drug and alcohol consumption and in cases of liver failure.

There are many different factors that can cause changes to the brain, creating distinct types of dementia. Some examples include Alzheimer's disease, Huntington's disease, dementia caused by alcohol or exposure to heavy metals, brain tumors, depression, and hyperthyroidism. Depending on the cause, dementia can occasionally be reversible but is usually irreversible. It can happen at any age but is significantly more common in the population over 65 years of age. Dementia is the reason for half of all nursing home admissions.

Conventional medical treatments for dementia are limited. It is important to ensure the safety of those with dementia and arrange for caregivers to assist them in everyday duties. Elimination of any drugs that may be worsening symptoms is important, and drugs to help lessen symptoms may be prescribed.

Common Medicinal Herbs

Herbal medicines are often used by practitioners in combination with other herbs and/or other types of treatment. The following herb has been used in the management of memory loss and dementia:

🌿 *Ginkgo*

Clinical trials to treat memory loss involving ginkgo have shown varying results. It appears that ginkgo may help recover memory in people with memory loss, but it may not significantly increase memory in those without impairment. Further scientific studies are needed to confirm these results. Although many clinical trials have reported positive results when using ginkgo to treat symptoms associated with dementia, the patterns of changes in measures of outcomes have not been consistent; thus, additional trials are needed.

While many people take Ginkgo biloba *extract (GBE) made from the leaf to enhance memory, there is currently little scientific evidence that it will work unless you have significant memory impairment.*

Caution

If you are taking other medications or supplements, talk to a health-care professional before starting any herbal medicines. Consult a health-care professional for proper diagnosis of and a safe treatment plan for dementia.

Menopause

Medical Background

Menopause is defined as the period in a woman's life after menstruation has stopped. This happens because of a decrease in uterine function, leading to changes in hormone production. Impairment of uterine function can result either naturally from age or from medical intervention.

Menopause usually starts around the age of 50; however, it can happen anytime between 35 and 60 years of age.

Perimenopause is the period just before menopause, in which menstrual cycles start changing. Menstruation becomes shorter, more frequent, and irregular. During this period, estrogen levels in a woman's body fluctuate daily, which can cause unpleasant effects, including hot flashes, physical changes to the vagina, such as dryness or inflammation, and an increased risk for osteoporosis. Hot flashes are a very common symptom involving a raise in body temperature and sweating for up to 5 minutes that appears in 80% of women. There is an increased risk of osteoporosis because of an increased release of calcium from bones, and women are encouraged to get screened regularly for this disease after the age of 65. Symptoms of menopause can last up to a year after menstruation stops and can range from absent to severe in some women.

Common medical treatments for the unpleasant consequences of menopause include drugs to balance hormone levels and avoiding triggers for these consequences.

Common Medicinal Herbs

Herbal medicines are often used by practitioners in combination with other herbs and other types of treatment. The following herbs have been used in the management of symptoms associated with menopause:

❧ *Alfalfa*

Alfalfa has traditionally been used to treat symptoms of menopause. Scientific research is needed to investigate this use.

❧ *Black Cohosh*

Preliminary results from a number of clinical studies of using black cohosh to treat the unpleasant consequences of menopause have shown conflicting results. Further studies are needed to confirm or discount this use.

❧ *Chaste Tree*

Chaste tree has traditionally been used to treat symptoms of menopause. Scientific research is needed to investigate this use.

❧ *Dong Quai*

Within traditional Chinese medicine, dong quai has a long history of use in women's health, including for the treatment of the unpleasant consequences associated with menopause. However, attempts to quantify its effects in scientific clinical trials that have enrolled women with the Western diagnosis of menopausal symptoms have been largely unsuccessful.

❧ *Evening Primrose Oil*

Although evening primrose oil is often advertised for the symptoms of menopause, clinical trials do not find a significant benefit over a placebo.

❧ *Hops*

One clinical trial suggests that hops may decrease hot flashes and other menopausal discomforts. Animal studies, however, show conflicting results. Additional research is needed to investigate the use of hops for symptoms related to menopause.

❧ *Red Clover*

This herb has been examined for its use in prevention and treatment of cardiovascular disease resulting from the changes of menopause, but its action showed mixed results. Several trials have been done using red clover to treat hot flashes, again with mixed results. Further research is required to determine appropriate use of this herb.

Caution

If you are taking other medications or supplements, talk to a health-care professional before starting any herbal medicines.

Migraine

Medical Background

Migraines are a type of chronic headache. They can be differentiated from other types of headaches by the symptoms that accompany them, which can include nausea and vomiting, as well as sensitivity to light, sound, and strong odors. Occasionally, migraines can also be accompanied by an

> *Dong quai is arguably one of the oldest and most established therapeutic agents used in the traditional Chinese medicine healing model.*

aura of visions, flashes, or bright arcs. Migraine attacks can vary in intensity and disrupt daily life.

Up to 25% of the North American population experiences migraine headaches, and they appear five times more often in women. Pain is often worse on one side, described as a throbbing feeling that can last between 4 and 72 hours. Potential triggers for the onset of a migraine include alcohol, hunger, visual stimuli, such as bright flashing lights, head or neck injury, fatigue, and stress. Predisposition to migraines may be genetic.

Common medical treatments include drugs to manage pain. Migraines may be managed if a certain trigger is determined, so it is recommended that a headache diary be kept describing the environment, diet, and circumstances during which the migraines appear.

Common Medicinal Herbs

Herbal medicines are often used by practitioners in combination with other herbs, diet modifications, and other types of treatment. The following herbs have been used in the management of migraine headaches:

Feverfew

Three systematic reviews have concluded that feverfew may be more effective than a placebo in preventing migraines, but the study designs were poor and thus additional research is needed to confirm these preliminary findings. There is currently no evidence that feverfew will help to treat the symptoms of a migraine once it has already started.

> *Feverfew has been used medicinally for a variety of indications dating back to Ancient Greece, and its use has been documented in many of the* materia medica *written in the Middle Ages.*

Meadowsweet

This herb is commonly used to relieve pain and decrease inflammation. Clinical trials are needed to investigate this use.

Willow

Willow has traditionally been used as a painkiller, so it may benefit patients with migraines. Clinical trials are needed to investigate this use.

Caution

If you are taking other medications or supplements, talk to a health-care professional before starting any herbal medicines. Consult a health-care professional for a safe and effective treatment protocol for migraines.

Multiple Sclerosis

Medical Background

Most nerves in the body are covered by a substance called myelin, which speeds up the conduction of nerve impulses. Multiple sclerosis is a disease that affects the myelin covering the nerves of the central nervous system. Symptoms include impaired vision and abnormalities of the eye, abnormal touch sensations producing pain from contact with normal stimuli, overall weakness, urinary abnormalities, and mild intellectual difficulties. These symptoms tend to appear, worsen, and retreat in a cycle that can be different for each person.

The source of the myelin breakdown seems to be an attack by the immune system. The trigger for this attack is unknown, although one theory maintains that an overactive immune system can be caused by an infection. A genetic component is also suspected. Risk factors for this disease are also unknown, and it can appear in anyone, usually between the ages of 15 and 60. The prevalence of multiple sclerosis in temperate climates is much higher than in tropical climates, so less exposure to vitamin D from sunlight may be a factor.

Common medical treatments include drugs to manage symptom flare-ups, drugs to suppress the immune system to help prevent flare-ups, and painkillers. Regular exercise is also recommended.

Common Medicinal Herbs

Herbal medicines are often used by practitioners in combination with other herbs, dietary modifications, and other types of treatment. The following herb has been used in the management of multiple sclerosis:

Evening Primrose

It has been suggested that the essential fatty acids in evening primrose may be beneficial for patients with multiple sclerosis. These fats are thought to slow the progression and severity of returning symptoms. While theoretically plausible, scientific research is needed to confirm this use.

Evening primrose oil was one of the first nutritional and botanical supplements to gain popularity in the renaissance of alternative medicine. In 1993, a survey of complementary medicine use in Australia showed that more than 12% of women supplemented with this product.

Caution

If you are taking other medications or supplements, talk to a health-care professional before starting any herbal medicines. Consult a health-care professional if you are experiencing symptoms of multiple sclerosis.

Nausea and Vomiting

Medical Background

Nausea is the uncomfortable feeling of needing to vomit. Vomiting is the involuntary expulsion of food from the stomach as the result of uncontrollable abdominal muscle contractions. Nausea and vomiting can result from many common situations, such as motion sickness, pregnancy, common viral infections, such as the flu, overeating, stress, or drug therapy. However, it can also be a symptom of a more serious condition, such as food poisoning, if accompanied with diarrhea. Food poisoning can be especially dangerous for children because of the resulting significant loss of fluids.

Vomiting can occur in people of all ages. Vomiting as a result of motion sickness is most common in children between the ages of 2 and 12 and is also more common in women than in men. In addition, 8 out of 10 women experience nausea and vomiting in the form of morning sickness in their first 3 months of pregnancy. Individuals of all ages may also experience nausea and vomiting as side effects of medication. Most vomiting episodes resolve themselves, but if they do not, dehydration and malnutrition can result.

Conventional treatments include many over-the-counter medications that suppress symptoms of nausea and stop vomiting, as well as rehydration fluids. Prescription medication is also available for specific causes of nausea and vomiting.

Motion Sickness

Motion sickness is a feeling of physical discomfort that is brought on by motion. Symptoms can include nausea, vomiting, pale skin color, yawning, and dizziness. The motion that causes these symptoms is often one that moves the passenger forward and backward or up and down repetitively. This can be experienced when traveling in any kind of moving vehicle, most commonly airplanes or ships. Visual stimulation or poorly ventilated air can also cause symptoms of motion sickness.

Motion sickness can be experienced by anyone at any age. It is more common in females than males and is frequently found in children between the ages of 2 and 12. The cause of motion sickness is excessive stimulation of an area in the ear that controls our sensation of balance. This excessive stimulation can also be produced when our brain expects a different movement than the kind the body experiences. It is possible for the body to adjust to such patterns of motion over a long trip if the intensity and rhythm are constant.

Common medical treatments for motion sickness include prescription and non-prescription medications that come in pill or patch forms. It is often recommended that individuals who are susceptible to motion sickness take these medications as a preventative measure before being exposed to the motion. Susceptible individuals can also decrease their chances of experiencing symptoms by positioning themselves where there is the least movement and making sure the area is adequately ventilated. Focusing on stationary objects in the distance and avoiding reading while in movement may also help.

Morning Sickness (Nausea from Pregnancy)

Nausea and vomiting are common early symptoms of pregnancy and are caused by a large increase in estrogen levels. This is often experienced in the morning and thus called morning sickness, but it is possible to experience nausea and vomiting at any time of the day during pregnancy.

Morning sickness is most common in the first 3 months of pregnancy and is experienced at some point by 80% of pregnant women. The severity of morning sickness varies, and it affects every woman differently. It usually lasts between a few days and weeks and is not accompanied by abdominal discomfort. If vomiting becomes severe or lasts longer than a few weeks, a health-care professional should be consulted.

Conventional treatments for morning sickness do not often include drugs, except in severe cases, because of the risk of harming the fetus. Recommended practices to control nausea and vomiting during pregnancy include ensuring there is fresh air in the room during sleep and when food is eaten, eating a few crackers in the morning before rising, and eating up to five sparse meals throughout the day instead of three large meals.

Common Medicinal Herbs

Individual herbal medicines are often used by practitioners in combination with other herbs and other types of treatment. The following herbs have been used in the management of nausea and vomiting:

Ginger

Clinical trials have produced mixed results about the oral ingestion of ginger for motion sickness, as well as for postoperative nausea and vomiting. Further scientific research is needed to confirm this use. The use of ginger during pregnancy to relieve morning sickness is controversial, but preliminary clinical trials show encouraging results. More research is needed.

> *Very few herbs have more of a medicinal history than ginger. Its use originated in the healing models of the East and quickly spread to the ancient cultures of Europe and the Middle East.*

❧ *Peppermint*

Oral consumption of peppermint is traditionally used in the treatment of nausea and vomiting. Clinical research is needed to investigate the use of peppermint in preventing motion sickness.

Caution

If you are taking other medications or supplements, talk to a health-care professional before starting any herbal medicines. If you have recurring or prolonged periods of vomiting, contact a qualified health-care professional. Consult a health-care professional before taking herbs during pregnancy to establish a safe and effective protocol for morning sickness.

Nerve Pain

Medical Background

Nerve pain, also known as neuralgia, neuropathy, or neuropathic pain, is caused by damage to either the central or the peripheral nervous system. Symptoms include a tingling or burning sensation, an altered sense of touch that can produce pain from ordinary stimuli, and complete or partial loss of sensation.

Nerve damage can result in several ways, including direct injury to the nerve, as in the case of amputation or a deep wound, compression of the nerve by inflamed tissues, damage to the spinal cord, and factors associated with diabetes. Anyone who undergoes these events is vulnerable to nerve damage.

Common treatments include drugs to help manage pain, including oral and topical applications in some cases, treatment to manage anxiety and depression if it is present, or surgery if compression of the nerve is causing the pain. Treatment with drugs does not usually eliminate all the pain.

Common Medicinal Herbs

Herbal medicines are often used by practitioners in combination with other herbs and other types of treatment. The following herbs have been used in the management of nerve pain:

❧ *Capsicum*

An extract from capsicum called capsaicin has been applied topically in several clinical trials for treatment of diabetic neuropathy, with positive results. Capsicum seems to be a safe and effective treatment for diabetic neuralgia. More research is needed to investigate using capsicum to treat other forms of neuralgia.

❧ *Evening Primrose*

Evening primrose has traditionally been used to treat neuralgia. Several clinical trials have shown positive results using evening primrose oil to treat diabetic neuropathy. The high fatty acid content of the oil may be responsible for this effect.

> *Evening primrose has been used for many medical purposes in the past, giving rise to the plant being commonly referred to as the king's cure-all.*

❧ *St. John's Wort*

Although St. John's wort has traditionally been used both orally and topically to treat neuralgia, no scientific studies have investigated this use.

Caution

If you are taking other medications or supplements, talk to a health-care professional before starting any herbal medicines. If symptoms of neuralgia are present, consult a health-care professional for a diagnosis and a safe and effective treatment plan. To assess health risks and develop a treatment plan, it is important to diagnose the source of pain.

Obesity

Medical Background

Obesity is characterized by severely excessive body fat, as determined using the body mass index (BMI) and waist measurements. Obesity is influenced by a combination of genetic disposition, sedentary lifestyle, and chronic overeating. Complications of obesity can include diabetes, several cancers, cardiovascular disorders, liver disorders, and osteoarthritis. Obesity contributes to 300,000 premature deaths a year.

The prevalence of obesity in North America is high, with approximately one-third of the population identified as obese. Obesity shows a clear trend of increasing prevalence with age and a higher prevalence in women who are poorer or less educated. There is also a rising prevalence of obesity in childhood — the rates have doubled in the last 30 years for children between the ages of 6 and 19. The rise in prevalence of obesity in the general population may be influenced by environmental factors, such as the availability of food, portion sizes, and inactive leisure-time activities.

Current treatments for obesity include a combination of dietary changes — including altered proportions, proper food choices, and caloric restrictions — exercise, and behavioral therapy.

Common Medicinal Herbs

Individual herbal medicines are often used by practitioners in combination with other herbs and other types of treatment. The following herbs have been used in the management of obesity:

Bitter Orange

Several clinical trials have been conducted using combination products containing bitter orange to promote weight loss. These studies have produced mixed results and some reports of cardiovascular (heart) side effects, so more high-quality trials are needed before this product can be recommended.

Hoodia

One unpublished clinical trial and several animal studies have been conducted examining the use of hoodia in promoting weight loss. It has been reported to suppress appetite, although proper data from the clinical trial are not available. Further studies are needed to study its effects in humans.

> *Hoodia has become popular because of stories of the Kalahari bushmen of sub-Saharan Africa using this plant to ward off hunger and thirst when they were traveling in the desert.*

Licorice

One clinical trial reported that individuals taking licorice oil lost more weight than those taking a placebo in a 12-week trial. Additional studies are needed to confirm these preliminary findings.

Ma Huang

Although a component of ma huang, ephedrine, has been found in some clinical trials to help people lose weight when it is combined with caffeine, this combination has dangerous side effects, including negative effects on the heart and even death. Ma huang (and ephedrine) cannot be legally sold in Canada for use in weight loss because of these potentially dangerous side effects.

Caution

If you are taking other medications or supplements, talk to a health-care professional before starting any herbal medicines. Untreated obesity can have serious long-term health consequences. A qualified health-care professional can help you design a safe plan for losing weight.

Pain

Medical Background

The most common reason that people seek medical attention is for the treatment of pain, which exists in a range of severities and can be classified as chronic or acute, local or general. Pain has both an emotional and physical component and can affect the lives of each individual differently. Tolerance to pain, which determines how severe a person thinks the pain is, can influence the individual's experience of pain.

Acute pain is often the result of an injury and is caused by short-term activation of pain receptors. Chronic pain may be a result of constant activation of pain receptors or damage to the nervous system. Repeated injury in the same location can increase sensitivity in the tissues and cause emphasized pain perception, leading to chronic pain. Chronic pain can also lead to more serious symptoms, including appetite loss, insomnia, weight loss, and depression.

Conventional medical treatment depends on the type and cause of the pain. It is important to consult a health-care professional to determine the cause of the pain before self-treating it. Acute pain is often treated with medication. Chronic pain can be treated with drugs that affect the nervous system, nerve stimulation, and antidepressants. Behavioral and relationship counseling are also recommended.

Common Medicinal Herbs

Herbal medicines are often used by practitioners in combination with other herbs and other types of treatment. The following herbs have been used generically in the management of pain:

Cat's Claw

Cat's claw has been used traditionally for a number of painful conditions. Animal studies indicate it has an anti-inflammatory action. Additional clinical research is needed.

> *The Peruvian government has recently invested in an extensive planting campaign for cat's claw as an alternative (and more suitable) crop to replace the illegal cultivation of coca.*

Ginger

Several clinical trials suggest that ginger may be helpful in the management of musculoskeletal pain.

Meadowsweet

Meadowsweet has traditionally been used as a painkiller. Although constituents found in this herb have demonstrated analgesic properties, trials are needed to evaluate clinical use.

Willow

Willow contains many compounds that can help in the management of pain, and clinical trials have shown positive results in patients with lower back pain. Further research is needed to confirm these results.

Caution

If you are taking other medications or supplements, talk to a health-care professional before starting any herbal medicines. It is important to diagnose a source of pain. Consult a health-care professional if pain symptoms persist or worsen.

Peptic Ulcers

Medical Background

Peptic ulcers are caused when the mucosal lining of the stomach or small intestine is worn away by either *Helicobacter pylori* bacteria or frequent use of non-steroidal anti-inflammatory drugs (NSAIDs) such as aspirin and ibuprofen. Peptic ulcers present no symptoms in half of all patients, but they can cause a gnawing or burning sensation felt in the upper abdomen. This pain can be relieved by food or antacids. Some individuals with peptic ulcers in the stomach experience increased pain with eating or nausea and vomiting.

About 5% to 10% of the population is estimated to experience a peptic ulcer at some point in their lives. They can be present at any age, but they are most common among middle-aged adults. Smokers have an increased risk of peptic ulcers and a slower ulcer healing rate.

Conventional medical treatments for peptic ulcers include antibiotics, if *H. pylori* bacteria are present, and anti-secretory drugs to prevent further damage by stomach acid. Avoidance of NSAIDs and aggravating foods is also recommended. In severe cases, surgery may be appropriate.

Common Medicinal Herbs

Herbal medicines are often used by practitioners in combination with other herbs, dietary and lifestyle modifications, and other types of treatment. The following herbs have been used in the management of peptic ulcers:

Chamomile

Chamomile is traditionally used as a digestive agent and is thought to be healing to the gut tissues, so it may be helpful in treating peptic ulcers. Further scientific research is needed.

Licorice

A modified form of licorice extract called deglycyrrhizinated licorice, or DGL, which contains only small amounts of glycyrrhizinic acid, has been shown in a number of clinical studies to speed the healing of peptic ulcers. Licorice in general may help support mucosal cells and produce more protective mucus. Given that most of the supporting scientific evidence deals with DGL as an extract, further research on licorice's protective properties is needed to confirm the use of the herb itself.

> *Licorice is extensively cultivated as a medicinal herb and to produce a distinctively flavored sugar for making candy. Most of the licorice candy available in North America, however, is not flavored with licorice but with anise oil.*

Meadowsweet

Meadowsweet is traditionally used to treat gastrointestinal conditions, including peptic ulcers. Scientific research is needed to verify this use.

Slippery Elm

While yet to be proven in clinical studies, slippery elm is traditionally used to treat inflammations of mucous membranes, which may be useful in soothing peptic ulcers. Scientific research is needed to verify this use.

Caution

If you are taking other medications or supplements, talk to a health-care professional before starting any herbal medicines. Proper diagnosis of ulcers is important, so consult a health-care professional if symptoms of a peptic ulcer are present.

Premenstrual Syndrome

Medical Background

Premenstrual syndrome is a collection of symptoms that a woman may experience in the week before menstruation, ending shortly after menstruation starts. Symptoms include irritability, depression, moodiness, cravings, bloating, headaches, and breast tenderness. The symptoms may vary in form and intensity each month. Premenstrual syndrome appears to be caused by the normal fluctuation in hormones that affect a woman's body preceding menstruation.

Up to 80% of women experience some kind of mood change or physical symptoms within 10 days before their period. Not all women experience these changes every month, and many report that the change can be positive, increasing energy or creativity. Both genetic and environmental stressors can have an influence on whether premenstrual syndrome symptoms are experienced each month. Women who smoke are four times more likely to be diagnosed with severe forms of premenstrual syndrome than women who don't smoke. Symptoms are absent when ovulation has stopped, during pregnancy, for example.

Conventional medical treatments for premenstrual syndrome are mainly concentrated on relieving individual symptoms. Initial treatments include dietary changes, exercise, and stress management techniques. Non-prescription medications are also used. Severe cases of premenstrual syndrome are treated with hormone therapy and drugs that modify the menstrual cycle.

Common Medicinal Herbs

Herbal medicines are often used by practitioners in combination with other herbs, diet modification, and other types of treatment. Please talk to a health-care professional before starting any herbal medicines if you are taking other medications or supplements. The following herbs have been used in the management of premenstrual syndrome:

❧ *Black Cohosh*

Black cohosh has traditionally been used to treat women's health issues; however, there is little scientific research that confirms its effectiveness for premenstrual symptoms. More studies are needed.

> *The Cherokee and Iroquois First Nations used a tea made from black cohosh root to alleviate rheumatic pains and to promote lactation and menses.*

❧ *Chaste Tree*

Small clinical trials support the traditional use of this herb to manage both physical and psychological symptoms associated with premenstrual syndrome. More research is needed to confirm these preliminary findings.

❧ *Evening Primrose*

Some studies have indicated that evening primrose can help improve premenstrual symptoms; others have found no significant effects. Further scientific research is needed.

❧ *Red Clover*

One small study found that red clover might decrease premenstrual breast pain, but further studies are needed to confirm this preliminary finding.

❧ *St. John's Wort*

A couple of small clinical studies suggest that St. John's wort may decrease premenstrual symptoms. Additional research is needed to confirm these preliminary findings.

🌺 *Wild Yam*

The root of wild yam is traditionally used to treat painful menses (periods). Scientific research is needed to explore this use of wild yam.

Caution

If you are taking other medications or supplements, talk to a health-care professional before starting any herbal medicines. If symptoms of premenstrual syndrome are particularity severe or persistent, consult a health-care professional for a safe and effective treatment plan.

Prostate Conditions

Medical Background

The prostate is a walnut-sized ring of glandular tissue positioned at the top of the penis. Its only known function is to produce seminal fluid that will be ejaculated with sperm. The prostate surrounds the urethra at its entry to the penis, and abnormalities of the prostate can affect urination.

The prevalence of prostate conditions increases with age, and the risk significantly increases over 65 years of age. The three most common diseases of the prostate are benign prostate hyperplasia, prostatitis, and prostate cancer. Symptoms of these three conditions include incontinence, inconsistent urine flow, frequent urination, and hesitancy when urinating because of pressure put on the urethra.

It is difficult to distinguish between prostate conditions because their symptoms are similar. A health-care professional should be consulted to determine a proper diagnosis and treatment plan. Conventional medical treatments for prostate diseases depend on the diagnosis. These treatments include insertion of a urinary catheter and treatment of infections with antibiotics, drug therapy, or radiation therapy. Prostate cancer can also be treated with hormone therapy or surgery.

Common Medicinal Herbs

Herbal medicines are often used by practitioners in combination with other herbs and/or other types of treatments. The following herbs have been used in the management of prostate conditions:

🌺 *Nettle*

Clinical trials have shown nettle root to be an effective way to treat benign prostate hyperplasia. This herb has been tested alone and in combination with saw palmetto.

🌺 *Red Clover*

Two clinical trials have suggested that red clover may help prevent prostate cancer, although a conflicting trial has also been published. Further research is needed.

🌺 *Saw Palmetto*

Clinical trails have shown that saw palmetto helps mediate symptoms of benign prostate hyperplasia, such as weak urine stream and urination at night. This herb can be used alone or in combination with other herbs, such as nettle.

> *Historically, the ripe fruit of saw palmetto was partially dried and used for a variety of conditions of the bladder, urethra, and prostate. It was called the plant catheter.*

Caution

If you are taking other medications or supplements, talk to a health-care professional before starting any herbal medicines. Consult a health-care professional for a proper diagnosis before taking herbs for prostate conditions and for information about interactions between herbs and drugs if you are already on other medications.

Psoriasis

Medical Background

Psoriasis is an inflammatory disease that produces dry, scaly lesions on the skin. These raised patches of pink or red skin are surrounded by a well-defined border and covered by a pale layer of dead skin. There are usually no other symptoms, although the lesions can be slightly itchy. The lesions can appear on any part of the body but are usually found on the elbows, knees, buttocks, scalp, or penis. They are often symmetrical. There are several forms of psoriasis, distinguished by the size and shape of lesions, the most common appearing as several smaller patches that expand and eventually join.

Psoriasis affects between 1% and 5% of people worldwide. While it usually begins between the ages of 16 to 20 or 57 to 60, it is possible to develop psoriasis at any age. Remissions and outbreaks of lesions are often unpredictable. Psoriasis is not contagious, and the cause is unknown, although it is most common in fair-skinned people and a genetic component is suspected. Potential environmental triggers that may cause a flare-up of lesions include injury to the skin, sunburn, stress, and certain drugs.

Conventional medical treatments consist of anti-inflammatory topical drugs, oral drugs, and phototherapy in more severe cases. Moisturizing the area after showers or baths is also recommended.

Common Medicinal Herbs

Herbal medicines are often used by practitioners in combination with other herbs and other types of treatment. The following herbs have been used in the management of psoriasis:

🌺 Evening Primrose

Although evening primrose acts as an anti-inflammatory agent, it has proven to be unsuccessful in treating psoriasis in clinical trials.

🌺 Milk Thistle

It has been suggested that milk thistle may benefit patients with psoriasis because it has moderate anti-inflammatory affects and it supports the liver. Scientific research is needed to confirm this theory.

> *While the Greeks and Romans noted the medicinal properties of milk thistle, current interest in this product did not begin until the late 1960s, when silymarin was first isolated from the ripe seeds of this herb.*

Caution

If you are taking other medications or supplements, talk to a health-care professional before starting any herbal medicines. In cases in which lesions cover more than 10% of the body or in the case of small children, consult a health-care professional for an appropriate treatment plan.

Skin Rashes and Irritations

Medical Background

Skin rashes and irritations include a wide variety of acute, seasonal, and chronic skin conditions. A skin rash can be described as any kind of visible irritation on the skin, in most cases appearing as a shade of pink or red. Symptoms often include an itching sensation around the area. Rashes are characterized by their shape, size, color, texture, location, and distribution. They can be developed by people of all ages but become more common after 65 years of age.

Rashes and irritations can be triggered by many things. A common type of irritation is called contact dermatitis, which is an acutely inflamed, itchy, red response to contact with an irritant or allergen. Common irritants include commercial soaps and chemicals, while allergens may be almost anything and can be different for everyone. Rashes can also be caused by infections, and it is recommended that these be diagnosed and treated by a health-care professional.

Conventional medical treatments for rashes vary according to the cause of the rash. Some skin irritations, such as dermatitis, can be managed through hydration and avoidance of environmental triggers. Rashes are also commonly treated with topical medications, such as hydrocortisone, which acts as an anti-inflammatory and relieves itching.

Common Medicinal Herbs

Individual herbal medicines are often used by practitioners in combination with other herbs and other types of treatment. The following herbs have been used in the management of skin rashes and irritations:

Aloe Vera

Studies suggest that aloe vera possesses an anti-inflammatory effect that may be helpful in treating rashes. Further studies are needed to confirm this result.

> *The clear mucilaginous gel from the cells in the inner portion of the aloe leaves is the part of the plant used medicinally for skin abrasions, rashes, and infections. This aloe gel is distinct from the bitter yellow juice found in the rind of the leaves, which is a potent laxative.*

Burdock

Burdock has traditionally been used internally and externally to treat skin conditions. Further scientific research is needed to confirm this use.

Calendula

Animal studies have demonstrated that calendula has an anti-inflammatory effect when applied topically. While these findings are promising, more clinical trials are needed to verify this effect.

Chamomile

Clinical trials indicate that topically applied chamomile has an anti-inflammatory effect. This herb can be used to treat rashes resulting from dermatitis and in conjunction with other treatments to treat more serious skin conditions.

Echinacea

Traditionally, echinacea has been used topically for wound healing, and animal studies have supported the anti-inflammatory effect of this herb. Further clinical trials are needed to confirm this action.

Licorice

Licorice has been shown to inhibit inflammatory responses from the immune system. This can be beneficial for rashes and may also help control allergic responses. Further clinical research is needed to confirm these actions.

Caution

If you are taking other medications or supplements, talk to a health-care professional before starting any herbal medicines. It is best to have a skin irritation assessed by a health-care professional to determine the source and an appropriate treatment, especially if the condition lasts more than a few days or appears to be worsening over time. These herbs are not recommended for treating complicated skin disorders.

Sore Throat

Medical Background

A sore throat is often the first sign of the common cold and is characterized as a scratchy, raw, sometimes tender feeling along the throat. The part of the throat seen when the mouth is wide open is usually a flushed red color during the period of irritation. If any white plaques or patches are seen in the back of the mouth, it may be an indication of an infection or more serious throat illness that should be brought to the attention of a health-care professional. For example, a sore throat can also result from infection by other agents, such as the bacterium that causes strep throat. The best way to protect against all infectious bacteria and viruses is to wash your hands regularly and keep food preparation areas as sterile as possible.

Current conventional medical treatments for a sore throat include anesthetic throat sprays and lozenges. Gargling with salt water is also recommended.

Common Medicinal Herbs

Individual herbal medicines are often used by practitioners in combination with other herbs and other types of treatment. Before starting any herbal medicine, please talk to a health-care professional if you are taking other medications or supplements. The following herbs have been used in the management of a sore throat:

Echinacea

Although this is a popular herb for preventing and treating cold symptoms, clinical studies have shown conflicting evidence. Generally, the research suggests that echinacea will not help prevent cold symptoms, including a sore throat, but some forms of echinacea may be beneficial if taken within the first 48 hours of the onset of symptoms.

Elder

This herb has traditionally been used in the form of a gargle to soothe sore, irritated throats. Clinical trials are needed to investigate this use.

Slippery Elm

Slippery elm is traditionally used in the form of a liquid or lozenge to soothe minor sore throat irritations. It is thought that this herb may help soothe the throat by calming irritated mucous membranes.

Goldenseal

Goldenseal may help support the immune system, allowing it to fight off any infections that are causing a common cold or a sore throat. Further research is needed to clarify its usefulness for treating the symptoms of the common cold.

> *Goldenseal has enjoyed a long medicinal history and is often referred to by herbalists as king of the tonics of the mucous membranes.*

Caution

If you are taking other medications or supplements, talk to a health-care professional before starting any herbal medicines. If symptoms of a sore throat worsen or persist, contact a health-care professional. These herbs are not recommended for treating advanced throat illnesses.

Stress

Medical Background

Psychological stress can be caused by a number of factors, including the stress of responsibility, financial and educational concerns, conflict within relationships, memories of disturbing experiences, anticipation, or pressure. Stressors can be psychological or physical and vary between individuals — something that evokes stress in one person may not bother another person.

The stress response is an instinctive reaction to an immediately stressful situation. It is also called the "flight or fight" response, because humans have evolved to respond to stressful situations by either preparing to defend themselves (by fighting the source of the stress) or leaving the situation as quickly as possible (taking flight from the source of the stress). This response is triggered by specific hormones released by the body when experiencing a stressful situation. Unfortunately, these innate responses are not particularly suited to modern-day stressors. Psychological adaptations to longer-term stress can cause anxiety or depression.

Current conventional medical treatments for stress include coping techniques, such as breathing exercises, meditation, and time management. Prescription medication to help decrease the anxiety or depression that can be associated with long-term stress is also available.

Common Medicinal Herbs

Individual herbal medicines are often used by practitioners in combination with other herbs and other types of treatment. The following herbs have been used in the management of stress:

Ashwagandha

Several animal studies suggest ashwagandha may prevent or decrease reactions to stress. However, more research is needed to confirm these preliminary findings.

Ginseng (Asian)

Several small studies have shown Asian ginseng to enhance coping abilities in the face of both mental and physical stressors. Further research is necessary to confirm whether Asian ginseng may be helpful for stress-related issues.

Ginseng (Siberian)

One clinical trial suggested that Siberian ginseng increases general stress resistance. Further research is needed to confirm this finding.

> *Interest in the medicinal use of Siberian ginseng began only in the 1960s, when researchers in the Soviet Union became aware of its potential as a substitute for the more expensive and difficult to obtain Asian ginseng and American/Canadian ginseng.*

Lemon Balm

Inhalation of lemon balm in the form of an essential oil acts on the nervous system and instills calmness. Further research is needed on the use of lemon balm to alleviate stress.

Licorice

Licorice is used in traditional Chinese medicine to treat both physical and mental stress. Some of the constituents are known to stimulate adrenal function. More scientific research is needed to investigate this use.

Caution

If you are taking other medications or supplements, talk to a health-care professional before starting any herbal medicines. Consult a health-care professional for a safe and effective plan for coping with stress. These herbs are not recommended for treating specific stress disorders, including acute stress disorder and post-traumatic stress disorder.

Tinnitus
(Ringing in the Ears)

Medical Background

Tinnitus is described as a noise in the ears that can only be heard by the individual experiencing it. The noise can be explained in many different ways, often as a ringing, roaring, or hissing sound. The intensity of the sound can be mild to severely disturbing and may be constant or may come and go. Tinnitus may be more prevalent during periods of stress.

Approximately 10% to 15% of the population experiences tinnitus. It can be caused by a blockage of the ear canal, ear infections, periods of loud noise, trauma to the eardrum, or drug toxicity. Occasionally, sounds in the ears can be caused by turbulent blood flow through arteries in the neck. Tinnitus can also occur as a side effect of antibiotics and usually disappears when use of the antibiotic is discontinued.

Half of all patients experiencing tinnitus find relief with devices that restore hearing, such as hearing aids. Others wear devices that make low noises to drown out the tinnitus, to aid in sleep. If it is a symptom associated with another condition, treating the underlying cause can cure tinnitus. Non-prescription drugs do not effectively treat tinnitus, so professional help is advised.

Common Medicinal Herbs

Individual herbal medicines are often used by practitioners in combination with other herbs and other types of treatment. Please talk to a health-care professional before starting any herbal medicines if you are taking other medications or supplements. The following herb has been used in the management of tinnitus:

Ginkgo

Clinical trials have shown mixed results on using ginkgo to treat tinnitus. While initial studies are promising, additional research is needed.

> Ginkgo trees are now extensively cultivated to meet the growing medicinal demand, and they continue to be favored by city planners because they flourish in adverse conditions in urban environments.

Caution

If you are taking other medications or supplements, talk to a health-care professional before starting any herbal medicines. Because tinnitus could indicate hearing disorders, consult a health-care professional for evaluation if you are experiencing symptoms of tinnitus.

Tobacco (Cigarette) Addiction

Medical Background

Tobacco addiction is the psychological and physical dependence on nicotine, which is the main component in cigarettes. Nicotine is highly addictive and is inhaled along with hundreds of cancer-causing chemicals found in cigarette smoke. Most individuals with a nicotine addiction experience withdrawal symptoms, such as irritability, anxiety, loss of concentration, fatigue, and anger, when their body is deprived of nicotine for a length of time. Although the negative health effects associated with smoking cigarettes have been public knowledge for at least 20 years, approximately 20% of the population in North America currently smokes cigarettes. Health issues directly and indirectly caused by smoking are a leading cause of death in North America.

More than half of all smokers start smoking before they are 18 years old. Factors that influence children to start smoking include peer influences and observing smoking habits in role models. In teenagers, smoking may also be correlated with poor grades in school and other risky behaviors, such as extreme dieting or drinking alcohol. Smoking is more common in men, and prevalence increases in people with less education and people who are living near the poverty line.

Conventional medical treatments include counseling and both prescription and non-prescription drugs.

Common Medicinal Herbs

Individual herbal medicines are often used by practitioners in combination with other herbs and other types of treatment. The following herb has been used in the management of tobacco addiction:

🌿 Lobelia

Several human trials have shown an extract from lobelia to be effective in treating tobacco addiction. Natural health products containing lobelia extracts are sold in Canada to treat tobacco addiction.

Lobeline is a constituent of lobelia, and lobeline products are often used in treating tobacco addictions because lobeline is chemically similar to nicotine.

Caution

If you are taking other medications or supplements, talk to a health-care professional before starting any herbal medicines. Tobacco addiction can have fatal long-term consequences. Consult a health-care professional for counseling and guidance about how to quit smoking.

Urinary Tract Infection

Medical Background

A urinary tract infection (UTI) is a growth of bacteria or fungi affecting the urinary system. Approximately four million yearly patient visits to health-care practitioners are related to urinary tract infections. This type of infection usually presents with a frequent urge to urinate, pain in the lower abdomen, and possibly blood in the urine. Urinary tract infections can also be present even if there are no symptoms.

Bacterial urinary tract infections most commonly result from contamination of the sterile ureter with foreign bacteria. Occasionally, the infection can be caused by blood-borne bacteria. Bacterial urinary tract infections can be especially threatening for the elderly because of an increased risk of bacterial transfer to the bloodstream that could cause a more serious, widespread infection. Fungal infections most often disturb the bladder and kidneys, and are usually found in conjunction with bacterial infections.

Urinary tract infections are 50 times more common in women than in men between the ages of 20 and 50. This is because women have a physically shorter ureter, so it is easier for bacteria to enter and travel into the body toward the bladder, where they can multiply. After the age of 50, the incidence of urinary tract infections in men increases because of a higher rate of prostate disorders. Risk of acquiring a urinary tract infection is increased by pregnancy, urinary stones or other objects obstructing the urinary tract, swelling of the prostate, presence of medical equipment, such as a urinary or bladder catheter, and a previous history of urinary tract infections. Practices to decrease the chance of contracting a UTI if these risk factors are present include urinating shortly after sexual intercourse, increasing total fluid intake, wearing loose-fitting cotton clothing, and wiping the elimination area from front to back.

Conventional medical treatments of urinary tract infections involve antibiotics, either acutely or sometimes in regular low doses for individuals with recurring infections.

Common Medicinal Herbs

Individual herbal medicines are often used by practitioners in combination with other herbs and other types of treatment. The following herbs have been used in the management of UTIs:

🌿 *Cranberry*

Clinical trials indicate that cranberry juice and cranberry extract are helpful for *preventing* urinary tract infections. It is clear, however, that cranberry juice is not effective in *treating* urinary tract infections.

🌿 *Goldenseal*

Goldenseal is traditionally used to treat urinary tract infections. While some of the herb's constituents, such as berberine, have antimicrobial effects, this use has yet to be confirmed by scientific evidence.

🌿 *Juniper*

Juniper is traditionally used as a urinary antiseptic to treat uncomplicated infections that do not involve the kidney. Further research is needed on the use of juniper in urinary tract infections.

> *Juniper berries are the principal flavoring agent in gin. However, gin contains insufficient amounts of the essential oil to afford it any medicinal properties.*

🌿 *Uva-ursi*

Uva-ursi is a urinary antiseptic containing antimicrobial agents. It can be used to treat uncomplicated urinary tract infections that do not involve the kidneys. More research is needed to confirm the effectiveness of this herb as a treatment for UTIs.

Caution

If you are taking other medications or supplements, talk to a health-care professional before starting any herbal medicines. If you are experiencing symptoms of a urinary tract infection, consult a health-care professional to determine a safe and effective treatment plan. An untreated urinary tract infection can have long-term consequences, such as kidney infections.

Varicose Veins

Medical Background

Varicose veins are characterized by enlarged, possibly protruding veins in the leg that are especially visible when standing. They can result from weakness and dilation of veins in the leg and insufficient blood return to the upper body. Varicose veins may not be associated with any symptoms, but in some cases a feeling of pressure, pain, and swelling may be experienced in the affected area, accompanied by general fatigue. Varicose veins are close to the surface of the skin and in severe cases can produce ulcers after a minor injury or may potentially aid in the formation of blood clots.

Both men and women can have varicose veins, although this condition is more common in women because over time estrogen has a thinning effect on the structure of veins. Pregnancy can also create pressure that makes blood return from the lower limbs difficult. Although there may be a genetic component to varicose veins, there are no other known risk factors.

Treatments for varicose veins include socks or stockings that put pressure on the lower legs to help compress and support the protruding veins. Surgery is needed in the case of blood clots, and ulcers are treated locally.

Common Medicinal Herbs

Individual herbal medicines are often used by practitioners in combination with other herbs and other types of treatment. Before starting any herbal medicines, please talk to a health-care professional if you are taking other medications or supplements. The following herb has been used in the management of varicose veins:

❧ Horsechestnut

Horsechestnut seed extract has been found to strengthen veins in the lower leg and increase the return of blood to the upper body. It has been shown to act preventatively by decreasing the destruction of venous walls that cause the weakness.

> *In the United Kingdom, the hard fruits of the horsechestnut tree are referred to by many small boys as conkers and are used in a traditional game. Unlike the chestnut tree, the fruit is not edible, though it can be used as fodder for animals.*

Caution

If you are taking other medications or supplements, talk to a health-care professional before starting any herbal medicines. Consult a health-care professional for guidance about how to safely treat varicose veins. Although horsechestnut seed extract is safe to consume, the leaves, raw seeds, and twigs are toxic and can potentially have harmful side effects.

Vertigo (Dizziness)

Medical Background

Vertigo is a condition caused by lesions in the inner ear that produce a false spinning, whirling, or leaning sensation. Lesions in the ear can also cause feelings of dizziness, feelings of being light-headed, and loss of coordination. Dizziness can result from a variety of situations, including changes in atmospheric pressure, prolonged headaches, or ear infections. This symptom could also signal more serious conditions, such as heart disease, a sudden drop in blood pressure, or possibly a tumor.

Symptoms of dizziness can affect people of all ages. Ear infections are a common cause of dizziness in children. The elderly may also be particularly susceptible to dizziness as a side effect of medications or as a result of naturally aging inner ear components.

Current treatments for vertigo and dizziness include symptom-suppressing drugs, but it is important to determine the cause of the symptoms to ensure that the treatment is appropriate.

Common Medicinal Herbs

Individual herbal medicines are often used by practitioners in combination with other herbs and other types of treatment. The following herb has been used in the management of vertigo and dizziness:

❧ Ginkgo

One clinical trial found that ginkgo decreased the intensity and severity of vertigo symptoms compared to a placebo. This finding is supported by several animal studies. Further research is needed to confirm these results.

> *Ginkgo has also been used in traditional Chinese medicine for "benefiting the brain," as an astringent to the lungs, and for relief of asthma symptoms.*

Caution

If you are taking other medications or supplements, talk to a health-care professional before starting any herbal medicines. Consult a health-care professional if you are experiencing recurrent vertigo or dizziness, which could be a sign of more serious conditions.

Yeast Infections
(Skin and Nails)

Medical Background

Yeast infections are caused by a species of yeast called *Candida*, a natural fungus that normally lies dormant on the skin. This yeast can become overgrown in damp, warm environments, especially if the immune system is not working properly. Yeast infections are characterized by red, itchy patches of varying sizes on the skin. These patches can also include bumps that contain discharge. Two common types of yeast infections are yeast infections in skin folds that provide the required conditions — such as armpits, the groin, finger webbings, beneath the breasts, or on mucous membranes, including the mouth — and yeast infections of the nails, which may appear after an improper manicure or among those whose hands are chronically exposed to water.

Yeast infections can appear in people of all ages and are generally initiated by warm temperatures, tight clothing, and poor hygiene. Children and the elderly are at risk for yeast infections in the form of diaper rash, which is a condition resulting from infrequently changed diapers or undergarments. Diabetes, pregnancy, use of immunosuppressive drugs, and a range of hormone-based conditions can also increase the probability of yeast infections by altering the immune system.

Conventional treatments for yeast infections include drying agents and topical and oral antifungals.

Common Medicinal Herbs

Individual herbal medicines are often used by practitioners in combination with other herbs and other types of treatment. The following herb has been used in the management of skin and nail yeast infections:

🌿 *Tea Tree Oil*

The results from two clinical trials suggest that topical tea tree oil products may be effective in treating fungal nail infections. Further research is needed into the use of tea tree oil on other sites of yeast infection.

> *Due to increased popular demand, the commercial production of Australian tea tree oil increased in the early 1990s from 20 tons to 140 tons per annum. In addition to its medicinal applications, it is now used extensively in the cosmetic and skin-care industries.*

Caution

If you are taking other medications or supplements, talk to a health-care professional before starting any herbal medicines. If you are unsure whether you have a skin or nail yeast infection, or if your infection does not improve, contact a qualified health-care professional. Tea tree oil is a strong irritant and should not be ingested or applied to broken skin or mucous membranes. This herb should not be used for vaginal yeast infections.

Selected References

Berardi RR, Kroon LA, McDermott JH, et al. Handbook of Nonprescription Drugs: An Interactive Approach to Self-Care, 15th ed. Washington, DC: American Pharmacists Association, 2006.

Gray J (ed). Therapeutic Choices, 5th ed. Ottawa, ON: Canadian Pharmacists Association, 2007.

The Merck Manual for Healthcare Professionals, online version, www.merck.com/mmpe/index.html.

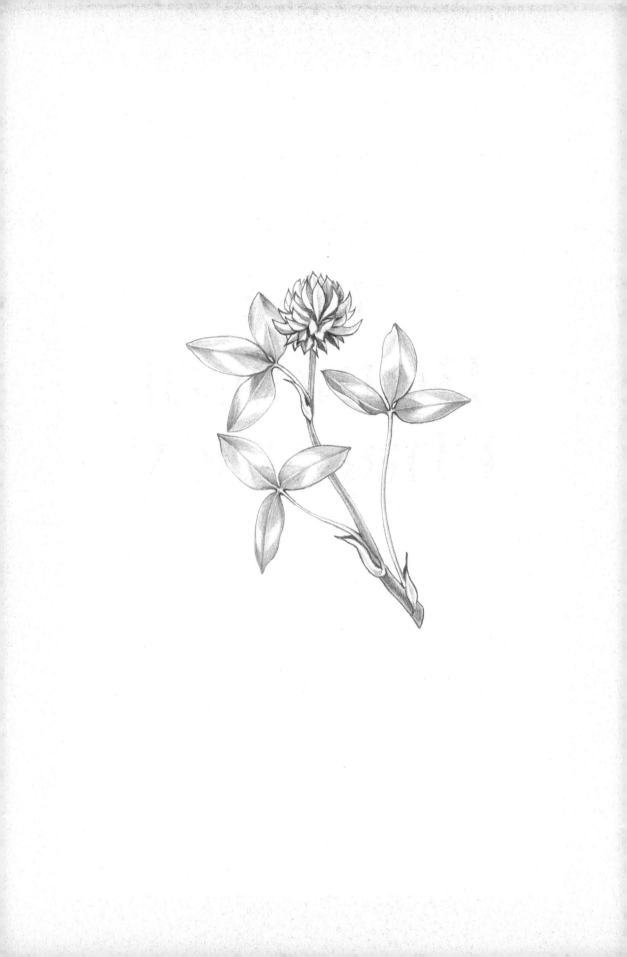

PART 2

The Botanical Pharmacy

Preface

The literature reviews in this section are organized in a standardized, accessible format, despite the fact that the nature and quantity of information vary from herb to herb. The reviews of each herb follow a basic outline: a thumbnail sketch; a sidebar indicating the herb's family, synonyms, and medicinal forms; an introduction (description, parts used, traditional use, current medicinal use); and relevant research on preventative and therapeutic effects (constituents, effects, adverse effects, cautions/contraindications, drug interactions, dosage regimens). Given the different types of information — scientific, anecdotal, cross-cultural — available for each herb, as well as the quality and quantity of the available information, the preventative and therapeutic effects section may be organized in different ways.

In all cases, a systematic search of the available English language literature was conducted. We have focused the review summaries on human studies where possible (i.e., when human studies exist), but also discuss key animal (in vivo) and test tube (in vitro) studies to provide added clarification or to explain common uses that have not yet been studied in humans. These reviews place an emphasis on human studies that are double-blind, randomized, and controlled, because this is considered the "gold standard" of scientific evidence.

In a double-blind study, neither the researchers nor the participants know who is taking the herb and who is taking the comparator substance. This helps to eliminate possible biases and the "placebo" or expectancy effect that can occur when people think they know what will happen when they ingest a product. Randomization simply means that every participant in a trial has an equal chance of ending up in each treatment group. A controlled trial has a comparator group — either a placebo group or an active treatment group — where the herbal treatment is compared with another treatment thought to be effective. In placebo-controlled trials, one is testing to see if the herbal treatment is better than the placebo; in a trial with an active treatment control, one is testing to see if the herbal treatment is at least as good as the active treatment (this is sometimes called an equivalency trial).

These reviews place an emphasis on human studies that are double-blind, randomized, and controlled, because this is considered the "gold standard" of scientific evidence.

The herbal summaries also review evidence from human studies of other designs, which although not as rigorous as double-blind, randomized, controlled trials, do provide important information about what happens when humans ingest herbs. The phrase "open label" refers to a trial that is not blinded (i.e., the participants and the researchers know that the participants in the trial are taking the herbal product). In this trial design, it is difficult to separate out the effect of the herb from the placebo effect. However, if no effect at all is identified in this kind of trial, it is a pretty good indication that the product doesn't work for the condition being tested.

Uncontrolled trials do not use comparator groups, which makes it hard to distinguish between the effects of the herb and the natural course of the condition (i.e., the participants just get better or worse on their own). Observational is a description given to a group of designs in which the researchers do not actively intervene, but simply document what people are doing. This provides useful information about the use of herbal medicines in "real life" contexts. Case reports are individual observations, usually from clinicians, about what happened to a specific patient. Although case reports rarely provide "proof" that an herb caused a specific effect, they are excellent ways to generate research hypotheses that can be tested in more rigorous study designs.

In each case, the herbal reviews in this book highlight the best available evidence for the uses most commonly associated with each herb. Cases of conflicting evidence or problems with the study designs (e.g., the dose studied was much lower than usually used or the number of participants in the trial was too small) are noted. Where possible, summary conclusions are provided to indicate where the evidence is the strongest and where more research is needed before a firm conclusion can be drawn.

Glossary of Common Botanical Medicine Terms

Anti-emetic
An agent that decreases nausea and vomiting.

Adaptogen
An agent that supports the body's ability to accommodate varying physical and emotional stresses.

Alterative
An agent with the ability to restore normal body function(s) from an initial unhealthy state. This includes a variety of herbal medicine categories, including antimicrobials and digestive or hepatic tonics.

Astringent
An agent, normally rich in tannins, that can precipitate proteins, resulting in a contraction of tissues.

Bitter
An agent that aids and supports the digestive process, promoting salivation and the secretion of stomach acid and digestive enzymes.

Carminative
A primarily digestive agent that supports and soothes the digestive system, relieving gas, spasm, and distention.

Cathartic (Purgative)
An agent with a pronounced laxative effect, resulting in dramatic evacuation, or purging, of the bowels.

Cholagogue
An agent that promotes secretion of bile by causing contraction of the gallbladder.

Choleretic
An agent that promotes the production and secretion of bile.

Demulcent
A normally mucilaginous agent that soothes irritated tissues, notably mucous membranes.

Diaphoretic
An agent that promotes detoxification by promoting perspiration.

Emmenagogue
An agent that stimulates or harmonizes menstrual flow.

Febrifuge
A fever-lowering agent.

Galactagogue
An agent that promotes lactation.

Glycoside
A botanical constituent consisting of sugar and non-sugar (aglycone) components.

Hepatic
A general term used to describe an agent that supports healthy liver function.

Nervine
An agent that affects the nervous system, either tonifying, sedating, or stimulating.

Phytoestrogen
Compounds, usually flavonoids, that have a weak affinity for estrogen receptors.

Stomachic
An agent that supports gastric functions and promotes appetite.

Tonic
A nurturing agent that invigorates either specific organs or the entire individual.

Vulnerary
An agent that supports healing of wounds.

Alfalfa
Medicago sativa L.

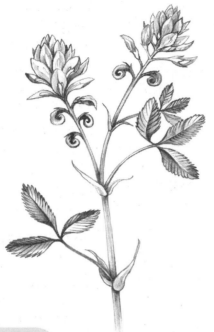

Introduction

Family
- Fabaceae (also known as Leguminosae)

Synonyms
- Lucerne
- Buffalo herb
- Chilean clover
- Purple medick

Medicinal Forms
- Dried leaves
- Seeds
- Liquid extract

Description

Alfalfa is native to eastern Mediterranean Europe and the Middle East and was first described in literature by Pliny (AD 23–79) as being introduced to Greece by Darius, King of Persia (550–486 BC). Alfalfa can now be found throughout the world. Originally cultivated by the Greeks and Romans, alfalfa is currently produced primarily as a fodder crop in North America. This perennial herb with clover-like, three-lobe leaves and spiraling seed pods grows to approximately 36 inches (1 meter). Its flowers range in color from purplish blue to yellow.

Parts Used

While sprouted seeds are commonly eaten, the aerial parts are most commonly used medicinally.

Traditional Use

Although alfalfa has been used medicinally in traditional Chinese medicine (to treat digestive disorders) and Ayurvedic medicine (for digestive conditions, as a diuretic, and in the treatment of arthritis), it is not often mentioned in North American textbooks of herbal medicine.

Current Medicinal Use

Modern-day herbalists consider alfalfa to be a good general tonic, due largely to its reputation as an excellent source of vitamins, minerals, and protein. While more research is needed, alfalfa may be effective in reducing high cholesterol levels. Evidence from traditional use suggests that alfalfa may also be helpful in managing menopause and menstrual discomfort.

Relevant Research

Preventative and Therapeutic Effects

Constituents

- Amino acids: canavanine.
- Saponins with the aglycone medicagenic acid.
- Isoflavone flavonoids: genistein, daidzein, formononetin.
- Coumarins: coumestans, medicagol.
- Alkaloids.
- Miscellaneous: carbohydrates, peptides, pigments, acids, vitamins (especially vitamins A, B_1, B_6, B_{12}, C, E, K).

Effects on Cholesterol

Several studies have demonstrated that the addition of alfalfa meal to cholesterol-containing diets prevented hypercholesterolemia (high cholesterol levels in blood) in rats and prevented hypercholesterolemia, decreased hypertriglyceridemia (high fatty acid levels in blood), and prevented atherosclerosis (thickening of blood vessel walls) in rabbits and monkeys. In addition, it has been shown that alfalfa decreased hypercholesterolemia, decreased plasma phospholipids, normalized plasma lipoproteins, and reduced the extent of aortic and coronary atherosclerosis in monkeys when it was added to their high-cholesterol diet.

One uncontrolled, open-label clinical trial included 11 patients diagnosed with type II and 4 patients diagnosed with type IV hyperlipoproteinemia (high lipid levels in blood) who were given 40 g of heat-prepared alfalfa seeds three times daily at mealtimes for 8 weeks (remainder of diet unchanged). Of the patients with type II hyperlipoproteinemia, 9 showed significantly lowered total plasma cholesterol, low-density lipoprotein (LDL), and apolipoprotein B, while apolipoprotein A-1 did not change. The 4 patients with type IV did not appear to experience the same beneficial effects; however, the small number made it difficult to detect statistically significant effects.

Several researchers have suggested that the alfalfa saponins are the active component of the plant. Rat experiments have indicated that saponins from alfalfa decrease the absorption of cholesterol from the intestine. This is partially supported by the finding that alfalfa increases the excretion of fecal neutral steroids in rabbits and monkeys, which implies that alfalfa interferes with the absorption of cholesterol. In addition, in vitro (test tube) experiments showed that alfalfa plant saponins bound significant amounts of cholesterol from both ethanol solution and from micellar suspension. The cholesterol-lowering action of alfalfa was thought to be a combination of the saponin-cholesterol interaction and an interaction with bile acids.

Miscellaneous
Cardiovascular Effects
Alfalfa has been used in the management of clotting disorders, primarily due to its high vitamin K content; however, the clinical relevance of this indication is questionable. It may be of use in situations arising from vitamin K deficiency.

Women's Health Care
The isoflavones found in alfalfa (genistein, daidzein) have also been extracted from other plants and shown to have phytoestrogenic properties (i.e., to have effects similar to human estrogen in the body). Consequently, many complementary practitioners have suggested that alfalfa is useful in the management of menopause and menstrual discomfort. However, a study using a natural health product containing alfalfa and nine other herbs to manage hot flashes found no effect on the number of symptoms or intensity of symptoms over a 12-month period. It is hard to determine the effect of alfalfa from this study because there were multiple herbs included in the supplement.

> *Many complementary practitioners have suggested that alfalfa is useful in the management of menopause and menstrual discomfort.*

Immune System Effects
A Chinese study suggests that polysaccharides isolated from alfalfa may have beneficial effects on the immune system. This has yet to be confirmed.

Adverse Effects
Allergic reactions to alfalfa powder have been reported. In addition, diarrhea and stomach upset may occasionally occur. Photosensitivity reactions have been noted in animals, and, very rarely, skin reactions are seen in humans.

Early animal studies found no toxicity associated with alfalfa or alfalfa saponins; however, there was some evidence of growth inhibition in studies where alfalfa was ingested without the addition of cholesterol to the diet. Ames mutagenicity testing was negative for a variety of extracts from alfalfa.

Alfalfa may have more severe adverse effects, as was noted in a 1981 case study in which a man who ingested 80 to 160 g of alfalfa seeds daily on eight occasions for up to 6 weeks at a time (as part of a study) developed pancytopenia (decrease in blood cells). This was followed by a report of systemic lupus erythematosus (SLE)-like syndrome in monkeys fed alfalfa sprouts and a letter reporting two cases in which patients with SLE, which was clinically and serologically in remission, had reactivations of their disease in association with the ingestion of alfalfa tablets. L-canavanine (LCN) is the component of alfalfa that appears to be responsible for these unwanted effects, not the saponins that are considered to be the active ingredient needed for positive cholesterol-lowering effects.

Ingestion of a diet consisting of 1.0% to 1.2% of alfalfa saponins by monkeys and rabbits is considered harmless. Humans currently ingest saponins from a variety of sources, including alfalfa sprouts, soybeans, chickpeas, spinach, asparagus, and sunflower seeds, without any ill effects.

Cautions/Contraindications

Patients with a history of systemic lupus erythematosus should avoid alfalfa. Seeds should be avoided during pregnancy and lactation.

Drug Interactions

Given the possible anticoagulant action of the vitamin K and the coumarins (e.g., medicagol) found in alfalfa, excessive doses may interfere with jointly administered anticoagu-

> *Given the possible anticoagulant action of the vitamin K and the coumarins (e.g., medicagol) found in alfalfa, excessive doses may interfere with jointly administered anticoagulant therapy.*

lant therapy. However, simple coumarins have more toxicity to rodents and dogs than they do to humans. A more significant risk occurs when the plant becomes infected with mold and the coumarin is converted to the more potent anticoagulant dicoumarol. Thus, quality control for mold-free products is a significant issue here.

In addition, the estrogenic nature of the isoflavones present may interfere with hormone replacement therapy and birth control pills if taken in excessive doses.

Dosage Regimens
- Dried leaves: 5–10 g three times daily.
- Liquid extract (1:1 in 25% alcohol): 5–10 mL three times daily.

Selected References

Briggs C. Herbal medicine: Alfalfa. Canadian Pharmaceutical Journal 1994;127(2):84–86.

Malinow MR, et al. Pancytopenia during ingestion of alfalfa seeds. Lancet 1981;i:615.

Mölgaard J, et al. Alfalfa seeds lower low density lipoprotein cholesterol and apolipoprotein B concentrations in patients with type II hyperlipoproteinemia. Atherosclerosis 1987;65:173–79.

Aloe Vera

A. vera (L.) Burm. f.

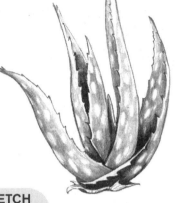

Common Uses
- *Aloe vera gel:* Minor skin irritation, wounds, and burns
- *Aloes:* Laxative

Active Constituents
- *Aloe vera gel:* Polysaccharides (including acemannan)
- *Aloes:* Anthraquinones

Adverse Effects
Aloe vera gel
- Allergic-type reactions (rare)

Aloes
- Abdominal cramping (severe)
- Reversible pigmentation of colonic mucosa
- Urine discoloration
- Nephritis, gastritis, vomiting, bloody diarrhea, watery diarrhea

Cautions/Contraindications
Aloe vera gel
- *External:* Known allergy
- *Internal:* Trace anthraquinone glycosides may be of concern in pregnancy and lactation

Aloes
- Contraindicated in pregnancy and menstruation, as well as appendicitis and abdominal pain of unknown origin. Not recommended for treatment of chronic constipation or in the presence of hemorrhoids.

Drug Interactions
Aloe vera gel (topical): None known
Aloes: Possible interaction with cardiac glycosides

Doses
Aloe vera gel
- *Externally:* A minimum of 70% concentration of aloe vera is necessary for wound healing and anti-inflammatory effects. Pure aloe vera gel is also available.
- *Internally:* No standard dosing
- *Antiviral:* Oral doses of 800–1600 mg of acemannan

Aloes
- *Laxative:* 50–200 mg aloes (dried sap) three times daily
- *Hypoglycemic agent:* 2.5 mL of the dried sap (aloes) daily

Introduction

Family
- Aloeaceae (aloe was formerly included in the Liliaceae family)

Synonyms
- Curacao aloe
- *A. barbadensis* P. Miller
- *A. vulgaris* Lam.

Medicinal Forms
- *Aloe vera:* Gel, ointment, lotion
- *Aloes:* Dried exudate (latex or juice)

Description

Aloe is a perennial succulent, native to East and South Africa, that grows wild in the tropics and is now cultivated extensively worldwide. There are more than 300 species of aloe plants; however, the species used primarily for medicinal purposes is now known as *A. vera* (L.) Burm.f. Previously, it was identified as *A. barbadensis* P. Miller or *A. vulgaris* Lam. The aloe vera plant grows in a rosette from a base that reaches 8 centimeters ($2\frac{1}{2}$ inches) or more in diameter at maturity. The leaves, which protrude from the base, are long and spear-like with thorny ridges. They can reach 0.5 meters (18 inches) in length and 8 to 10 centimeters (3 to $3\frac{1}{2}$ inches) across at the base, tapering to a point.

Parts Used

The clear mucilaginous gel from the cells in the inner portion of the aloe leaves, or parenchyma, is the part of the plant used medicinally for skin abrasions and infections. This gel, often referred to simply as aloe gel, is distinct from the bitter yellow juice found in the rind of the leaves (just beneath the epidermis), which is a potent laxative. Aloe vera has been cultivated since the 1950s for this bitter yellow juice, which was an important source of the drug aloes, or "aloin," known for its ability to stimulate bowel movements. Aloes' use as a laxative has been all but discontinued in North America. However, the plant continues to be cultivated for the gel, which is primarily used externally to treat a variety of skin conditions. Although these two products (aloes and aloe vera gel) are obtained from the leaves of the same plant, their chemistry, pharmacology, and uses are very different; thus, they will be described separately.

Aloes (or aloe) is the dried exudate (latex or juice) collected from freshly cut leaves. Aloes is often sold as a reddish-black or dark brown solid mass, which tastes bitter and has a characteristic unpleasant odor. This concentrated form was originally produced by boiling the latex in a copper kettle until it reached the required consistency, and then it was left to harden. Today, the liquid is more often vacuum-dried, which produces a powdered product.

In contrast, the colorless aloe vera gel is collected from the center of the leaf. It is very sensitive to light and heat, and thus is removed from the leaf mechanically and preserved, buffered, and stabilized immediately. This process may differ from manufacturer to manufacturer, which means that the quality of aloe vera gel is highly variable.

Traditional Use

Aloe vera gel has been widely used in the treatment of wounds since before 550 BC. The Greek physician Dioscorides, for example, claimed that aloe vera gel could be used to heal skin infections, chapping, and hemorrhoids. There are many legends about the powers of aloe vera, including that it was the secret of Cleopatra's beauty, which may account for its use in a variety of health and beauty aids, and that it was applied to the body of Jesus Christ after his crucifixion. Aloe vera has been widely used in India to relieve constipation, to aid digestion, and to attempt to treat parasitic worms; in China as a common dermatological remedy; and in Mexico to treat minor skin irritations. It is also a common folk remedy in most of North America and the West Indies.

Current Medicinal Use

Research has shown that aloe vera gel promotes healing of minor wounds, such as lacerations and burns, possibly through its immune system–enhancing, antibacterial, or anti-inflammatory activity. While more research is needed, topical aloe vera products may be useful in the treatment of psoriasis and dental conditions. Even though aloes has been shown to have antiviral and hypoglycemic properties, the fact that it is a strong purgative means that it has only limited clinical uses.

Relevant Research

Preventative and Therapeutic Effects

Constituents

Aloe Vera Gel

- Polysaccharides: celluolose, glucose, mannose, L-rhamnose, aldopentose, acemannan.

- Enzymes: oxidase, amylase, catalase, lipase, alkaline phosphatase, glutathione peroxidase; cyclooxygenase.

- Vitamins: B_1, B_2, B_6, choline, folic acid, C, alpha-tocopherol, beta carotene.

- Essential amino acids: lysine, threonine, valine, methionine, leucine, isoleucine, phenylalanine.

- Inorganic: calcium, sodium, chlorine, manganese, magnesium, zinc, copper, chromium, potassium sorbate.

- Aloinosides, including barbaloin (aloins A and B) emodin, aloe-emodin (trace amounts only).

Aloes

- Aloinosides, including barbaloin (aloins A and B), aloe-emodin, emodin, chrysophanol.

- Chromone derivatives: aloeresin A, B, C.

Aloe Vera Gel

Wound Healing

Most of the medicinal use of aloe vera gel centers around claims that it increases wound healing. In North America, where it is a common household plant, many individuals apply aloe vera gel obtained by breaking the leaves to minor cuts, abrasions, and burns. However, there is some controversy surrounding its effectiveness and mechanism of action.

The first case report of the use of aloe vera for wound healing was published in 1935. Fresh aloe vera gel provided rapid relief from the itching and burning of a woman's acute radiodermatitis (a skin condition caused by a depilatory X-ray dose to her scalp 8 months earlier). Three similar cases have been reported in the literature. Many

> In North America, where it is a common household plant, many individuals apply aloe vera gel obtained by breaking the leaves to minor cuts, abrasions, and burns.

studies of the effects of aloe vera on wound healing have been published since the 1930s. For example, researchers using topical application of the fresh leaf demonstrated effective treatment of eczema and pruritus vulvae (external itching of the female genitalia). In addition, a controlled, open-label study with 12 subjects found that finger abrasions treated with 50% fresh aloe vera gel in petroleum jelly healed faster than those treated with petroleum jelly alone. Most of these early studies were not blinded or controlled and involved only very small numbers of participants.

> Not all the published studies are positive. Some studies have found that aloe vera gel actually hinders the healing process.

A recent review of clinical trials using aloe vera to treat thermal burn wounds concluded that topical application may provide healing benefits for first- and second-degree burns. Four studies were reviewed in which patients were treated with either an aloe vera preparation, a common burn treatment, such as a vaseline gauze or silver sulfadinazine, or both treatments, depending on the study. Positive results concerning aloe vera's healing benefits were found in all the studies selected. Flaws in the studies' design, however, such as not standardizing the active ingredient and choosing subjective outcome measures, mean that the results need to be confirmed with larger, more rigorous studies.

However, not all the published studies are positive. Some studies have found that aloe vera gel actually hinders the healing process. Several controlled (but open-label) studies funded by the US army found no difference in experiments comparing the effects of aloe gel and no treatment on rates of wound healing (in rats and rabbits). A small study in 6 people with second- and third-degree thermal burns also found no improvement with aloe vera treatment. Unfortunately,

these researchers did not use the fresh herb and do not identify the commercial preparations used.

In addition, studies into the effects of aloe vera on the healing of full thickness wounds have found either insignificant or negative results. The most well known of these involved the treatment of 21 women with wound complications after cesarian delivery or laparotomy for gynecologic surgery. In this non-blinded study, wounds treated with standard management healed significantly faster than those treated with aloe vera. In contrast, a recent controlled study assessing the effect of a commercial preparation of aloe vera on partial thickness wounds showed a significant increase in healing. It has been suggested that aloe vera should not be used to treat full thickness wounds because it causes the top skin layer to fuse too quickly, inhibiting the wound from healing properly; however, its use in partial thickness wounds continues to be supported by many authors.

Gloves coated with aloe vera have recently become available in the health-care and factory industries in an attempt to prevent dry, cracked skin on hands. A recent review of this topic examined one open-label study involving 29 factory assembly-line workers and two animal studies. The assembly-line workers showed a statistically significant improvement to the condition of the skin on their hands when using the gloves, although the authors of the review noted that this effect may be attributed to simply wearing gloves. The effect of manufacturing the gloves and the influence of aloe vera on the integrity of the gloves was also questioned. The authors concluded that aloe vera–lined gloves are probably not detrimental to users, although more studies need to be done surrounding their use.

Several mechanisms of action for the wound-healing properties of aloe vera gel have been suggested. The first is that aloe vera may simply act as a protective barrier. Other researchers have demonstrated increased capillary dilation after the topical application of aloe vera and suggest that this may provide further insight into the mechanism of action of aloe vera.

Effects on the Immune System

It has been suggested that some of the physiological actions of aloe vera may result from direct simulation of the immune system. Studies investigating this theory involve the oral ingestion or injection of acemannan, an active ingredient isolated from aloe vera gel. Acemannan has been shown to enhance the body's ability to kill bacteria in a dose-dependent fashion; increase numbers of circulating monocytes and macrophages (immune system components); enhance T-cell (an immune cell) response; increase white blood cell response to forein antigens; enhance the release of cytokines (immune system components), including interleukin-1, interleukin-6, interferon, and tumor necrosis factor; and activate macrophages (immune cells).

Antibacterial Activity

In the early 1950s, it was suggested that aloe vera gel had an antibiotic action. Early studies found that aloe vera gel inhibited *Myobacterium tuberculosis* and *Bacillus subtilis* in vitro (in test tubes). In addition, aloe vera juice was shown to inhibit the growth of *Staphylococcus aureus*, *Streptococcus pyogenes*, and *Salmonella paratyphi*. However, the juice was also reported to be unstable (medicinal components may become inactive over time). More recent studies provide similar results. Aloe vera extracts have been found to kill a variety of bacteria, including *Streptococcus agalctiae*, *Enterobacter cloacae*, *Citrobacter* species, *Serratia marcescens*, *Klebsiella pneumoniae*, *Pseudomonas aeruginosa*, *Staphylococcus aureus*, *Escherichia coli*, *Streptococcus faecali*, and a yeast, *Candida albicans*. Other studies have not found any antibacterial activity against *Staphylococcus aureus* or *E. coli*.

> *Aloe vera extracts have been found to kill a variety of bacteria, including* Streptococcus agalctiae, Enterobacter cloacae, Citrobacter *species,* Serratia marcescens, Klebsiella pneumoniae, Pseudomonas aeruginosa, Staphylococcus aureus, Escherichia coli, Streptococcus faecali, *and a yeast,* Candida albicans.

Anti-Inflammatory Activity

Many studies have demonstrated the anti-inflammatory properties of aloe vera and other aloe species. Researchers have shown, for example, that aloe vera gel and hydrocortisone decrease inflammation in an additive, dose-related manner when they are used concurrently. Another study found direct anti-inflammatory activity that could be attributed to known sterols isolated from aloe vera gel (e.g., lupeol, campesterol). In this study, aloe vera gel also appeared to block hydrocortisone's inhibitory effects on wound healing. Another research team demonstrated that constituents of a water-based gel extract of aloe vera inhibited the release of reactive oxygen species by human white blood cells, reducing the harmful effects of this release at the site of inflammation.

Three primary mechanisms of action for the anti-inflammatory effects of aloe vera have been postulated: 1) anti-bradykinin activity has been found in some aloe species (e.g., *A. arborescens*, *A. saponaria*); 2) emodin, aloe-emodin, and aloin were shown to produce salicylates when metabolized, which appear to inhibit thromboxane production by competitive inhibition through stereochemical means; and 3) magnesium lactate, a constituent of aloe vera, is a known inhibitor of histidine decarboxylase and thus may prevent the formation of histamine in mast cells. The first hypothesis has been demonstrated in other aloe species, but there is little evidence of such action in studies with aloe vera. The second hypothesis has more support in the literature. A clinical case report in which a commercial preparation of aloe vera was applied to a monkey who was accidentally scalded provides some support because the amount of thromboxane A2 produced by the monkey was decreased. Other studies also provide support for this finding. However, one researcher noted that many of the other ingredients used in commercial aloe vera preparations, such as petrolatum, mineral oil, and aquaphor, could be causing the effect by inhibiting prostaglandin. This emphasizes the need for well-designed (i.e., controlling for other ingredients) studies of aloe vera.

It has been reported that decolorized (anthraquinone-free) aloe vera gel is a more potent inhibitor of inflammation than the colorized form. One study in support of this hypothesis found that high concentrations of anthraquinones increased the production of prostaglandins, while trace amounts appeared to decrease the inflammatory response. However, another study found that an aloe vera gel extract containing anthraquinone was more effective than an anthraquinone-free product. In addition, one researcher demonstrated that anthraquinone is necessary for the absorption of aloe vera given orally.

Protection Against Radiation

Investigation of the effectiveness of aloe vera gel in the treatment of radiation burns began in the late 1930s, when radiation-induced burns or ulcers were a common model to test the ability of aloe vera to increase wound healing. Several early studies demonstrated an increased rate of healing. One of the best was a study with 20 albino rabbits in which 4 different treatments (fresh aloe vera gel, commercial aloe vera ointment, dry gauze bandage, and nothing) were applied to the four quadrants of a wound caused by beta radiation. Visual assessment over a period of 58 days led to the findings that both aloe vera treatments resulted in statistically significant accelerated healing.

> *Investigation of the effectiveness of aloe vera gel in the treatment of radiation burns began in the late 1930s, when radiation-induced burns or ulcers were a common model to test the ability of aloe vera to increase wound healing.*

Several review papers have focused on the use of aloe vera for protection against radiation. One review published in 2005 examined topical aloe vera application in cancer patients receiving radiation therapy. Five clinical trials were evaluated, each comparing a product containing aloe vera gel with a variety of control treatments, including a standard topical water-based cream and an unscented soap. The authors concluded that there is no evidence demonstrating that aloe vera effectively prevents or treats skin reactions due to radiation in cancer patients. This contradicts findings of another review published the same year, which examined three of the same trials and concluded that aloe vera gel may benefit burn wounds by offering moisturization without the side effects of 1% hydrocortisone cream. More clinical trials are needed to further investigate this topic.

Diabetes

Aloe vera has been traditionally used in diabetes for its enhancement of wound healing. Researchers have demonstrated in a controlled, open-label study of mice that aloe vera increases the rate of healing, provides pain relief, and decreases edema (swelling) as compared to a saline control in both normal mice and those with streptozotocin-induced diabetes. A recent study has suggested that oral ingestion of an aloe vera extract may also be useful in treating insulin resistance. This study examined the effects of oral administration of polyphenol-rich extract from aloe vera given to mice with experimentally induced insulin resistance. The extract successfully decreased both body weight and blood sugar level in the mice, implying a decrease in insulin resistance.

Miscellaneous

Anticancer

Acemannan, a compound isolated from aloe vera, has been reported to have antitumor activity. For example, it has been used in the treatment of fibrosarcomas in dogs and cats. In addition, Roidex (a formulation of squalene, vitamin A, vitamin E, and aloe vera) demonstrated more chemopreventive and curative properties than squalene alone in the prevention and treatment of mouse skin tumors. Aloe juice has also been reported to have antimetastatic activity (it prevents spreading of cancer) and to enhance the activity of 6-fluorouracil and cyclophosphamide.

Antiviral

Acemannan has also been reported to have antiviral activity, and it has been suggested that it may play a role as an adjuvant treatment in HIV/AIDS. Although most of these experiments have been test tube studies, the concentrations of acemannan used appear to be achievable in animals and humans. One study demonstrated that the immune response of chickens to Newcastle disease virus was increased by adding acemannan to a Newcastle vaccine. A study of avian polyomavirus in birds with similar results has also been published.

Psoriasis

There is conflicting evidence about whether aloe vera will be helpful for psoriasis. One double-blind, placebo-controlled clinical study of 60 patients diagnosed with psoriasis vulgaris found that treatment with 0.5% aloe vera extract (without occlusion, or covering) was a significantly better treatment than the placebo. Another double-blind, placebo-controlled clinical study of 35 patients with stable plaque psoriasis on their arms and legs found no difference between treatment with

aloe vera gel or the placebo after 12 weeks. The authors commented that the improvement rate for the placebo gel was particularly high, implying that it may have contained an active ingredient. This contradictory evidence means that more research is needed before a firm conclusion can be drawn about this use for aloe vera.

Peptic Ulcer

Aloe vera gel has been taken internally for the treatment of peptic ulcers. One group of authors claims several complete cures among 12 patients diagnosed with duodenal lesions (X-ray confirmation). However, no follow-up clinical studies appear to have been performed.

Dental Conditions

Several studies report the effectiveness of aloe vera gel in increasing the rate of healing after dental procedures.

Veterinary Use

Effective use of aloe vera has been reported for the treatment of ringworm, allergies, abscesses, fungal infections and different types of inflammation in animals. Although aloe vera has been questioned as a "cure-all" in veterinary medicine, a detailed investigation of two cases using the commercial preparation Dermaide Aloe to treat the severe accidental thermal burns of two dogs showed that aloe vera accelerated the rate of healing, decreased the production of prostaglandins, and inhibited infection by *Pseudomonas aeruginosa*. Its use was also reported to be beneficial in the treatment of a monkey who was accidentally scalded.

Final Notes

Variation in the quality of aloe vera has been documented and may account for some of the negative or inconclusive studies. In addition, aloe vera has been reported to be biochemically unstable and may deteriorate in a short time, which may also explain some of the conflicting study results. More good-quality clinical trials are needed to provide conclusive evidence of aloe vera's effectiveness in the management of skin conditions.

> *More good-quality clinical trials are needed to provide conclusive evidence of aloe vera's effectiveness in the management of skin conditions.*

Aloes

Laxative

Anthraquinone glycosides are the compounds responsible for the well-documented laxative effect of aloes. These glycosides induce the intestinal secretion of water and electrolytes and modify intestinal motility. Laxative effects occur approximately 8 hours after the ingestion of aloes, which is metabolized by intestinal bacteria to form the active compound aloe-emodin-9-anthrone. This substance has been shown to inhibit rat colonic Na+, K+-ATPase in vitro and to increase the paracellular permeability of rat colonic mucosa. Due to its strong purgative effect, aloes is not commonly recommended for use as a routine laxative (see Adverse Effects).

Diabetes

Aloes' use as a hypoglycemic agent has been demonstrated in 5 non-insulin-dependent patients and in an animal model (mice) of diabetes. The mechanism of action for this effect has yet to be determined, although it is hypothesized that it may have positive effects by stimulating the synthesis and/or release of insulin from the beta cells of the islets of Langerhans.

Miscellaneous Effects

Aloes has been used to flavor products used to discourage nail biting (it has a very bitter taste). Several hydroxyanthracene derivatives have been shown to inhibit a variety of viruses in vitro, including herpes simplex (types 1 and 2), varicella-zoster, pseudorabies and influenza. It was not active against adenovirus or rhinovirus.

Adverse Effects
Aloe Vera Gel

External: Adverse effects associated with the external application of aloe vera gel have been very rarely reported in the literature. Contact dermatitis, possibly due to an allergic reaction, has been reported in several cases. There is one report of widespread dermatitis after the topical application of aloe vera gel to stasis dermatitis and one report of an acute allergic reaction. One case of cathartic effects (stimulating bowel movements) after topical application of aloe vera gel to the mucosal surface has also been reported.

Internal: Adverse effects associated with oral ingestion of aloe vera seem to be more serious. Two cases of Henoch-Schönlein purpura have been reported in individuals who ingested aloe vera, and both experienced kidney involvement. A case of hepatitis thought to be related to the ingestion of aloe vera capsules has also been reported.

> *Adverse effects are most common with chronic use of aloes, which tends to result in tolerance.*

Aloes

Adverse effects are most common with chronic use of aloes, which tends to result in tolerance. In addition, chronic use may lead to a reversible pigmentation of the colonic mucosa. After aloes use is discontinued, the pigmentation disappears in 4 to 12 months. Urine may become orange (if pH is acidic) or reddish purple (if pH is alkaline). This is caused by the renal elimination of the hydroxyanthracene derivatives. Severe abdominal cramping is common. Nephritis (kidney problems), gastritis (stomach irritation), vomiting, bloody diarrhea with mucus, and watery diarrhea leading to osmotic imbalances have been reported.

Cautions/Contraindications

Aloe Vera Gel
External: Known allergies.
Internal: Trace anthraquinone glycosides may be of concern in pregnancy and lactation.

Aloes

Aloes are contraindicated in pregnancy, lactation, and menstruation; appendicitis and abdominal pain of unknown origin; and spasmodic obstipation (intestinal blockage). They are not recommended for treatment of chronic constipation in the presence of hemorrhoids or chronic renal disease.

Drug Interactions

Aloe Vera Gel: None known.

Aloes: Although no clinical examples appear to have been published, the anthraquinone glycosides have been known to induce hypokalemia (low potassium levels in the blood), which may interfere with the action of cardiac glycosides.

Dosage Regimens
Aloe Vera Gel
- **Externally:** A minimum of 70% concentration of aloe vera is necessary for wound healing and anti-inflammatory effects. Pure aloe vera gel is also available.
- **Internally:** No standard dosing.
- **Antiviral:** Oral doses of 800–1600 mg of acemannan.

Aloes
- **Laxative:** 50–200 mg aloes (dried sap) three times daily.
- **Hypoglycemic agent:** 2.5 mL of the dried sap (aloes) daily.

Selected References

Canigueral S, Vila R. Aloe. British Journal of Phytotherapy 1994;3(2):67–75.

Maenthaisong R, Chaiyakunapruk N, Niruntraporn S, Kongkaew C. The efficacy of aloe vera used for burn wound healing: A systematic review. Burns 2007;33:713–18.

Richardson J, Smith JE, McIntyre M, Thomas R, Pilkington, K. Aloe vera for preventing radiation-induced skin reactions: A systematic literature review. Clinical Oncology 2005;17:478–84.

Shelton RW. Aloe vera, its chemical and therapeutic properties. International Journal of Dermatology 1991;30(10):679–83.

Ashwagandha
Withania somnifera

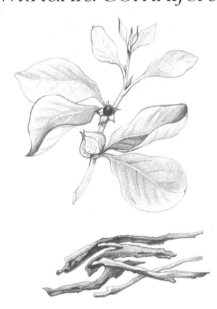

THUMBNAIL SKETCH

Common Uses
- Diabetes (type 2)
- Longevity and anti-aging

Active Constituents
- Alkaloids
- Steroidal lactones (withanolides, especially withafern A)
- Saponins

Adverse Effects
- Gastrointestinal upset (mild)

Cautions/Contraindications
- Pregnancy

Drug Interactions
- None reported clinically

Doses
Adult dose
- *General guidelines:* 1–6 g of the whole herb is consumed daily in capsule or tea form. Tea is made by boiling ashwagandha roots in water for 15 minutes and allowing it to cool. The usual dose is 750 mL daily. Tincture or fluid extracts are dosed 2–4 mL three times daily.
- *Hypercholesterolemia and diabetes (type 2):* 3 g daily

Children's Dose
- 1–2 g daily of powdered ashwagandha fortified in 100 mL of milk was given to children aged 8 to 12 years to stimulate growth in one trial. Caution in using ashwagandha in children is recommended due to the lack of studies in this population.

Introduction

Family
- Solanaceae

Synonyms
- Ajagandha
- Amangura
- Amukkirag
- Asan
- Asgand
- Asgandh
- Asgandha
- Ashagandha
- Ashvagandha
- Ashwaganda
- Ashwanga
- Asoda
- Asundha
- Asvagandha
- Aswagandha
- Avarada
- Ayurvedic ginseng
- Clustered winter cherry
- Ghoda asoda
- Hayahvaya
- Indian ginseng
- Kanaje Hindi
- Kuthmithi
- Samm al ferakh
- Turangi-Ghanda
- Vajigandha
- Winter cherry
- Withania

Medicinal Forms
Investigations of ashwagandha have used a variety of doses, dosage forms, and preparation methods without specification or quantification of the bioactive constituents. Oral preparations include aqueous extracts, dried powders, juices, teas, and cooked forms of ashwagandha. Commercially available ashwagandha supplements are usually found in the form of dried powder in capsules or as teas.

Description
Ashwagandha shrubs grow to approximately 1.25 meters (4 feet) tall. This evergreen is found primarily in the Middle East, India, and some parts of Africa. The name may be based on the Sanskrit *ashva* (horse) and *gandha* (smell), which likely refers to the strong smell of the roots. Others argue that the name refers to the belief that ingesting the plant will give one the strength of a horse.

Parts Used
The root of the ashwagandha plant is used medicinally.

Traditional Use
Ashwagandha has been used in Ayurveda, the Indian traditional medicine system, to improve musculoskeletal function and as a tonic to improve overall health. The whole plant, but especially the leaves and the root bark, have traditionally been used for their adaptogenic, antibiotic, aphrodisiac, deobstruent, diuretic, narcotic, strongly sedative, and rejuvenating properties. Ashwagandha is also traditionally used to increase the firmness of the uterus after a miscarriage and in treating postpartum difficulties. Other uses include treating nervous exhaustion, debility, insomnia, wasting diseases, failure to thrive in children, impotence, infertility, and multiple sclerosis. This herb has been applied as a soft, moist mass to boils, swellings, and other painful parts. The fruit is diuretic, while the seed is both diuretic and hypnotic. Ashwagandha has also been traditionally used to improve memory.

Current Medicinal Use
Ashwagandha is used for its purported overall effects on health, including helping the body resist physical and psychological stress. It is thought to tonify and normalize a wide range of bodily functions.

Relevant Research

Preventative and Therapeutic Effects

Constituents

- **Alkaloids:** isopelletierine, anaferine, withanine, somniferine, tropine, psuedotropine.
- **Steroidal lactones:** withanolides, withaferins.
- **Saponins:** sitoindoside VII and VIII.
- **Others:** flavonoids, iron, choline, acylsteryl glucosides, coumarins (scopoletin and aesculetin), triterpene (beta-amyrin), phytosterols (stigmasterol and beta-sitosterol), essential oils (ipuranol, withaniol).

Diabetes (Type 2)

A number of animal studies suggest that ashwagandha may have beneficial effects for diabetes, but there is only one published human study investigating the effects of this herb on type 2 diabetes. In a case series, 12 participants aged 40 to 60 with mild type 2 diabetes were recruited. Half were treated with the roots of ashwagandha (six 500-mg capsules daily) in powder form for 30 days and half were given an oral hypoglycemic drug, Daonil (glibenclamide). There was a 12% decrease in blood glucose for the ashwagandha group, which was comparable to that of the group treated with Daonil. Although the diets of all subjects did not change substantially during the study, there was a higher mean caloric intake in those ingesting ashwagandha than in those in the Daonil group. In addition, there was a significant decrease in serum cholesterol, triglycerides, low-density lipoproteins, and very low-density lipoproteins in the hypercholesterolemic patients treated with ashwagandha as compared with those in the control group. This was a small study, and its results may not be representative of the effects of ashwagandha on a broader population of type 2 diabetes patients. There was no information given about whether individuals were randomized to the treatment and placebo groups.

There are four animal studies that support ashwagandha's positive role in diabetic hyperglycemic pathogenesis. Two of these studies used polyherbal formulations that contained this herb. The findings of animal research must be interpreted with caution, however, when attempting to extrapolate these data to humans.

Growth Stimulation (in Children)

One human study has been performed to examine the effects of ashwagandha on the growth of children. In a randomized, double-blind case series, 60 healthy children aged 8 to 12 years were divided into 5 groups of 12. Group 1 received 2 g daily of purified and powdered ashwagandha fortified in 100 mL of cow's milk (no details about purification and powdering methods were stated). Group 2 was given 2 g daily of a mixture of equal parts ashwagandha and punarnava (*Boerhaavia diffusa*). Groups 3 and 4 received ferrous fumarate (5 mg and 30 mg daily, respectively), while Group 5 was given a placebo. At the end of 60 days, Group 1 experienced a slight increase in hemoglobin, packed cell volume, mean corpuscular volume, serum iron, body weight, and hand grip, and significant increases compared to the baseline levels, as well as compared to the placebo group, in mean corpuscular hemoglobin and total proteins. There was a greater increase in body weight in all groups than in the placebo group. Further research is needed to confirm this use for ashwagandha.

Inflammation

There is one published human trial that noted the effects of ashwagandha on inflammation, and several animal studies suggest that this herb may play a role in decreasing inflammation. In the double-blind trial, 101 men in India were treated with an ashwagandha preparation to investigate its anti-aging effects. Lower erythrocyte sedimentation rate (a measure of chronic inflammation) was observed for men in the treatment group than for those in the control. The methods used were poorly described, however, and the number of participants in each group was not available in the abstracts found for this review.

Seven animal studies have looked at the effectiveness of this herb for inflammation, and all have shown positive results. The findings of animal research must be interpreted with caution when efforts are made to extrapolate these data to humans. Additional human studies are necessary before definitive conclusions regarding ashwagandha's anti-inflammatory effects are possible.

Withanolides (steroidal lactones) are believed to have anti-inflammatory effects. Several withanolides in ashwagandha demonstrate selective cyclooxygenase-2 (COX-2) enzyme inhibition, and this herb has also been reported to decrease alpha-2 macroglobulin, a liver-synthesized plasma protein that increases during inflammation.

> *The findings of animal research must be interpreted with caution when efforts are made to extrapolate these data to humans. Additional human studies are necessary before definitive conclusions regarding ashwagandha's anti-inflammatory effects are possible.*

Longevity and Anti-Aging

There are two published human studies, one of a polyherbal preparation containing ashwagandha, that explored ashwagandha's ability to extend human life and/or delay the aging process. Both reported positive effects associated with the ingestion of ashwagandha, but neither is of high methodological quality and thus no definitive conclusions can be drawn about this use.

In the double-blind trial, 141 healthy men in India, 101 of whom completed the treatment, were randomized into control and treatment groups and given either two tablets (0.5 g per tablet) of placebo or ashwagandha three times daily with milk (type unspecified) for 1 year. Hair melanin content, hemoglobin, and seated stature measurements were used as parameters to determine the effectiveness of delaying aging. The authors reported positive effects for ashwagandha. The exact number of participants in each group was not clearly indicated, however, and the outcome measures used are not necessarily clear indicators of longevity or aging.

Miscellaneous Effects

Athletic Performance

The only published human study investigating the effects of ashwagandha on athletic performance investigated a herbal product containing ashwagandha in addition to other herbal medicines. Although the positive effects of this trial are supported by some preliminary animal work, additional research is needed to explore the specific properties of ashwagandha as a single agent.

In one review, ashwagandha was noted to have shown ergogenic effects in animal tests, including swim times and anabolic activity, that were equal to or more improved than the outcomes achieved by Korean ginseng (*Panax ginseng*). Both herbal powders were found to contain starch, however, and since it was present in high doses, the reported results may have been caused by carbohydrate supplementation rather than the inherent effects of the herbal constituents. Furthermore, the findings of animal research must be interpreted with caution when efforts are made to extrapolate these data to humans.

Cancer

There are no published clinical trials to date for ashwagandha's effects on cancer. However, multiple studies involving animals or cell cultures found positive results, suggesting that this herb may be an effective anticancer agent. There have been 20 animal studies published on the effects of ashwagandha on cancer. Overall, 18 of these studies show positive results and two studies concluded that this herb is ineffective. One of the positive studies used cell cultures, while one of the negative studies used a polyherbal product. The findings of animal research must be interpreted with caution when attempting to extrapolate these data to humans, so more human studies are necessary before definitive conclusions regarding ashwagandha's effects on bone marrow are possible.

Ashwagandha's antitumor activity is reportedly due to its action as a radiosensitizer. Its effects are thought to be enhanced by heat to decrease glutathione content. It is also possible that its anticancer effects are mediated by the recruitment of cytotoxic T cells. Mechanistically, it has been proposed that withaferin A induces apoptosis in androgen-responsive and androgen-refractory prostate cancer cells via a prostate apoptosis response-4 (Par-4) gene-dependent pathway. It is also a possibility that withaferin A inhibits proteasomal chymotrypsin-like activity, which is believed to be responsible for tumor proliferation, as well as inhibiting the activation of NF-kB, a constitutively active transcription factor that is partly responsible for tumor proliferation. Ashwagandha has also been reported to inhibit suppression of macrophage chemotaxis by a carcinogenic toxin and to have anti-angiogenesis properties, which could contribute to its anticancer effects. Animal studies suggest that increased hematopoeisis may also play a role.

Cardiovascular System

To date, 11 animal studies investigating ashwagandha's cardiovascular effects support the clinical evidence described above. All but one of the animal studies found for this review indicate that ashwagandha has positive effects on the cardiovascular system. These include decreasing total blood lipid level and blood pressure, sustaining heart function in the presence of toxins, increasing HDL concentration and concentration of endogenous antioxidants, promoting cardiac function after induced ischemia, and reperfusion of the heart. However, the findings of animal research must be interpreted with caution when efforts are made to extrapolate these data to humans. The one negative study found that this herb has no protective effect against stroke. Additional human studies are necessary before definitive conclusions regarding ashwagandha's cardiovascular effects can be drawn.

With respect to cardiovascular effects, decreased blood pressure and heart rate may be due to the sedative nature of alkaloids in ashwagandha. The chemical structures of its withanolides resemble those of cardiac glycosides and have demonstrated mild ionotropic and chronotropic effects on the heart. It is possible that ashwagandha's cardioprotective properties could be attributed to its ability to reduce lipid peroxidation and scavenge free radicals. The withanolides in the plant also exhibit calcium channel-blocking activity on isolated smooth muscle preparations, which might contribute to the cardiovascular effects.

> *All but one of the animal studies found for this review indicate that ashwagandha has positive effects on the cardiovascular system.*

Neurological Disease

There is only one human study of a combination product containing ashwagandha administered in cow's milk that reported a positive effect on symptoms associated with Parkinson's disease when combined with an Ayurvedic cleansing program. Several animal studies and one in vitro study suggest that this herb may be effective in neurodegenerative diseases, while one animal study counters these claims. There are 15 published animal studies concerning ashwagandha treatment for neurodegenerative diseases or their symptoms, and 14 — two of which used cell lines — show positive results. Of these reports, three investigated ashwagandha's effects on Alzheimer's disease and three looked at Parkinson's disease. One study indicated that this herb has no prophylactic effect on chlorpyrifos-induced neurotoxicity. The findings of animal research must be interpreted with caution when efforts are made to extrapolate these data to humans.

Osteoporosis

One human study has investigated the effects of ashwagandha on osteoporosis using a herb-mineral formulation containing ashwagandha with positive results. The results of three animal studies support the suggestion that ashwagandha may have protective effects against osteoporosis. The findings of animal research must be interpreted with caution when efforts are made to extrapolate these data to humans.

Stress

There are no published studies on the effect of ashwagandha on stress in humans. There are 16 animal studies on this topic, and all but one gave positive results. The research showed that ashwagandha was effective in ameliorating and preventing induced stress. Treated animals showed increased endurance in swimming tests, increased levels of antioxidant defense enzymes, greater protection against lipid peroxidation, improved gastric motility, less neurocellular degeneration, decreased suppression of male sexual behaviour and reduced immunosuppression. The single negative trial found that ashwagandha treatment did not improve the endurance of rats in swimming tests. The findings of animal research must be interpreted with caution when efforts are made to extrapolate these data to humans.

Adverse Effects

Generally, adverse effects associated with ashwagandha have been minor. However, products containing ashwagandha have been reported to cause dermatitis; excessive salivation; gastrointestinal upset; and severe hyperthyroidism (thyrotoxicosis). Since the herbal products contained a range of different active agents in addition to ashwagandha, it is not possible to conclude with certainty that these adverse effects were associated with consuming ashwagandha.

Cautions/Contraindications

Ashwagandha is contraindicated in pregnancy because of its reputed abortifacient activity.

Drug Interactions

No drug interactions have been reported in humans. Theoretically, however, ashwagandha may interact with the following:

- Amphetamines
- Anticoagulants (additive effects)
- Cholinesterase inhibitors (possible additive effect)
- Digoxin (alkaloids in ashwagandha are structurally similar to digoxin, so ashwagandha may interact with the therapeutic action of this drug, possibly contributing falsely elevated levels of digoxin readings in assays)
- Haloperidol (may decrease tardive dyskinesia symptoms caused by haloperidol)
- Immunosuppressant drugs (may decrease effectiveness)
- Morphine (may decrease morphine tolerance and dependence)
- Paclitaxel (may increase Paclitaxel's effectiveness in lung cancer)
- Sedative or hypnotic agents, such as barbiturates and benzodiazepines (may have additive effects)
- Thyroid medications (may interact)

Dosage Regimens

Adult dose

- General guidelines: 1–6 g of the whole herb consumed daily in capsule or tea form. Tea is made by boiling ashwagandha roots in water for 15 minutes and allowing it to cool. The usual dose is 750 mL daily. Tincture or fluid extracts are dosed 2–4 mL three times per day.
- Hypercholesterolemia and diabetes (type 2): 3 g daily.

Children's Dose

- 1–2 g daily of powdered ashwagandha fortified in 100 mL of milk was given to children aged 8 to 12 years to stimulate growth in one trial. Caution is recommended in using ashwagandha in children due to the lack of studies in this population.

Selected References

Andallu B, Radhika B. Hypoglycemic, diuretic and hypocholesterolemic effect of winter cherry (*Withania somnifera* Dunal) root. Indian Journal of Experimental Biology 2000;38(6): 607–9.

Kuppurajan K, Rajagopalan SS, Sitoraman R. Effect of ashwagandha (*Withania somnifera* Dunal) on the process of ageing on human volunteers. Journal of Research in Ayurveda and Siddha 1980;1(2):247–58.

Venkataraghavan S, Seshadri C, Sundaresan TP. The comparative effect of milk fortified with Aswagandha, Aswagandha and Punarnava in children — a double-blind study. Journal of Research in Ayurveda and Siddha 1980;1: 370–85.

Astragalus

Astragalus membranaceus Moench

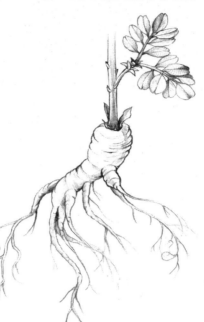

THUMBNAIL SKETCH

Common Uses
- Resistance to disease
- Stress ailments (including viral infections and fatigue)
- Adjunctive therapy to chemotherapy and radiation treatment

Active Constituents
- Astragalan
- Astragalosides

Adverse Effects
- None known

Cautions/Contraindications
- None known

Drug Interactions
- None known

Doses
- *Dried root (or as tea):* Adult dose normally 9–15 g daily in divided doses
- *Tincture (1:5):* 2–6 mL three times daily
- *Powdered solid extract (2:1):* 250–500 mg three times daily
- *Formulas:* Astragalus is often seen in combination formulas with other similar herbs, such as Chinese privet (*Ligustrum lucidum* Ait. Oleaceae), codonopsis (*Codonopsis pilosula* (Franch) Nannf., Campanulaceae), and Asian ginseng (*Panax ginseng* C.A. Meyer, Araliaceae), and is often mixed with Chinese licorice.

Introduction

- Fabaceae
  (also known as
  Leguminosae)

Synonyms
- Milk-vetch root
- Membranous vetch
- Yellow vetch
- Huang qi

Medicinal Forms
- Dried root
  (as a tea)
- Tincture
- Powdered solid
  extract

Description
Astragalus is an herbaceous perennial, with hairy stems and 12 to 18 pairs of leaflets on each leaf, that grows up to 1 meter (39 inches) in height. It is native to northern China and Tibet, growing both in the grassland and in lightly forested areas that are well drained.

Parts Used
The part of the plant used medicinally is the root, which is harvested from 4- to 7-year-old plants and dried. In Asia, the seeds of *Astragalus complanatus* R. Br. have also been used medicinally.

Traditional Use
Astragalus has long been a part of traditional Chinese medicine. In fact, it was included in the classic *Shen Nong Ben Cao Jing*, which was written 2,000 years ago. It is thought to strengthen the body's vital energy, or *qi*, and was often used in conditions of physical weakness and during chronic illness. It was believed to both strengthen and invigorate. It is one of the most widely used herbs in fu-zheng therapy — the use of herbs to augment the host defense mechanisms. The species of astragalus that has been used for medicinal purposes, *Astragalus membranaceus* Moench (and its variety mongholicus), has been extensively studied in Asia. Within traditional Chinese medicine, astragalus is considered a sweet and warming tonic used to increase stamina, endurance, and resistance to disease. As a classic tonic, it is considered superior to Asian ginseng for young adults.

Current Medicinal Use
In many instances, the traditional and current medicinal uses are one and the same. For example, astragalus is currently used as an immune stimulant and is thought to be helpful for the common cold. Research into its use as an adjunctive therapy for cancer patients is just beginning. It is important that cancer patients considering taking astragalus should consult with an appropriately trained health-care provider first.

Relevant Research

Preventative and Therapeutic Effects

Constituents

- Triterpene glycosides (saponins): astragalosides, acetylastragalosides, isoastragalosides, astramembrannins.

- Polysaccharides: astragalans.

- Flavonoids: kaempferol, quercetin, isorhamnetin, astragalin g-aminobutyric acid.

- Miscellaneous: free amino acids (including arginine, glutamic acid, canavanine, alanine), trace minerals (including zinc, manganese, magnesium), sterols.

Effects on the Immune System

The immunity effects of astragalus have been investigated in a multitude of in vitro and in vivo studies. Astragalus has been shown to significantly increase the spontaneous incorporation of [3H] thymidine in mononuclear cells; increase the proliferation of lymphocytes (white blood cells); potentiate IL-2 (a signaling molecule of the immune system) production and activity; activate T cell blastogenesis (replication of immune cells); increase T cell cytotoxicity (defense abilities); enhance the secretion of tumor necrosis factor (TNF), which can cause the death of tumors; potentiate the function of the reticuloendothelial system (RES), a group of cells capable of ingesting bacteria and particles in the body; increase natural killer (NK) cells' cytoxicity; and increase the activity of peritoneal macrophages. Astragalus has also been shown to augment the interferon (immune) response of mice who are exposed to viruses.

In addition, many studies have investigated the effects of astragalus when it is given in situations of immunosuppression. For example, in a large clinical study, 572 cancer patients were given fu-zheng therapy that included astragalus, in combination with standard medical treatment for 2 months. The study results suggested that patients experienced protection of adrenal cortical function during radiation and chemotherapy treatment, as well as reduction of bone marrow depression and gastrointestinal effects. This is supported by a controlled study in which mice were given astragalus concurrently with mitomycin C. In this study, astragalus showed protective effects against immunosuppression in the mice. The authors of the study hypothesized that this resistance to immunosuppression may be correlated with the observed stimulation of the reticuloendothethial system (RES), activation of T cell blastogenesis, and increased NK cell cytotoxicity.

Two Chinese randomized controlled trials have examined the use of an astragalus extract in patients with systemic lupus. The English abstracts of these studies indicate that all patients were treated with conventional treatments, and half of the patients in each study were also administered astragulus extract through injection or IV administration. The authors reported that the treatment

> Many studies have investigated the effects of astragalus when it is given in situations of immunosuppression.

group had decreased death rates of white blood cells, decreased clinical symptoms, a decreased infection rate, and an increased red blood cell count compared to the group receiving only conventional treatment. In addition, a randomized controlled clinical trial of 115 patients with leukopenia (a decrease in white blood cells) who were treated with two concentrations of astragalus preparation (15 g twice daily vs. 5 g daily) for 8 weeks found that there was an obvious rise in the white blood cell counts of both groups but that the group with the larger dose had a significantly greater increase, suggesting a dose-dependent effect. Not all studies, however, were positive. In another controlled study, an extract of astragalus in combination with the herb *Ligustrum lucidum* W.T. Aiton (Oleaceae) did not prevent cyclophosphamide-induced myelosuppression (decreased bone marrow activity) in mice.

Cardiac Effects

A variety of trials have investigated the effect of astragalus in patients or animal models with Coxsackie B virus (CBV) myocarditis, an inflammation of heart muscles caused by an infection. One controlled clinical trial of patients (10 in the treatment group; 8 controls) with CBV myocarditis who were treated with astragalus by intramuscular injection (8 g/day) for 3 to 4 months or given only conventional treatment found that the clinical condition of those treated with astragalus was improved in comparison to the control group. Another study found that astragalus treatment increased the survival rate and decreased the percentage of abnormal action potential in mice infected with Coxsackie B3 virus when compared with controls. In searching for the mechanism of action of these effects, researchers have found that astragalus significantly enhanced the OKT3, OKT4, and OKT4/OKT8 antibody ratio in patients with viral myocarditis; appeared to inhibit the replication of Coxsackie B3 virus RNA in the myocardial tissue of mice in vivo (in a living specimin) and in vitro (in a test tube), and significantly inhibited the Ca^{2+} influx across the myocardial plasma membrane in vitro. Several researchers have suggested that astragalus is a rational treatment choice for patients with viral myocarditis.

In other studies of cardiac effects, components of astragalus have been shown to be effective as positive inotropes, which can improve the condition of patients with congestive heart failure by altering heart contractions. In one uncontrolled study, 19 patients were given intravenous astragaloside IV (an active component of astragalus) for 2 weeks, at which point their symptoms of chest distress and dyspnea (shortness of breath) were relieved and their capacity for exercise was increased. In another study, 22 patients with positive ventricular late potentials (abnormal heart rhythm) were treated with a 24-g IV drip of astragalus (the control group was given lidocaine) for 2 weeks. The researchers reported that treatment with astragalus successfully shortened the duration of late potentials significantly more than lidocaine. Astragalus treatment has also been shown to be more effective than nifedipine (a calcium channel antagonist) in the treatment of 92 patients suffering from ischemic heart disease and was effective in increasing cardiac output in 20 patients with angina pectoris.

A Chinese study has been conducted in which 83 congestive heart failure patients were randomized to receive either conventional treatment or a concentrated astragalus injection once a day for 15 days. The abstract of this article reported an improvement in cardiac output and cardiac index, and a lessened incidence of a repeated cardiac event in the group receiving astragalus treatment. One team of researchers suggested that the heart-toning abilities of astragalus may be partially due to its antioxygen free radical action, based on their study of 43 patients suffering from their first acute myocardial infarction.

> *Astragalus treatment has also been shown to be more effective than nifedipine (a calcium channel antagonist) in the treatment of 92 patients suffering from ischemic heart disease and was effective in increasing cardiac output in 20 patients with angina pectoris.*

Miscellaneous Effects

Antiviral Effects

Several researchers have reported that astragalus has an antiviral effect.

Anticancer Effects

An in vitro study showed that astragalus increased the secretion of both tumor necrosis factor-a and tumor necrosis factor-b. A clinical study of 54 consecutive cases of small cell lung cancer treated with both standard medical treatment and traditional Chinese medicine (including astragalus) reported increased survival when compared to the average survival statistics of conventional medical treatment alone. This is supported by a controlled in vivo study of mice with renal cell carcinoma. The group receiving 500 mcg each of astragalus and *Ligustrum lucidum* intraperitoneally (into the abdomen) daily for 10 days had a significantly higher cure rate than did saline controls. It has been hypothesized that the antitumor effects of astragalus are the result of an augmentation of phagocyte and LAK cell activities.

Prevention of Ototoxicity
(Damage to the Ear Caused by a Toxin)

A study in guinea pigs found that a mixture of astragalus and *Pyrola rotundifolia* L. (Pyrolaceae) significantly reduced the ototoxicity and nephrotoxicity (damage to the kidney caused by a toxin) of the antibiotic gentamicin. The ototoxic effects of aminoglycoside antibiotics are thought to be related to a decrease of cAMP, and astragalus has been shown by other researchers to increase cAMP.

Miscellaneous

One study demonstrated that an aqueous solution of astragalus was able to significantly increase the motility of human sperm in vitro. The active constituents responsible for this effect are as yet unknown. Another study reported that a decoction of astragalus root was an effective treatment of senile benign renal arteriolosclerosis. Additional studies are needed to confirm these effects.

Adverse Effects

None known.

Cautions/Contraindications

Since astragalus has been reported to increase tumor necrosis factor, its use may theoretically be of concern in the management of HIV. Clarification of this potential effect is necessary.

Drug Interactions

None known.

Dosage Regimens

- Dried root (or as tea): Adult dose normally 9–15 g daily in divided doses; however, doses from 30–60 g daily are also seen occasionally.
- Tincture (1:5): 2–6 mL three times daily.
- Powdered solid extract (2:1): 250–500 mg three times daily.
- Formulas: Astragalus is often seen in combination formulas with other similar herbs, such as Chinese privet (*Ligustrum lucidum* Ait. Oleaceae), codonopsis (*Codonopsis pilosula* (Franch) Nannf., Campanulaceae) and Asian ginseng (*Panax ginseng* C.A. Meyer, Araliaceae). It is also often mixed with Chinese licorice.

Selected References

Cay XY, Xu YL, Lin XJ. Effects of radix Astragali injection on apoptosis of lymphocytes and immune function in patients with systemic lupus erythematosus. Chinese Journal of Integrated Traditional and Western Medicine 2006;26(5):443–45.

Rui T, Yang Y, Zhou T, Zhang J, Yang X, Chen H. Effect of *Astralagus membranaceus* on electrophysiological activities of acute experimental Coxsackie B-3 viral myocarditis in mice. Chinese Medical Sciences Journal 1993; 8(4):203–6.

Zhou ZL, Yu P, Lin D. Study on effect of *Astralagus* injection in treating congestive heart failure. Chinese Journal of Integrated Traditional and Western Medicine 2001; 21(10):747–59.

Bitter Orange
Citrus aurantium

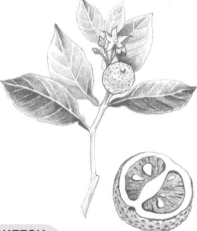

Common Uses
- Weight loss
- Antifungal

Active Constituents
- Essential oils (including linalool, linalyl acetate, limonene, myrcene)
- Synephrine (chemically similar to ephedrine)

Adverse Effects
- Cardiovascular reactions (including death)
- Headaches
- Rhabdomyolysis
- Skin reactions

Cautions/Contraindications
- High doses or long-term use is not recommended
- Pre-existing cardiovascular disease
- Hypertension
- Pregnancy or breastfeeding

Drug Interactions
- Antihypertensives
- Caffeine
- Cytochrome P450 metabolized agents (e.g., destromethorphan, cyclosporine, felodipine, indinivir)
- Monoamine oxidase inhibitors
- *Panax ginseng*
- Thyroid hormones
- Weight-loss formulas (e.g., containing ephedra, guarana, and/or green tea with caffeine)

Doses
- *Dried (capsules or tablets):* 100–1,000 mg daily (equivalent to 2–20 mg/kg body weight/day). Do not take more medicine or take it more often than recommended.
- *Tea:* For treating dyspepsia (indigestion) or lack of appetite, the German Commission E recommends a total daily dose of 4–6 g of dried bitter orange peel made into tea, taken three times daily.
- *Topical oil:* For treating fungal infections, 25% emulsion of bitter orange oil three times daily, 20% bitter orange oil in alcohol three times daily, and 100% bitter orange (bergamot) oil once daily have been used.

Introduction

Family
- Rutaceae

Synonyms
- *Aurantii pericarpium*
- Chao zhi ke
- *Citrus amara*
- *Citrus bergamia*
- *Citrus bigarradia*
- *Citrus silension*
- *Citrus sinensis*
- *Citrus vulgaris*
- Daidai
- *Fructus aurantii*
- *Fructus aurantii immaturus*
- Goutou orange
- Green orange
- Kijitsu
- Seville orange
- Shangzhou zhiqiao
- Sour orange
- Xiangcheng
- Xiucheng zhi ke
- Zhi qino
- Zhi qiao
- Zhi shi

Medicinal Forms
- Capsules or tablets
- Tea
- Topical oil
- Bitter orange used for weight loss is most commonly found in combination with other herbal products

Description

Bitter orange is an evergreen tree native to the tropical parts of Asia.

Parts Used

Supplements are made from the fruit.

Traditional Use

Bitter orange has historically been used for a wide range of conditions, including gastrointestinal upset, and as a digestive aid. Most often it is used as part of an herbal formula rather than as a single agent.

Current Medicinal Use

Bitter orange products are most commonly used as appetite suppressants or for weight loss; however, this use is questionable and associated with safety concerns.

Relevant Research

Preventative and Therapeutic Effects

Constituents

- Leaf: essential oils, including monoterpene hydrocarbons, alcohols, flavonoid glycosides, aldehydes, ketone-free acids, esters, coumarins, tetranotriterpenoids (limonin).

- Flower: methyl anthranilate, limonoids (triterpenoide bitter principles), flavonoid, essential oils (linalool, linalyl acetate, alpha-pinenes, limonene, nerol), synephrine, 5,8-epidioxyergosta-6, 22-dien-3ß-ol, adenosine, asparagine, tyrosine, valine, isoleucine, alanine, ß-sitosterol, ß-daucosterol.

- Fruit: synephrine, octopamine, tyramine, naringin, neohesperidin.

- Seeds: 17-ß-D-glucopyranosides.

- Peel: flavonoids (neohesperidin, dyhydrochalcone, naringin, sinensetin, nobiletin, tangertein), furocoumarins, essential oils (monoterpene hydrocarbons, bitter and non-bitter flavonoids, furanocoumarins, flavonoid glycosides, mineral salts, pectin, organic acids, vitamins (A, B_1, C), carotenoid pigments).

Weight Loss

Three systematic reviews have been done on the safety and efficacy of bitter orange for the treatment of obesity. All these reviews concluded that the effect of bitter orange for weight loss is still questionable due to the limited amount of available data. Although there are a few more trials reporting positive findings than negative ones, most of the trials are brief and small. In addition, since all the human studies are based on the combined effect of bitter orange and other ingredients, more evidence is needed to strengthen these results.

There have been five randomized controlled trials in humans examining the effects of bitter orange in combination with other ingredients on body weight, three of which demonstrated positive results. However, there has not been any evidence examining and supporting the effects of bitter orange alone on weight loss. Each clinical trial is described below.

One randomized controlled trial showed that administering an herbal preparation (ma huang, bitter orange, and guarana) in combination with exercise can significantly reduce fat mass. In a double-blind, randomized, placebo-controlled trial, subjects receiving an herbal mixture (bitter orange, St. John's wort, and caffeine) in combination with strict diet and exercise for 6 weeks reported significant loss in body weight and body fat. Another study demonstrated that consuming a nutritionally enriched JavaFit coffee (caffeine, garcinia cambogia, bitter orange extract, and chromium polynicotinate) may provide enhanced metabolic rates and increase resting energy expenditure only in individuals who are sensitive to the caffeine and herbal combination.

Despite these positive results, one double-blind, placebo-controlled trial found that the use of a commercial formula (extracts of bitter orange, green tea, and guarana) did not significantly affect the metabolic rate and ATP utilization in overweight adult males, both at rest and during treadmill walking.

Another randomized controlled trial evaluated the effect of a dietary herbal supplement (pantothenic acid, green tea leaf extract, guarana extract, bitter orange, white willow bark extract, ginger root, proprietary charge thermoblend) in the treatment of obesity. Results indicated that this dietary supplement actually caused weight gain, compared with the placebo. Even at full non-prescription doses, no significant weight loss was observed.

These studies not only used different herb and vitamin combinations, but also included varying levels of caffeine, exercise, and dietary modification. In addition, the weight-loss products were investigated in different populations (e.g., overweight vs. obese), making comparison difficult. Therefore, more high-quality clinical trials are required to make any conclusions on the effect of bitter orange on weight loss.

> *The effect of bitter orange for weight loss is still questionable due to the limited amount of available data.*

Three animal studies have been done on rats to examine the efficacy of bitter orange or in combination with other ingredients for weight loss. Two studies examined the use of bitter orange alone, while one looked at the use of bitter orange in combination with caffeine and tea catechins. The first two studies found that administration of bitter orange in rats not only reduces food intake and body weight gain but also lowers perirenal fat pad weight. The last study, however, found that the intake of bitter orange combined with a usual level of caffeine and tea catechins failed to suppress body fat accumulation.

The most active components in the fruit of bitter orange are synephrine and octopamine. Synephrine alkaloids are believed to be alpha-adrenergic agonists with some beta-adrenergic agonist properties. As a sympathomimetic agent, these synephrine alkaloids can potentially increase energy expenditure and decrease food intake. A double-blind, placebo-controlled trial determining the effects of a synephrine-based compound in healthy overweight adults also suggested a significantly greater weight loss compared with the placebo group. However, only high concentrations of synephrine (0.1–1 mM) can significantly stimulate lipolysis in the fat cells of humans and animals. Octopamine has shown lipolytic effects in adipocytes of rats, hamsters, and other animals, but the effect is not significant in humans.

Antifungal

There has only been one human study that evaluated the antifungal effect of bitter orange. These results are supported by an in vitro study. A clinical trial of bitter orange oil was conducted in 70 patients with tinea corporis, cruris, and pedis. Group 1 (N=20) was treated with 25% emulsion of bitter orange oil three times daily; group 2 (N=20) was treated with 20% bitter orange oil in alcohol three times daily; group 3 (N=20) was treated with 100% pure bitter orange oil once daily; and group 4 (N=10) received an imidazole derivative, dosing schedule unknown. In group 3, 25% of patients dropped out of the trial for reasons not specified. Of the remaining patients in group 3, 33.3% were cured in 1 week. More than 90% of patients who completed the treatment with pure bitter orange oil achieved clinical cures in 2 weeks, whereas 80% of those who received imidazole required 4 weeks of treatment. This study had many obvious flaws, including lack of randomization and blinding, small sample size, and different dosing schedules for the three treatments. In addition, no statistical analysis was conducted and the reason for dropping out was not described.

An in vitro study was conducted on the oils of bergamot orange (bitter orange). Three bergamot oils (natural essence, distilled extracts, and furocoumarin-free extracts) were tested against seven species of dermatophytes. Compared to conventional treatments, such

as itraconazole or griseofulvin, all three preparations had equal or lower minimum inhibitory concentrations, indicating in vitro activity against several common dermatophytes and suggesting potential use for topical treatment of fungal infections. Another study demonstrated that bitter orange can inhibit the growth of a range of fungi, especially *Trichophyton rubrum*. There was no difference in the minimum fungicidal concentration between bitter orange and an imidazole derivative. However, its mechanism of action has not been elucidated.

Overall, bitter orange appears to have some promise as an antifungal, but additional high-quality randomized controlled trials in humans are required to confirm these preliminary findings.

> *Overall, bitter orange appears to have some promise as an antifungal, but additional high-quality randomized controlled trials in humans are required to confirm these preliminary findings.*

Miscellaneous Effects

Antibacterial

An in vitro study examined the antibacterial properties of various plants against *Escherichia coli*, *Staphylococcus aureus*, and 15 other bacteria. Bitter orange extract was the only plant that inhibited all 17 bacteria tested.

Antiviral

One study examined the inhibitory effect of 34 kinds of herbal medicines on rotavirus infection and reported that the fruit of bitter orange had the most potent inhibitory activity. Additional high-quality randomized controlled trials in humans are required to confirm these preliminary findings.

Anxiolytic

Two related animal studies examined the anxiolytic effect of bitter orange on mice. Since there are no human clinical trials, it is not clear whether bitter orange will be helpful in the management of anxiety. Two main compounds present in the essential oil from bitter orange, limonene (97.8%) and myrcene (1.4%), have biological activity related to depression of the central nervous system. This may explain the sedative and anxiolytic effect reported in the rodents.

Adverse Effects

Cardiovascular Reactions

From January 1, 1998, to February 28, 2004, Health Canada received 16 reports in which products containing bitter orange (synephrine) were suspected of being associated with serious cardiovascular adverse reactions, including tachycardia, cardiac arrest, ventricular fibrillation, transient collapse, and blackout. Of the 16 patients, two died, both of whom had taken products containing ephedrine and caffeine in addition to bitter orange. Certain groups of individuals may have an increased risk of adverse reactions associated with the use of synephrine-containing products. These groups may include

- People with heart conditions, diabetes, thyroid disease, central nervous system disorders, glaucoma, pheochromocytoma, hypertension, known risk factors for cardiovascular disease, or an enlarged prostate.

- Peopele who are underweight.

- People taking thyroid hormones, monoamine oxidase inhibitors, medications to control heart rate or blood pressure, and products containing caffeine.

One double-blind, placebo-controlled, randomized study found that although bitter orange alone had no effect on blood pressure, a combination product with other active herbal ingredients, such as caffeine, significantly increased blood pressure. Multiple case reports also provide evidence that bitter orange–containing combination products may be associated with cardiovascular reactions. Although no large epidemiologic studies of the safety of bitter orange exist, it contains synephrine, which is structurally similar to ephedrine. Synephrine has vasoconstrictor properties and can increase blood pressure in humans. The details of four key reported cases are provided below.

A three-arm crossover study examined the cardiovascular effect of bitter orange and its combination products. Ten healthy, non-smoking adults were administered Advantra Z (synephrine from bitter orange), Xenadrine EFX (vitamin C, vitamin B_6, pantothenic acid, magnesium, Tyroplex, green tea extract, Seropro, yerba mate, d-methionine, gingerroot, isotherm, bitter orange, 2-dimethylamino-ethanol, and grape seed extract), or a placebo. Compared with the placebo, Xenadrine EFX (but not Advantra Z) significantly increased the systolic and diastolic blood pressure and heart rate. Another case report described exercise-induced syncope associated with QT prolongation in a healthy 22-year-old patient after a second dose of Xenadrine EFX. Cardiovascular stimulatory actions are not likely caused by bitter orange alone but may be affected by caffeine or other stimulants in the multi-component formulation.

> *Multiple case reports also provide evidence that bitter orange–containing combination products may be associated with cardiovascular reactions.*

One case report described a possible incidence of acute lateral-wall myocardial infarction as a result of using Edita's Skinny Pill (a dietary supplement containing 300 mg bitter orange as well as carnitine, chromium, citrimax, chitosan, herbal diuretic complex, guarananine, green tea, and calcium) for 1 year. The authors noted that although citrimax, guarananine, and green tea are reported to have stimulatory effects, adverse reactions are not likely at the dosages contained in the supplement. However, when taken together, individual ingredients may interact in ways that are difficult to predict. Also, the patient had several risk factors for myocardial infarction, including a history of smoking, physical inactivity, and a heart murmur. Another patient experienced variant angina after initiation of CortiSlim (an ephedra-free weight-loss supplement containing vitamin C, calcium, chromium polynicotinate, bitter orange peel extract, green tea leaf extract, banana leaf extract, vanadyl sulfate, magnolia bark extract, beta-sitoserol, and suntheanine).

In addition to the cases reported in humans, a study of rats treated with bitter orange demonstrated dose-related cardiotoxicity, specifically ventricular arrhythmias with enlargement of QRS complex. Since the amount of bitter orange used in this study was approximately equivalent to the recommended daily intake in many dietary supplements for weight loss, the possible association between bitter orange intake and cardiotoxicity remains to be examined in more detail.

Evaluation of these reports is challenging because of many factors, such as the lack of information on the ingested dose of bitter orange, the contributory effects of multiple ingredients, and the ambiguity of the reported information. Therefore, additional studies and case reports are required to validate this conclusion.

Headaches

Two studies reported the most common side effect with bitter orange extract was headaches. Bitter orange contains tyramine, synephrine, and octopamine, all of which may worsen migraines and other types of primary headaches.

Ischemic Colitis

One case reported a patient who developed ischemic colitis 1 week after initiation of NaturalMax Skinny Fast (a weight-loss supplement containing bitter orange, *Garcinia cambogia*, L-carnitine, chitosan, and chromium arginate). The patient had no other predisposing factors, and discontinuation of the supplement led to immediate improvement and resolution of her symptoms.

Ischemic Stroke

A recent case report described an association between ischemic stroke and short-term daily use of a product containing synephrine derived from bitter orange. The patient, with no notable medical history and taking no other medications, experienced memory loss and unsteady gait after taking the supplement for 1 week. Nearly all the patient's symptoms, except for residual, mild, subjective impairment of concentration, were resolved after 1 week of treatment with aspirin and immediate release dipyridamole.

Rhabdomyolysis

One case report documented a previously healthy male who developed rhabdomyolysis after ingestion of a synephrine-containing dietary supplement (other ingredients in the supplement were not identified in the report). In addition, he experienced pulmonary edema, acute renal failure, disseminated intravascular coagulation, and bilateral compartment syndromes in his lower extremities. The patient required prolonged hospitalization for hemodialysis and developed permanent sensory and motor neurological deficits in his distal lower extremities. Although it was not clearly specified whether this supplement contained bitter orange, synephrine is one of the major components of bitter orange peel, so the association between bitter orange and rhabdomyolysis should not be excluded.

Skin Reactions

Two cases of localized phototoxic reactions associated with topical application of aromatherapy oil made from bitter orange have been reported. Bitter orange peel contains furocoumarins, which can produce possible phototoxic effects, resulting in erythema, swelling, blisters, pustules, dermatoses leading to scab formation, and pigment spots.

Cautions/Contraindications

Allergy or hypersensitivity to the Rutaceae family: Since bitter orange is classified in the Rutaceae family (e.g., lemons, oranges, mandarins, tangerines, limes, kumquats, etc.), people with known allergy or hypersensitivity to the Rutaceae family should avoid its use.

Narrow-angle glaucoma: Theoretically, the synephrine in bitter orange fruit, peel, or juice might worsen narrow-angle glaucoma.

High dosage or prolonged use: Ingestion of large amounts (the specific amount was not stated) of bitter orange peel in children has been reported to cause intestinal colic, convulsions, and even death. Although no clinical studies have been done on the long-term effects of bitter orange usage, theoretically bitter orange is not safe for prolonged use because of its synephrine content. Long-term use should be avoided due to a lack of sufficient evidence.

Hypertension: One study suggested that most healthy individuals have baroreceptor buffering capacity that limits the extent of blood pressure alterations secondary to sympathomimetics, but people with muted buffering ability (e.g., elderly persons, patients with hypertension, or patients with cardiovascular problems) have markedly greater blood pressure increases than healthy individuals in response to sympathomimetics. Although no studies have been done on the effects of bitter orange on patients with pre-existing cardiovascular or hypertension problems, bitter orange can theoretically worsen hypertension.

Pregnancy and breastfeeding: Bitter orange is generally safe when used orally in amounts normally contained in food, but various cases of adverse reactions have been reported when used orally for medicinal purposes. Since the effects of bitter orange on a fetus or a breastfeeding infant are not known, its use should be avoided.

Sun exposure: Applying bitter orange oil to the skin and exposing that area to sunlight or to artificial light (e.g., sun tanning booths) is more likely to result in skin reactions, such as erythema, swelling, blisters, pustules, and dermatoses, leading to scab formation and pigment spots. A similar effect has not been reported by individuals who took bitter orange by mouth.

Underweight people: One case report described the use of bitter orange–containing dietary supplement for weight loss in a 16-year-old adolescent with anorexia nervosa. Bitter orange contains adrenergic agonist properties that can mask the symptoms of anorexia nervosa (e.g., bradycardia and hypotension) and exacerbate weight loss, and its use in underweight people can make it difficult for clinicians to monitor a patient's clinical progress.

> *Theoretically, bitter orange is not safe for prolonged use because of its synephrine content. Long-term use should be avoided due to a lack of sufficient evidence.*

Drug Interactions

Antihypertensives

Synephrine (found in bitter orange) has the potential to raise blood pressure and cause vasoconstriction, which may counteract the blood pressure-lowering effects of antihypertensives. One human study reported a significant increase in systolic blood pressure, diastolic blood pressure, and heart rate after a single dose of bitter orange. Although bitter orange extract has not been tested in clinical studies, bitter orange contains synephrine, which has been found to increase mean arterial pressure in rats.

Caffeine

There has been one double-blind, placebo-controlled, randomized study showing that a combination product with bitter orange and caffeine significantly increased blood pressure. Administration of bitter orange and caffeine can potentially aggravate hemodynamic effects in humans, but more evidence is required to support this conclusion.

Drugs Metabolized by Cytochrome P450 3A4

Several studies report that bitter orange juice can potentially inhibit the metabolism of drugs via the cytochrome P450 3A4 pathway, increasing the drug levels and their adverse effects. Agents that are metabolized by cytochrome P450 3A4 include but are not limited to anti-anxiety, blood pressure, cholesterol, decongestant, depression, allergy, antifungal, HIV, sedation, antinausea, steroid, and erectile dysfunction medications. Some possible drug interactions with bitter orange, such as dextromethorphan (antitussive), cyclosporine (immunosuppressant), calcium channel blockers, and indinavir (antiviral), are listed below.

In a study of 11 healthy volunteers, use of 30 mg dextromethorphan with 200 mL of Seville (bitter) orange juice increased drug bioavailability and inhibited gut cytochrome P450 3A4 metabolism. Concurrent use of dextromethorphan and bitter orange juice can potentially increase the risk of adverse effects. One study showed that coadministration of bitter orange fruit and cyclosporine enhanced the absorption of cyclosporine and resulted in acute toxicity. Therefore, the blood cyclosporine concentration should be carefully monitored when these two substances are used together.

In a randomized study, 10 healthy volunteers received a felodipine extended-release 10-mg tablet with 240 mL of Seville orange juice, dilute grapefruit juice, or common (sweet) orange juice (negative control). Results suggested that, compared to the negative control, felodipine in combination with Seville orange juice can cause toxic effects as a result of increased drug levels and inactivation of intestinal cytochrome P450 3A4 metabolism.

In an open-label study, 13 healthy volunteers received 800 mg of indinavir every 8 hours for 1 day and a single 800-mg dose the next morning with 240 mL of water or Seville orange juice. Bitter orange juice slightly increased indinavir levels, but the effect is not clinically significant.

Monoamine Oxidase Inhibitors

Bitter orange contains tyramine, octopamine, and synephrine, which are monoamine oxidase substrates. Concurrent use of bitter orange supplements with monoamine oxidase inhibitors (a class of antidepressant) can produce an indirect sympathomimetic response, resulting in dangerously high blood pressure. However, additional controlled studies are required to associate hypertensive reaction with the concurrent use of bitter orange and monoamine oxidase inhibitors.

Panax Ginseng

One study showed that *Panax ginseng* can prolong the QTc interval in healthy adults. Another case report described exercise-induced syncope associated with QT prolongation in a healthy 22-year-old patient after a second dose of Xenadrine EFX (vitamin C, vitamin B$_6$, pantothenic acid, magnesium, Tyroplex, green tea extract, Seropro, yerba mate, d-methionine, gingerroot, isotherm, bitter orange, 2-dimethylaminoethanol, and grape seed extract). Theoretically, combining *Panax ginseng* and bitter orange might have an additive effect on the QT interval and may increase the risk for cardiovascular events.

Thyroid Hormones

A 52-year-old woman experienced tachycardia on the same day as she began taking a dry herbal extract of an unripe fruit of bitter orange as a dietary supplement for weight loss. She had been taking 50 mcg thyroxine daily for hypothyroidism for the last 10 years and maintained good health during that time. It was not clear whether thyroxine interacted with the bitter orange supplement, but the adverse reaction resolved once the patient stopped taking the herbal treatment. Bitter orange can potentially interact with thyroid medications or worsen hyperthyroidism due to its synephrine content.

Weight-Loss Formulas

Herbs and supplements with multiple stimulant properties used for weight loss, such as ephedra and guarana, seem to increase the risk of hypertension and adverse cardiovascular effects when used with bitter orange. Multiple case reports also provide evidence that products containing bitter orange may be associated with cardiovascular reactions (see Relevant Research).

Selected References

Bent S, Padula A, Neuhaus J. Safety and efficacy of *Citrus aurantium* for weight loss. The American Journal of Cardiology 2004;94: 1359–60.

Fugh-Berman A, Myers A. *Citrus aurantium*, an ingredient of dietary supplements marketed for weight loss: Current status of clinical and basic research. Experimental Biology and Medicine 2004;229(8):698–704.

Haaz S, Fontaine KR, Cutter G, Limdi N, Perumean-Chaney S, Allison DB. *Citrus aurantium* and synephrine alkaloids in the treatment of overweight and obesity: An update. Obesity Reviews 2006 Feb;7(1):79–88.

Dosage Regimens

- **General guidelines:** Recommended doses of 100–1,000 mg daily are based on those most commonly used in available trials. Do not take more or more often than recommended. Bitter orange is not safe when used in doses higher than recommended because it contains the stimulant synephrine.
- **Dried (capsules or tablets):** 100–1,000 mg daily (equivalent to 2–20 mg/kg body weight/day). Synephrine content ranges from 0.33 mg/g contained in the pulp of whole fruit to 20 mg/g in some dietary supplements and 35 mg/g in extracts.
- **Tea:** For treating dyspepsia (indigestion) or lack of appetite, the German Commission E recommends a total daily dose of 4–6 g of dried bitter orange peel made into tea, taken three times daily. Bitter orange tea is made by soaking 2 g of peel in 150 mL boiling water.
- **Topical oil:** For treating fungal infections, 25% emulsion of bitter orange oil three times daily, 20% bitter orange oil in alcohol three times daily, and 100% bitter orange (bergamot) oil once daily have been used.
- **Children:** There is insufficient available evidence to recommend bitter orange for use in children.

Black Cohosh

Cimicifuga racemosa (L.) Nutt.

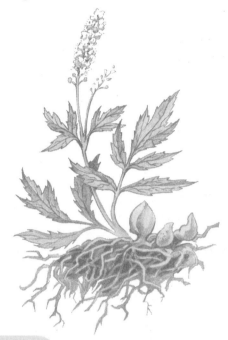

THUMBNAIL SKETCH

Common Uses
- Menopause symptoms (hot flashes, anxiety, depression)
- Premenstrual syndrome and dysmenorrhea (painful periods)

Active Constituents
- Terpenoids
- Formononetin

Adverse Effects
- Rare, limited to stomach upset.
- Historical evidence suggests that throbbing headaches and nervous system and cardiovascular depression can occur at high doses.

Cautions/Contraindications
- Pregnancy and breastfeeding

Drug Interactions
- None known

Doses
- *Dried root:* 40–200 mg taken by decoction or as a solid dose daily
- *Extract (40%–60% alcohol):* Equivalent to 40 mg of herb daily
- *Tincture (1:10 in 60% ethanol):* 0.4–2 mL daily

Note: In the case of menopause treatment, the onset of action of this plant can take up to 2 weeks to occur.

Introduction

Family
- Ranunculaceae

Synonyms
- Bugbane
- Bugwort
- Rattleroot
- Rattletop
- Richweed
- Rattlesnake root
- Rattleweed
- Macrotys
- Squaw root
- Papoose root
- Christopher weed
- Cimicifuga
- *Actaea racemosa* L.
- *Macrotys actaeoides*

Medicinal Forms
- Dried root
- Extract
- Tincture

Description

Black cohosh is an upright perennial with large compound, tooth-edged leaves. It grows up to 2 meters (80 inches) high, producing numerous small white flowers on a wand-like raceme. Black cohosh is native to the temperate climates of the northern hemisphere, including North America, where it is found from Maine to Ontario in the north and from Georgia and Missouri in the south. Even though black cohosh has been cultivated in Europe and is especially popular in Germany for its medicinal properties, all commercial stocks come from the United States and Canada. "Cohosh" is the Algonquin word for "rough," referring to its gnarled root, which is black in color when harvested and has an acrid taste and strong odor.

Parts Used

The plant grows from a thick fibrous root stock, which is the part used medicinally.

Traditional Use

Black cohosh has long been used for its medicinal properties, especially by peoples of the First Nations. The Cherokee and Iroquois peoples used a tea made from the root to alleviate rheumatic pains and to promote lactation and menses. Its use was commonly accepted into the eclectic medical movement in the early to mid-19th century, where it was prized as an antispasmodic, analgesic, and gynecological agent. It has been called squaw root and the menopause herb. The botanical name for black cohosh, *Cimicifuga racemosa*, comes from the Latin *cimex*, meaning "bug," and *fuga*, meaning "to repel," referring to the fact that it appears to act as an effective insect repellent. Black cohosh is also known as bugbane and bugwort.

Current Medicinal Use

As with its traditional uses, black cohosh products are primarily used in women's health care. Research has shown that substances found in black cohosh have hormone-like properties that influence the endocrine system. A growing amount of research, including clinical trials, show that some black cohosh products may help alleviate the symptoms of menopause (hot flashes, anxiety, mild depression), premenstrual syndrome, dysmenorrhea, and uterine spasm.

Relevant Research

Preventative and Therapeutic Uses

Constituents

- **Triterpenoids:** a complex mixture including actein, cimigoside, 12-acetylactein, cimifugoside, 27-deoxyacetylacteol.

- **Flavonoids:** formononetin.

- **Acids:** isoferulic, salicylic, acetic, butyric, palmitic.

- **Miscellaneous:** phytosterols, hydrolysable tannins, cimicifugin, resinous material referred to as acteina.

Endocrine Effects (Menopausal Symptoms)

Black cohosh's exact mechanism of action is not clear, but early evidence suggested that it had estrogenic properties, and on this basis it was categorized as a phytoestrogen. Phyto-estrogens are generally defined as plant-based estrogen-like compounds. Estrogen itself is not typically found in plants, but common phytoestrogens are found in many plants, including soy (*Glycine max.* L.), red clover (*Trifolium pratense* L.), and chaste tree (*Vitex agnus-castus* L.). A growing body of research has focused on attempting to determine whether black cohosh actually has any estrogenic properties. It is consistently reported that black cohosh extracts and isolated compounds derived thereof *do not* possess estrogenic activity, regardless of source, extraction procedure, dose, or length of exposure.

The vast majority of clinical investigations regarding this plant's medicinal action have been carried out in Europe, notably Germany. A recent evidence-based review examining seven randomized controlled studies using black cohosh to treat post-menopause vasomotor symptoms concluded that black cohosh appears to be most effective in cases of mild to moderate symptoms. Another systematic review examining the use of black cohosh for general menopause symptoms included four randomized controlled trials and concluded that "in spite of plausible mechanisms of action of *C. racemosa*, its clinical efficacy has not been convincingly demonstrated through rigorous clinical trials. Additional rigorous RCTs and biochemical and chemical investigations are warranted." Several examples of key studies are reviewed below.

In a randomized study conducted over 6 months with 60 women over 40 years of age who had ovarian insufficiency following hysterectomy but with at least one functioning ovary, investigators compared the effectiveness of a commercial product of black cohosh (Remifemin) and conventional hormone-based therapies. At a dose of 2 tablets twice daily, Remifemin was shown to decrease menopausal symptoms (measured using the Kupperman Menopausal Index) comparable to the three conventional therapy groups (1 mg estriol daily; 1.25 mg conjugated estrogen; combined estrogen-gestagen therapy). In addition, one study demonstrated that Remifemin (40 drops twice daily) given over 12 weeks showed estrogen-like stimulation of the vaginal mucosa similar to conjugated estrogens (0.625 mg daily) and an improvement in neurovegetative symptoms comparable to 2 mg of diazepam daily.

Another randomized, placebo-controlled, double-blind study conducted over 12 weeks on 80 women suffering from the unpleasant consequences of menopause also noted positive results. Remifemin (2 tabs twice daily) was shown to increase proliferation of vaginal

> *It is consistently reported that black cohosh extracts and isolated compounds derived thereof do not possess estrogenic activity, regardless of source, extraction procedure, dose, or length of exposure.*

epithelium and decrease physical and mental symptoms (as measured on the Kuppermann Menopausal Index and the Hamilton Anxiety Index) in a fashion superior to both the placebo and conjugated estrogen. Similar results have been noted in other clinical studies of Remifemin, including effectiveness in cases where conventional therapy is contraindicated or refused and in a protocol removing conventional treatment.

A randomized, placebo-controlled trial involving 351 peri- and post-menopausal women examined the effect of four therapies on menopausal symptoms. Black cohosh was a component of two of these therapies, either given alone (160 mg daily of 2.5% triterpene glycosides, 70% ethanol extract) or in combination with nine other herbs in a multibotanical (200 mg/day of black cohosh) to women randomized to receive these treatments. The authors reported no difference in vaginal dryness, regularity of menstrual cycle, or serum concentrations of FSH, LH, estradiol, or sex hormone–binding protein after 12 months in postmenopausal women taking black cohosh products.

Another randomized, placebo-controlled trial assessed the use of black cohosh (brand not specified) in the management of hot flashes experienced by 85 women diagnosed with breast cancer who had completed their primary cancer treatment, including chemotherapy and radiation. Fifty-nine of the study participants were also taking tamoxifen, and they were equally distributed among the treatment and placebo groups. Participants were asked to take either black cohosh (dose not known) or a placebo twice daily with meals for 60 days. Women in both the black cohosh and placebo groups reported benefits in terms of reduced number and intensity of hot flashes. There were no significant differences in the seven outcome measures reported between the two groups except for sweating, with more improvement reported in the black cohosh group. No differences in FSH or LH were identified between the two groups. The authors con-

clude that black cohosh was not significantly more efficacious than the placebo against most menopausal symptoms, including number and intensity of hot flashes. Since the dose of black cohosh was not provided, however, it is difficult to compare these findings with the results of earlier studies.

It should be noted that many of the clinical trials described above have been carried out with one specific proprietary product, Remifemin, where the tablets are standardized to 27-deoxyacetein content (1 mg/unit dose).

Miscellaneous Effects
Cardiovascular Effects

The administration of the resinous material acteina has been shown to lower blood pressure in various animal models and to cause peripheral vasodilation and increased blood flow in humans. Triterpene compounds extracted from a plant described as Japanese Cimicifuga were shown to reduce cholesterol levels in vivo.

Adverse Effects

Adverse effects appear rare, usually being limited to occasional stomach pains. The consumption of large doses (amounts not specified) were noted by early eclectic physicians to cause severe "bursting" frontal headaches and sensory and circulatory depression.

More recently, patients and clinicians have been alarmed by warnings about the potential for liver toxicity associated with black cohosh. More than 40 case reports of liver injury possibly related to black cohosh have been collected from Europe's national competent authorities and literature case reports.

> *Currently, the association between liver reactions and black cohosh remains inconclusive.*

A recent review of these reports concluded that the published cases were most likely misdiagnosed cases of idiopathic hepatitis, mistakenly attributed to black cohosh. Of the unpublished reports collected by government authorities, only 16 were considered sufficiently documented to assess a link with black cohosh. Of those, 12 were excluded or considered unlikely to be related and only four were found to have a temporal association with use of black cohosh. The two of those that were considered probably associated with black cohosh use were published and were identified as containing several flaws. In all cases, for example, the presence of black cohosh in the products was not definitely established. In many cases, the name of the product and dosage taken were not specified. Some cases were combination products, for which certain ingredients were not identified, and for other cases, the patients were on other medications that could have been linked to the negative effects. The conclusions of this review were that confounding issues, such as the common adulteration of black cohosh products with products of Asian species of *Actea* and the coadministration of drugs known to cause liver damage, might have played a part in a number of these reports.

Currently, the association between liver reactions and black cohosh remains inconclusive.

Cautions/Contraindications

Black cohosh should be avoided during pregnancy and lactation.

Drug Interactions

No clinical cases of drug interactions could be found for this plant.

Dosage Regimens
- Dried root: 40–200 mg taken by decoction or as a solid dose daily.
- Extract (40%–60% alcohol): Equivalent to 40 mg of herb daily.
- Tincture (1:10 in 60% ethanol): 0.4–2 mL daily.

Note: In the case of menopause treatment, the onset of action of this plant can take up to 2 weeks.

Selected References

Bone K. Phytotherapy review and commentary. Townsend Letter for Doctors and Patients 2006; July:66–70.

Borrelli F, Ernst E. *Cimicifuga racemosa*: A systematic review of its clinical efficacy. European Journal of Clinical Pharmacology 2002;58: 235–41.

Jacobson JS, Troxel AB, Evans J, Klaus L, Vahdat L, Kinne D, et al. Randomized trial of black cohosh for the treatment of hot flashes among women with a history of breast cancer. Journal of Clinical Oncology 2001;19(10): 2739–45.

Pockaj BA, Gallagher JG, Loprinzi CL, Stena PJ, Barton DL. Phase III double-blind, randomized, placebo-controlled crossover trial of black cohosh in the management of hot flashes. Journal of Clinical Oncology 2006;24(18): 2836–41.

Uevelhack R, Blohmer, JU, Graubaum HJ, Busch R, Grunwald J, Wernecke KD. Black cohosh and St. John's wort for climacteric complaints: A randomized trial. Obstetrics and Gynecology 2006;107:247–55.

Burdock
Arctium lappa L.

THUMBNAIL SKETCH

Common Uses
- *Internal:* Skin conditions and rheumatic conditions resulting from toxins
- *External:* Eczema and skin ulcers

Active Constituents
- Inulin
- Polyacetylenes
- Volatile oil
- Arctiopicrin

Adverse Effects
- Temporary worsening of symptoms, possibly because of detoxifying action

Cautions/Contraindications
- Pregnancy
- Diabetes

Drug Interactions
- Oral medications that lower blood sugar levels (possible)

Doses
Internal
- *Dried root:* 2–6 g of dried root, or decoction, three times daily
- *Liquid extract (1:1 in 25% alcohol):* 2–6 mL three times daily
- *Tincture (1:10 in 45% alcohol):* 8–12 mL three times daily
- *Decoction:* 1 part in 20, 500 mL per day

External
- An infusion or tincture (1:5 in 25% alcohol) of the leaf can be used externally as a poultice

Introduction

Family
- Asteraceae (also known as Compositae)

Synonyms
- Great burdock
- Bardane
- Begger's buttons
- Thorny burr
- Bardana
- Gobo
- Lappa
- Edible burdock

Medicinal Forms
- Dried root
- Extract
- Tincture
- Decoction
- Infusion

Description
Burdock is a biennial plant native to both Asia and Europe but now naturalized across North America. The stems grow to 1.5 meters (5 feet), with oblong leaves, reddish flower heads, and hooked bracts or burrs. The root is white inside, becomes soft and sweet with chewing, and has a mucilagenous texture.

Parts Used
While the root is the primary part used therapeutically, the leaves and seeds are also said to have medicinal properties. The roots are more favored in the Western herbal tradition, but the seeds are often used in traditional Asian medicine.

Traditional Use
In Western herbalism, burdock is considered an important alterative herb — an agent capable of favorably altering unhealthy conditions of the body and tending to restore normal function. In Western and Chinese herbalism, burdock was used as a detoxifying agent to "cleanse" the blood, removing toxins from the body. Consequently, it was used internally and externally for many conditions of the skin, such as acne, boils, abscesses, and eczema and for situations of chronic inflammation, such as rheumatism and gout.

Current Medicinal Use
Based on traditional evidence, burdock is primarily used in treating chronic skin diseases (eczema and ulcers), rheumatic ailments, and infections.

Relevant Research

Preventative and Therapeutic Uses

Constituents

Root
- Carbohydrates: inulin (up to 50%), mucilage, pectin.
- Polyacetylenes: notably sulfur-containing thiophenes.
- Volatile acids: include acetic acid, propionic acid, butyric acids, isovaleric acids.
- Polyphenolic acids: caffeic acid, chlorogenic acid.
- Aldehydes: include acetaldhyde, benzaldehyde, valeraldehyde.
- Miscellaneous: arctiopicrin (sesquiterpene lactone), tannin, "bitters" (lappatin), quercetin (flavonoid), kaempferol (flavonoid).

Leaves
- Terpenoids: include arctiopicrin, sterols, and triterpenols.
- Miscellaneous: mucilage, essential oil, tannins, inulin.

Seeds
- Flavonoids.
- Essential oil.
- Fixed oils.

Traditional Uses

Burdock root is reputed to restore health, induce sweating, perform diuretic functions (i.e., promote water loss from the body via urination), have antimicrobial properties, control fever, have antitumor properties, and act as a mild laxative. Oral consumption is considered useful in the management of many conditions, including chronic skin diseases, inflammatory conditions, and infections. Historically, burdock was thought to support liver function and detoxification. Externally, it is used in the treatment of skin conditions, such as eczema and skin ulcers.

Antibacterial Effects

Extracts of the leaves, flowers, and roots have all been shown to possess antibacterial activity. The leaves are reported to be active against both gram-negative and -positive bacteria, while the flowers and roots are active only against gram-negative bacteria. Arctiopicrin, a constituent isolated from both the leaves and roots, has been shown to have an antimicrobial action against gram-negative bacteria. The clinical relevance of this antimicrobial action is questionable, since the constituents thought to be responsible for this action are not normally found in the dried commercial herb.

> Historically, burdock was thought to support liver function and detoxification. Externally, it is used in the treatment of skin conditions, such as eczema and skin ulcers.

Miscellaneous

One study demonstrated that extracts of *Arctium lappa* root could produce a "pronounced and long-lasting decrease in blood sugar" when administered to rats. It also improved carbohydrate tolerance, with negligible toxicity. The constituent(s) responsible for this action is/are unknown. Dietary fiber extracted from the traditional Japanese food called gobo (burdock root) and added to the basal diet of rats (5%) was shown to protect against the toxic effects of various food colorings (erthrosine, tartrazine, indigo carmine, new coccine, and brilliant blue).

One study has demonstrated burdock's potential to regenerate rat liver cells that were damaged in an experimentally induced simulation of alcohol damage. Another animal study has demonstrated the use of burdock inulin extract as an effective prebiotic. This compound was shown to increase the concentration of beneficial gut bacteria in mice over a 2-week period. Further research is needed to determine the clinical application of these animal studies in humans.

An antimutagenic factor has been isolated from burdock juice. Other investigators have also noted this potential to decrease incidence of DNA mutation.

Adverse Effects

A well-publicized instance of poisoning has been reported in a 26-year-old woman who consumed "burdock tea" purchased in a local health food store and subsequently arrived at the emergency room suffering from symptoms characteristic of atropine poisoning (i.e., blurred vision, inability to void, rapid pulse, dry mouth, and "bizarre" behavior). Since tropane alkaloids such as atropine are not normally found in burdock root, the product was analyzed and found to contain an atropine concentration of 300 mg/g. It was assumed that the plant had been adulterated with a member of the nightshade family, probably deadly nightshade (*Atropa belladonna* L., Solanaceae). Unfortunately, this appears not to be an isolated example, as other instances of probable atropine adulteration have been noted, and this is often cited as a example of the poor quality control surrounding herbal medicines and the need for stricter guidelines.

Three cases of contact irritation (one adolescent and two adults) have been noted following the application of medicinal plasters containing burdock root. There is no clinical evidence to suggest that the preparation made from the leaves will cause a similar problem. However, some sesquiterpene lactones are known to be allergenic and some polyacetylenes and thiophenes are known to be photosensitizers. Thus, there is a potential for skin irritation with plant parts containing these compounds, especially in the case of presensitized individuals or with inappropriate use (e.g., too concentrated, for too long, too frequently, or with sun exposure soon after use).

While little information is available, concerns have been raised regarding burdock's pronounced "detoxifying" action. It has been noted that treating these "toxic" states may cause the symptoms of the conditions being treated to worsen temporarily, causing undue distress to the patient.

Burdock root has been shown to possess no carcinogenic potential in mice even when given at a high dose for a prolonged time.

Cautions/Contraindications

Given the hypoglycemic factor shown in animal studies, caution should be used in cases of diabetes. An extensive review article suggested that burdock possesses uterine stimulant properties; thus, it should be contraindicated during pregnancy and breastfeeding.

Drug Interactions

While no instance of a drug interaction could be found, this plant's influence on blood sugar levels has given rise to concerns over using it together with oral medications that lower blood sugar, as it may have an additive effect.

Dosage Regimens

Internal

- Dried root: 2–6 g of dried root, or decoction, three times daily.
- Liquid extract (1:1 in 25% alcohol): 2–6 mL three times daily.
- Tincture (1:10 in 45% alcohol): 8–12 mL three times daily.
- Decoction: 1 part in 20, 500 mL per day.

External

- An infusion or tincture (1:5 in 25% alcohol) of the leaf can be used externally as a poultice.

Selected References

Chandler F, Osborne F. Burdock. Canadian Pharmaceutical Journal 1997;130(5):46–49.

Lin SC, Lin CH, Lin CC, Lin YH, Chen CF, Chen IC, Wang LY. Hepatoprotective effects of *Arctium lappa* Linne on liver injuries induced by chronic ethanol consumption and potentiated by carbon tetrachloride. Journal of Biomedical Science 2002;9:401–9.

Calendula

Calendula officinalis L.

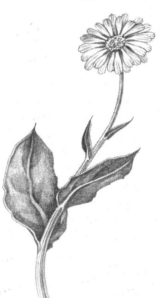

THUMBNAIL SKETCH

Common Uses
- *External:* Skin abrasions, minor burns, wounds
- *Internal:* Digestive irritation (minor)

Active Constituents
- Flavonoids
- Volatile oil
- Terpenoids

Adverse Effects
- Contact dermatitis (possibly)

Cautions/Contraindications
- Pregnancy
- Allergies to plants in the Asteraceae (Compositae) family

Drug Interactions
- None noted

Doses
Internal
- *Dried florets:* 1–4 g three times daily
- *Liquid extract (1:1 in 40% alcohol):* 0.5–1 mL three times daily
- *Tincture (1:5 in 90% alcohol):* 0.3–1.2 mL three times daily

External
- 5–10 mL of dried florets steeped in 240 mL boiling water for 10 minutes and allowed to cool; can be used as a gargle or to treat skin conditions

Formulas
- Calendula is often combined with other wound-healing herbs, such as *Symphytum officinale* L., Boraginaceae (Comfrey), *Matricaria recutita* L., Asteraceae (German chamomile) or *Echinacea* spp., Asteaceae (Coneflower), and may also be used in combination with phytomedicines with a reported antimicrobial action, such as *Hydrastis canadensis* L., Ranunculaceae (Goldenseal).

Introduction

Family
- Asteraceae (also known as Compositae)

Synonyms
- Gold-bloom
- Marigold
- Marybud
- Pot marigold
- Holigold
- Mary bud

Medicinal Forms
- Dried root
- Extract
- Tincture
- Calendula is also available, either alone or in combination, in many different dosage forms, including vaginal suppositories, creams, salves, toothpastes, and cosmetics

Description
Calendula is a common garden annual with a hairy stem and leaves. It stands 30 to 60 centimeters (1 to 2 feet) high and is easily recognizable by its brilliant orange single flowers with multiple, daisy-like florets. While native to Egypt, the Middle East, and Mediterranean Europe, it can now be found throughout the world. The attractive flowers are highly prized by horticulturists and landscapers and often form the centerpiece in ornamental gardens. Since the flowers are edible, it is also often found in culinary gardens. It is important to note that this plant is distinct from members of the *Tagetes* genus, which are also commonly called marigolds.

Parts Used
While the leaves and whole aerial part of the plant can be used medicinally, the whole flowers and petals (actually florets) are most commonly used.

Traditional Use
Calendula is one of the best-known plants in Western herbal medicine and has enjoyed a long medicinal history dating back to the early cultures of the Middle East and the Indian subcontinent. Its colorful flowers were thought to lift spirits and encourage cheerfulness. Calendula has been used as a cleansing and detoxifying herb. Creams, salves, and plasters were and are still used to treat skin conditions and promote wound healing. The flowers are edible and are often added to salads or made into teas and cordials.

Current Medicinal Use
Animal studies have found that calendula has anti-inflammatory, antiviral, and antibacterial properties. As with traditional uses, calendula products are primarily used externally as creams, gels, and even as a mouthwash in managing superficial wounds, minor scalds, skin abrasions, mouth sores, and mucosal irritations.

Relevant Research

Preventative and Therapeutic Uses

Constituents
- Terpenoids: lupeol, taraxerol, taraxasterol, faradiol, saponins, volatile oil component, campesterol, stigmasterol.
- Flavonoids: rutinoside, rutin, isoquercetin, narcissin, neohesperoside.
- Polysaccharides: rhamnoarabinogalactan, arabinogalactans.
- Miscellaneous: bitter principle called loiliolide (calendin), carotenoid pigments (beta carotene, lycopene, violaxanthin).

External Uses

Wounds

Salves or diluted tincture of calendula are reported to be useful in the management of superficial wounds, minor scalds, and skin abrasions. Calendula is also used as a gargle or mouthwash for mouth sores and mucosal irritation. Due to its astringent properties, calendula has been used to stop bleeding and "dry" discharges. Calendula has also been suggested in the treatment of fungal vaginal infections.

A recent controlled clinical trial has evaluated the use of a topical ointment containing calendula to treat venous leg ulcers. In total, 34 patients were randomized either to receive calendula ointment or a placebo, applied twice a day for three weeks. The authors reported a 41% decrease in total ulcer size in the treatment group compared to a 14% decrease in the control group. This study shows promising results and suggests that further research using calendula to treat ulcers is warranted. Another study reported that the addition of a compound herbal product containing calendula to 0.5% hydrocortisone decreased the healing times of abraded skin when compared to hydrocortisone alone. The clinical relevance specifically with regard to calendula is unknown because the compound product contained other herbal medicines with known wound-healing properties.

> *Salves or diluted tincture of calendula are reported to be useful in the management of superficial wounds, minor scalds, and skin abrasions.*

Calendula has also been proposed to prevent skin irritation resulting from radiation treatments. A single blind study has examined 225 postoperative breast cancer patients randomized to apply either trolamine (a common topical agent used to prevent radiation damage) or calendula twice a day to the treatment area during the period of radiation. The authors concluded that the ability of calendula to prevent radiation-induced irritation and toxicity was statistically superior to that of trolamine.

Unguentum lymphaticum — a topical agent that contains calendula, among other ingredients, and is regarded as being useful in the management of lymphedema (fluid collection in the lymphatic system) — was evaluated for efficacy in rats with induced acute lymphedema. Moderate relief was noted only in swelling occurring in the animal's legs. Again, because this is a combination herbal product, clinical relevance to the specific action of calendula is unknown. Physiological regeneration and growth of epithelium have been noted following topical application of calendula to surgically induced wounds in an animal study. It is thought to act by increasing the metabolism of various proteins during the regenerative phase.

Pain

A recent review has examined three studies using eardrops containing calendula to treat pain associated with ear infections in children. The authors of the review concluded that insufficient human evidence is available to recommend calendula to treat the pain of ear infections at this time.

Anti-inflammatory Effects

Calendula has been reported to have anti-inflammatory properties. Following topical application, both the triterpene and flavonoid fractions have been shown to possess an anti-inflammatory action. The most pronounced effect has been noted with the faridol esters extracted from the essential oil. In addition, it has been suggested that the anti-inflammatory action of the isorhamnetin flavonoid glycosides is due to an inhibition of lipoxygenase activity.

Miscellaneous Effects

As has been seen in other plants, the high-density polysaccharides are reported to have immunostimulant properties in vitro (test tube experiments). The clinical relevance of calendula products with high alcohol content has been questioned because these constituents are predominately water soluble. In addition, calendula has been reported to have antibacterial and antiviral activity. Calendula extracts made from various parts of the plant have been used in attempts to inhibit and destroy tumor cells and have been shown to possess cancer cell toxicity properties in vitro and antitumor activity in vivo (tests using live specimens). These actions appear not to be parallel, since the saponin-rich extract that exerted the most pronounced antitumor activity showed only weak potential for cell toxicity.

A related species, *Calendula arvensis* L., has been shown to destroy mollusks and is thought to be potentially useful in killing the snail vector that causes schistosomiasis.

Internal Uses

Calendula has traditionally been used in the management of indigestion and in the treatment of gastritis and other situations of digestive irritation. Calendula is also thought to stimulate blood flow to the pelvis and uterus, and is used in the treatment of delayed menstruation and dysmenorrhea (painful periods). However, no scientific evidence could be found to support these claims.

> *Calendula has traditionally been used in the management of indigestion and in the treatment of gastritis and other situations of digestive irritation.*

Adverse Effects

One study documents allergic responses, normally manifested as contact dermatitis, to members of the Asteraceae (or Compositae) family, including calendula. This is probably more likely to occur with topical products containing calendula than with those that are ingested as oral supplements.

Cautions/Contraindications

While no instances of allergic reactions could be found, it should be noted that other members of the Asteraceae family (e.g., German chamomile, feverfew) have been shown to have allergic potential. Calendula should be used with caution in pregnancy, due to a reputed action on the menstrual cycle.

Drug Interactions

No drug interactions have been reported in humans. Animal studies have indicated that calendula may have a sedative action and may reduce blood pressure. Because of the risk of additive effects, caution should be taken when consuming medications that also have these properties. Calendula may enhance the effect of medications that lower blood sugar and cholesterol. Calendula has also been noted to extend the duration of action of hexobarbitol in rats. The implications of these animal study findings for humans is not known.

Dosage Regimens

Internal

- Dried florets: 1–4 g (infusion) three times daily.
- Liquid extract (1:1 in 40% alcohol): 0.5–1.0 mL three times daily.
- Tincture (1:5 in 90% alcohol): 0.3–1.2 mL three times daily.

External

- 5–10 mL dried florets steeped in 240 mL boiling water for 10 minutes and allowed to cool; can be used as a gargle or to treat skin conditions.

Formulas

- Calendula is often combined with other wound-healing herbs, such as *Symphytum officinale* L., Boraginaceae (Comfrey), *Matricaria recutita* L., Asteraceae (German chamomile) or *Echinacea* spp., Asteaceae (Coneflower). It may also be used in combination with phytomedicines with a reported antimicrobial action, such as *Hydrastis canadensis* L., Ranunculaceae (Goldenseal).

Selected References

Basch E, Bent S, Foppa I, Haskmi S, Kroll D, Mele M, Szapary P, Ulbricht C, Vora M, Yong S. Marigold (*Calendula officinalis* L.): An evidence-based systematic review by the Natural Standard Research Collaboration. Journal of Herbal Pharmacotherapy 2006;6(3/4):135–59.

Duran V, Matic M, Jovanovc M, Mimica N, Gajinov Z, Poljacki M, Boza P. Results of the clinical examination of an ointment with marigold (*Calendula officinalis*) extract in the treatment of venous leg ulcers. International Journal of Tissue Reaction 2005;27(3):101–6.

Pommier P, Gomez F, Sunyach MP, D'Hombres A, Carrie C, Montbarbon X. Phase III randomized trial of *Calendula officinalis* compared with trolamine for the prevention of acute dermatitis during irradiation for breast cancer. Journal of Clinical Oncology 2004;22(8):1447–53.

Capsicum

Capsicum annuum L.

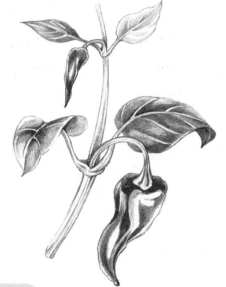

Introduction

Family
- Solanaceae

Synonyms
- Chile pepper
- Chili pepper
- Red pepper
- Cayenne pepper
- Tobasco pepper
- Hot pepper

Medicinal Forms
- Dried herb (fruit and seeds)
- Tincture
- Cream and ointment

Description

Recognized worldwide for its pungency, capsicum may have been cultivated as early as 7000 BC in Mexico and Peru. This perennial shrub grows to 1 meter (3 feet) in height, with bright red oblong fruit approximately 10 centimeters (4 inches) long, filled with white seeds. While there are more than 50 species of capsicum, the common sweet red, green, yellow, and orange peppers, as well as paprika and numerous types of chili peppers, are now all considered varieties of the same species.

Parts Used

The dried fruit and seeds are used medicinally.

Traditional Use

Capsicum is one the oldest and most widely used spices in the world. One author estimates that approximately 25% of the world's population uses capsicum on a daily basis. The spice itself has enjoyed a long history in many healing disciplines. Historically, it was used as a stimulant to the whole body and was thought to aid digestion, the nervous system and circulation. During the early part of the last century, it was a key herbal remedy used by the Thomsonian practitioners of North America. Within this "heroic" school of medicine, the aim was to stimulate the "vital energy" and expel pathogenic factors by inducing a "therapeutic" fever. In addition, capsaicin, the main active ingredient in capsicum, has been used for a variety of medicinal purposes, most often pain relief. Hot red peppers also have many culinary uses.

Current Medicinal Use

While capsicum is used for a number of conditions, its most common current use is topically for diabetic neuropathy, postherpetic neuralgia (nerve damage arising after shingles), and other painful conditions, such as rheumatoid and osteoarthritis. There are a number of excellent reviews on capsicum.

Relevant Research

Preventative and Therapeutic Effects

Constituents
- Capsaicinoids: capsaicin, dihydrocapsaicin, nordihydrocapsaicin, homocapsaicin, homodihydrocapsaicin.
- Carotenoids: lutein, carotein, capsanthin.
- Vitamins: A and C.

Notes: The nomenclature associated with capsicum is somewhat confusing. Capsicum is generally defined as the dried, ripe fruit of

Capsicum annuum L. and a large number of varieties and hybrids of this. In contrast, capsaicin is a compound purified from these species — chemical abstracts (CAS) registry 404-86-4, under the name N-[(4-hydroxy-3-methoxyphenyl)-methyl]-8-methyl-(E)-6-nonenamide. There are two possible stereoisomers of capsaicin, but only the *trans* isomer exists in nature. The *cis* isomer, civamide, is assigned a separate CAS registry number. To complicate matters even further, a third compound, often called synthetic capsaicin, has been synthesized and is often found as an adulterant in products labeled capsaicin. Synthetic capsaicin does not have the same chemical formula as either capsaicin or civamide and should not be used in their place. The official name of this adulterant is nonivamide, but it has also been called pelargonic acid vanillylamide. Nonivamide has never been found in capsicum fruit extracts. Because of widespread misrepresentation and adulteration of capsaicin products with nonivamide, efficient analytic systems have now been developed to unambiguously distinguish between the two. The active constituents of capsicum are considered to be the capsaicinoids. Of these, capsaicin is by far the most important.

Analgesic Effects
Diabetic Neuropathy
The use of topical applications of capsaicin for the relief of diabetic neuropathy has been extensively studied. The formation of the Capsaicin Study Group has resulted in numerous high-quality clinical trials. Most studies have employed 0.075% topical capsaicin in a cream base and have concluded that capsaicin is a safe and effective treatment for painful diabetic neuropathy. For example, one 8-week, double-blind, vehicle-controlled study of 0.075% capsaicin cream (Axsain) applied four times daily by 54 patients with moderate to severe diabetic neuropathy showed symptom improvement in 90% of capsaicin-treated patients, which was significantly better than the control group. A variety of other trials using the same protocol (0.075% capsaicin cream applied four times daily) have confirmed that 0.075% capsaicin cream was more effective than a vehicle control. This literature review found only one published negative trial with capsaicin.

> *The use of topical applications of capsaicin for the relief of diabetic neuropathy has been extensively studied.*

Post-Herpetic Neuralgia
A lower strength (0.025%) of capsaicin is used for the treatment of post-herpetic neuralgia (nerve damage arising after shingles) than for diabetic neuropathy (0.075%). In an uncontrolled study of 33 patients, 55% of the patients completing the study reported good or excellent pain relief; however, burning sensations after the application of capsaicin was so severe in one-third of the patients that the trial was discontinued prematurely. A large, open-label uncontrolled trial involving 208 patients concluded that topical capsaicin was a promising treatment for post-herpetic neuralgia. This supports the conclusions of several earlier studies. However, the percentage of patients with substantial pain relief varied from 39% to 75%. This variation may be due to different treatment schedules: one study used capsaicin 0.025% four times daily, while another study asked patients to apply capsaicin 0.025% five times daily for 1 week, followed by three times daily for an additional 3 weeks. Yet another study using a 5 times daily treatment regimen, but a 0.001% capsaicin cream, reported moderate pain relief in 62% of patients with post-herpetic neuralgia.

In addition, a case report suggests that the use of topical capsaicin (0.025% — Zostrix) in the mouth may be an effective treatment for post-herpetic vesicles in the oral cavity. One episode of xerostomia (dry mouth) forced the discontinuation of therapy for 1 day only. The signature burning sensation of capsaicin makes it very difficult to maintain a blinded trial; thus, to date, these findings have not been confirmed by a randomized, double-blind, controlled trial.

Miscellaneous Pain Indications

Capsaicin cream has reportedly been effective in the treatment of postmastectomy pain syndrome, rheumatoid arthritis, osteoarthritis, cluster headaches, reflex sympathetic dystrophy, relief of local stump pain, idiopathic trigeminal neuralgia, relief of sores of oral mucositis caused by chemotherapy or radiation, pain caused by Guillain-Barré syndrome, and painful psoriasis vulgaris. Capsicum plasters applied topically were found to relieve non-specific low back pain and, when applied at the Korean hand acupuncture point (K-D2) or the Chinese acupuncture point pericardium 6 (P6), or stomach 36 (St36), were found to reduce postoperative need for painkillers, as well as nausea and vomiting after abdominal hysterectomy. When applied to the Chinese acupuncture point stomach 36 (St36), capsaicin plaster was also seen to relieve postoperative pain after 6 hours in children who had undergone inguinal hernia repair surgery.

Pain Mediation

Capsaicin depletes substance P (SP), which mediates pain transmission from the peripheral nerves to the spinal cord. It does this via four stages: (1) SP is immediately released from both central and peripheral terminals; (2) SP fibers are functionally impaired; (3) the axoplasmic transport of SP is inhibited; and (4) SP is depleted (this starts after 1 day and may last for weeks). Although generally believed to be specific for type C nociceptive neurons (i.e., unmyelinated, slow-conducting fibers that transmit cutaneous pain information to the central nervous system), other research suggests that capsaicin causes damage to all unmyelinated sensory fibers. Myelinated fibers of the A delta category may also be damaged with high doses of capsaicin.

It has been suggested that capsaicin may be a useful neurochemical tool for research into the interaction of sensory neurons with other neuronal systems. Excellent reviews of capsaicin's action on a variety of systems, including the gastrointestinal, thermoregulatory, cardiovascular, respiratory, and nervous systems, have been published.

> *Excellent reviews of capsaicin's action on a variety of systems, including the gastrointestinal, thermoregulatory, cardiovascular, respiratory, and nervous systems, have been published.*

Miscellaneous Effects

One randomized controlled study demonstrated that the maximum tolerable oral dose of red pepper (capsicum) decreased energy intake and fat absorption in 16 male Japanese subjects. The red pepper was given in the form of a soup before a meal, and a dose-dependent effect was seen with different concentrations of red pepper in the soup. Oral administration of capsicum has also been shown to inhibit the rise of cholesterol in the liver and increase the fecal excretion of both cholesterol and bile acids in rats. Administration of capsaicin did not effect serum levels of cholesterol; however, it did appear to stimulate lipid mobilization from adipose tissue, and it lowered the serum triglyceride concentration in lard-fed rats.

A randomized, placebo-controlled, double-blind study involving 30 people found that ingestion of red pepper powder obtained by grinding the dried fruit of *Capsicum annuum* was more effective than a placebo in decreasing the intensity of dyspeptic symptoms. Participants in the study were asked to take capsules of the study drug 15 minutes before each meal, 1 capsule (500 mg) before breakfast, 2 capsules before lunch and 2 capsules before dinner for 5 weeks. Overall symptom scores, as well as epigastric pain, fullness, and nausea scores, of the red pepper group were significantly lower than the scores from the placebo group starting from the third week of treatment.

It has also been suggested that capsaicin may be useful in cancer treatment. A study using animal models has demonstrated that varying concentrations of capsaicin inhibit new blood vessel formation in a dose-dependent manner. This may be useful in the treatment of cancerous growths that depend on the growth of new blood vessels to spread, such as tumors. Further research into this application is needed.

Adverse Effects
Capsicum
Topical: Allergic contact dermatitis has been reported.

Internal: Sweating, generally confined to the head and neck; flushing of the face and upper body; salivation; watering of the eyes; nasal secretion. In addition, the principle agents in capsicum can be very irritating to the mucosal membranes, and these effects are used in the self-defense product commonly known as pepper spray. A toxicity study of chronic administration of capsicum extract to hamsters reported decreased vitamin A levels in liver tissue and eye toxicity, including a focal increase in corneal epithelial cells and hyalinisation and thickening of the substantia propria in the eyeballs. One report has described deep corneal and conjunctiva damage in 4 patients after exposure to pepper spray. In Canada, possession of pepper spray is prohibited for the general public. Other effects that have been reported in humans include increased fibrinolytic activity and decreased coagulation of blood. However, these effects have been reported after ingestion of capsicum in the diet, as opposed to medicinal effects.

Capsaicin
Topical: Erythema; burning and stinging sensations (no vesication) common at both the 0.025% and 0.075% concentrations when applied topically, but the intensity is diminished for most patients with continued use (i.e., after 2 weeks); some dry skin. Also, inhalation reactions, such as coughing and sneezing, occurred occasionally. Capsaicin is generally considered to be safe. No changes in cutaneous sensation of temperature or vibration were noted after administration of 0.075% capsaicin four times daily for up to 32 weeks continuously.

Internal: Increased gastric acid concentration is possible; however, two other studies found no increase in gastric acid secretion. In vitro experiments suggest that capsaicin is a potent inhibitor of platelet aggregation. Ingestion of large doses has been associated with necrosis, ulceration, and even carcinogenesis; however, small amounts appear to have few deleterious effects.

Cautions/Contraindications
Topical: Known allergy.

Internal: Contraindicated in cases of severe hypertension, and caution should be used in situations of acute gastric irritation. During pregnancy, capsicum should not be used at doses exceeding normal dietary levels. It has been shown that ingesting red pepper after anal fissure surgery can increase postoperative symptoms of pain, anal burning, and itching. There is no known risk associated with the occasional consumption of spicy peppers in individuals with hemorrhoids. Although not used medicinally, the leaves and stems of capsicum have been shown to be uterine stimulants in animal studies. In addition, due to capsicum's pungency, caution is recommended while breastfeeding.

Drug Interactions

No specific drug interactions appear to have been reported in the literature; however, since high doses of capsicum have been shown to increase the activity of two liver enzymes in rats (glucose-6-phosphate dehydrogenase and adipose lipoprotein lipase), the liver metabolism of some drugs may be affected. In addition, since catecholamine amine secretion is increased, caution is suggested with concomitant use of monoamine oxidase inhibitors (MAOIs) and antihypertensives.

Selected References

Dailey GE. Effect of treatment with capsaicin on daily activities of patients with diabetic neuropathy. Diabetes Care 1992;15(2):159–65.

Donofrio PD, Walker F, Hunt V, Tandan R, Fries T, Lewis G, et al. Treatment of painful diabetic neuropathy with topical capsaicin: A multicentre, double-blind, vehicle-controlled study. Archives of Internal Medicine 1991; 151:2225–29.

Tandan R, Lewis GA, Krusinski PB, Badger GB, Fries TJ. Topical capsaicin in painful diabetic neuropathy: Controlled study with long-term follow-up. Diabetes Care 1992;15(1):8–14.

Dosage Regimens

External

- Diabetic neuropathy: 0.075% capsaicin cream or ointment applied four times daily.
- Post-herpetic neuralgia: 0.025% capsaicin cream or ointment applied four times daily.

Internal

- Dried fruit: 30–120 mg three times daily.
- Capsicum tincture (BPC 1986): 0.3–1.0 mL daily.

Note: Capsicum is found in a variety of commercial external analgesic preparations, including Heet lotion, Infra-Rub ointment, Sloan's Liniment, Zostrix, Zostrix-HP, and Axsain.

Cat's Claw

Uncaria tomentosa
(Willd. Ex Roem. & Schult) DC *or*
Uncaria guianensis (Aubl.) J.F. Gmel.

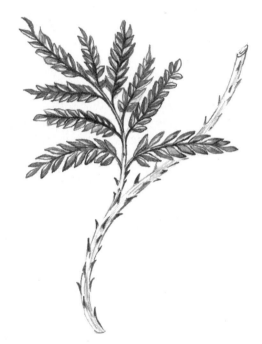

THUMBNAIL SKETCH

Common Uses
- Arthritis and other inflammatory conditions

Active Constituents
- Oxindole alkaloids
- Glycosides

Adverse Effects
- None noted

Cautions/Contraindications
- Pregnancy and breastfeeding

Drug Interactions
- None documented in humans
- Anticoagulants (theoretical)
- Immunostimmulants (theoretical)

Doses
- No established protocols were found. Products commonly available on the Canadian market contain 200–300 mg of concentrated extract of *U. tomentosa* bark standardized for oxindole alkaloid and polyphenol content.

Introduction

Family
- Rubiaceae

Synonyms
- Uña de gato
- Garabato
- Paraguayo

Medicinal Forms
- Dried bark and root (capsules, tablets, and teas)
- Tinctures

Description

Members of the genus *Uncaria* are found throughout tropical forests in Asia, Africa, South America, and Central America. The common name "cat's claw" comes from the curved thorns, or "hooks," used by the plant to fasten itself onto supporting plants. The species found in South America are woody climbing vines growing up to 30 meters (100 feet). While many South American plants are referred to as uña de gato, or cat's claw, the species *Uncaria tomentosa* (Willd. Ex Roem. & Schult) DC or *Uncaria guianensis* (Aubl.) J.F. Gmel. are the ones primarily used medicinally. These species are often considered to have identical therapeutic indications. They are also very similar in appearance, with only slight differences in the presentation of the leaves and the hooks. Since most cat's claw supplements available in North America appear to be made from *Uncaria tomentosa*, the following discussion will be limited primarily to this species.

Parts Used

The parts used medicinally are the root or the dried inner bark of the stem. It takes from 3 to 8 years for plants to reach a suitable size to harvest.

Traditional Use

Cat's claw has long been used by the indigenous peoples of South America to treat a wide range of ailments and diseases, including asthma, urinary tract infections, arthritis, and other inflammatory conditions. The herb has recently gained popularity in North America and Europe. Given this increase in demand, ecological concerns have been raised with regard to the sustainability of the crop. The Peruvian government has recently invested in an extensive planting campaign. Some consider that uña de gato may offer an alternative — and more suitable — crop to the illegal cultivation of coca.

Current Medicinal Use

There are very few human clinical studies of cat's claw. The current medicinal uses are very similar to the traditional uses, focusing primarily on its purported anti-inflammatory and immunostimulatory properties.

Relevant Research

Preventative and Therapeutic Effects

Constituents

- Oxindole alkaloids: include uncarine F, isopteropodine, pteropodine, isorhynchophylline, rhynchophylline, mitraphylline.
- Quinovic acid glycosides.
- Triterpenes: include oleanolic acid.
- Polyphenols: include catechins, rutin, quercetin.
- Miscellaneous: tannins.

Note: The alkaloid content of plants appears to vary appreciably from one year to the next.

Common Uses

Uncaria tomentosa has traditionally been used in the management of many conditions, notably rheumatism, peptic ulcers, intestinal disorders, certain cancers, asthma, inflammatory conditions, and menstrual irregularities. North American practitioners and patients have noted relief in cases of diverticulitis, diabetes, gastritis, colic, and leaky bowel syndrome.

Anti-inflammatory Effects

Although it has been suggested that cat's claw may be helpful for inflammatory conditions, such as arthritis, the majority of the evidence to date is limited to animal and in vitro studies. Three clinical trials have been published to date.

One randomized, double-blind, placebo-controlled clinical trial assessed the use of cat's claw in 40 patients with active rheumatoid arthritis who were already taking the conventional medicines sulfasalazine or hydroxychlorquine. After taking cat's claw for 24 weeks, the number of painful joints identified in the cat's claw group was significantly lower than in the placebo group. The second randomized, double-blind, placebo-controlled study included 45 people with osteoarthritis of the knee. After 4 weeks of treatment, those

in the cat's claw group, who were taking a freeze-dried extract of *Unicaria guinensis*, reported decreased pain. A third clinical trial reported that a natural herb-mineral combination containing cat's claw improved joint health and function with 1 to 2 weeks of treatment, but significant effects compared to a placebo were not sustained. Given that this was a combination product, it is not clear if any of these reported effects can be attributed to cat's claw. Additional clinical studies are needed to confirm these positive preliminary findings.

Many animal and in vitro studies have investigated the anti-inflammatory effects of cat's claw. This anti-inflammatory action could be due to agents with "intrinsic anti-inflammatory effect" or to the existence of a synergy between multiple constituents. It has been suggested that the mechanism of action is that cat's claw inhibits tumor necrosis factor-alpha (TNF-alpha) and exhibits anti-oxidant properties. It has also been suggested that cat's claw may limit cartilage degradation by suppressing catabolic processes and activating local IGF-1 anabolic pathways.

> *Although it has been suggested that cat's claw may be helpful for inflammatory conditions, such as arthritis, the majority of the evidence to date is limited to animal and in vitro studies.*

Miscellaneous Effects

Effects on the Immune System

A number of compounds extracted from cat's claw have been reported to have immunomodulatory properties. It appears to increase phagocytosis of human granulocytes and macrophages; stimulate the production of macrophages, interleukin-1 and interleukin-6; and suppress TNF-alpha.

Cancer Preventative Effects

A number of animal and in vitro studies have documented antitumor activity associated with cat's claw. Effects against leukemia cells have been noted in a number of studies.

Antiviral Effects

Glycosides extracted from the bark of *Uncaria tomentosa* have also been shown to possess antiviral properties. In a review article, a 6-year trial of 14 HIV-positive patients was described, in which administration of a "standardized cat's claw root extract rich in alkaloids" increased T helper cell counts and delayed or prevented the onset of symptoms.

Adverse Effects

Cat's claw appears to be generally well tolerated. Only one case of any adverse effects associated with cat's claw in humans has been reported. In this case, a patient with systemic lupus erythematosus who was taking a number of conventional medications developed acute renal (kidney) failure after taking cat's claw. Her symptoms improved when she discontinued the cat's claw.

Cautions/Contraindications

The safety of cat's claw products in pregnancy or lactation has not yet been established.

Drug Interactions

No cases of documented drug interactions could be found. However, a number of theoretical interactions are possible, including

- Anticoagulants and antiplatelet medications (e.g., warfarin and nonsteroidal anti-inflammatory medications, such as ibuprofen): Animal studies suggest compounds in cat's claw may increase the risk of bleeding by inhibiting platelet aggregation.

- Immunosuppressants, corticosteroids: Based on the animal and in vitro studies of cat's claw's immunostimulatory activity, it may theoretically decrease the effects of these drugs.

Dosage Regimens

- Little information could be found about the therapeutic dosage of *Uncaria tomentosa*. Products commonly available on the Canadian market contain 200–300 mg of concentrated extract of *U. tomentosa* bark, standardized for oxindole alkaloid and polyphenol content.

Selected References

Heitzman ME, Neto CC, Winiarz E, Vaisberg AJ, Hammond GB. Ethnobotany, phytochemistry and pharmacology of *Uncaria* (Rubiaceae). Phytochemistry 2005 Jan;66(1): 5–29.

Mur E, Hartig F, Eibl G, Schirmer M. Randomized double blind trial of an extract from the pentacyclic alkaloid-chemotype of *Uncaria tomentosa* for the treatment of rheumatoid arthritis. Journal of Rheumatology 2002; 29(4):678–81.

Piscoya J, Rodriguez Z, Bustamante SA, Okuhama NN, Miller MJ, Sandoval M. Efficacy and safety of freeze-dried cat's claw in osteoarthritis of the knee: Mechanisms of action of the species *Uncaria guianensis*. Inflammatory Research 2001;50(9):442–48.

Chamomile
(German)
Matricaria recutita L.

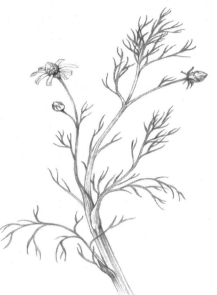

Common Uses
Internal
- Gastrointestinal discomfort, peptic ulcer, gastritis, indigestion, diarrhea
- Insomnia and anxiety (mild)
- Pediatric colic and teething

External
- Inflammatory skin conditions
- Canker sores and irritation of the gums and mouth

Active Constituents
- Volatile oil (chamazulene, (-)a-bisabolol, spiroethers)
- Apigenin and other flavonoids

Adverse Effects
- Contact dermatitis
- Vomiting (in very high doses)

Cautions/Contraindications
- Individuals with a known allergy to members of the sunflower (Compositae/Asteraceae) family

Drug Interactions
- None known

Doses
Internal
- *Dried flowers (usually as an infusion or tea):* 2–4 g three times daily
- *Liquid extract (1:1 in 45% ethanol):* 1–4 mL three times daily
- *Tincture (1:5 in 45% ethanol):* 3–10 mL three times daily

External
- Topical preparations are usually 3% to 10% chamomile by weight.

Introduction

Family
- Asteraceae (also known as Compositae)

Synonyms
- *Chamomile recutita*
- *Matricaria chamomilla* L.
- camomilla
- camomille Allemande
- chamomilla
- echte kamille
- feldkamille
- fleur de chamomile
- Hungarian chamomile
- Kamillen
- kleine kamille
- manzanilla
- matricaria
- matricariae flos
- pinheads
- single chamomile
- sweet false chamomile
- wild chamomile

Medicinal Forms
- Extract
- Tincture
- Solution
- Mouth spray
- Creams and ointments
- Dried flowers
- Tea bags

Description
German chamomile is one of two species of chamomile commonly used medicinally, the other being Roman or English chamomile (*Chamaemelum nobile* L. All.). The primary indications of both are similar, even though the constituents are slightly different. Outside the United Kingdom, German chamomile is the species that has been both evaluated most extensively and used therapeutically.

German chamomile is a relatively small, fragrant annual herb, 60 centimeters (16 inches) tall with a round, hollow stem and sharply cut leaves, native to most of Europe and western Asia and naturalized throughout North America. As a commercially viable crop, more than 4,000 tons of chamomile are produced annually, mainly in Eastern Europe, the Balkans, and parts of South America, and the bulk of this is German chamomile. Most of the cultivated crop is destined for Europe, especially Germany, rather than North America, where the herb has been relegated by the public to the role of a beverage.

Parts Used
The flowers, preferably picked a few days before opening, are the parts used medicinally.

Traditional Use
The fact that the Germans often refer to German chamomile as *alles zutraut*, meaning "capable of anything," gives some idea of the high regard in which this plant is held. Its panacea-like properties and numerous indications have led many people to refer to it, rather confusingly, as European ginseng. Chamomile tea has been used as a digestive, hypnotic, and antispasmodic, finding particular favor in the treatment of children's ailments. It should not be forgotten that chamomile helped Peter Rabbit get over a particularly overindulgent trip to Farmer McGregor's vegetable garden. It takes a brave skeptic to argue with evidence like that.

Current Medicinal Use
Components of this herb have been shown to have anti-anxiety, anti-inflammatory, antispasmodic, and antihistaminic properties. While what scientific evidence exists is promising, most of the supporting evidence for German chamomile comes from its traditional use. Based on this evidence, German chamomile is used to manage digestive upset (colic, indigestions, gastritis, diarrhea, peptic ulcer disease), mouth and skin irritations (insect bites, eczema, diaper rash), insomnia, and anxiety.

Relevant Research

Preventative and Therapeutic Uses

Constituents

Flowers

* Terpenoids: azulene, chamazulene, a-bisabolol, a-bisabololoxide A, B, C, matricin, farnesol.
* Flavonoids: apigenin, apiin, luteolin, quercetin, rutin.
* Coumarins: umbelliferone, herniarin.
* Miscellaneous: capric acid, polysaccharides, spiroethers, tannins.

Note: The yield of the medicinally important volatile oil fraction, rich in terpenoids and spiroethers, depends on both the age and locale of the plant. Matricin is converted to chamazulene in the extraction process. While standardization is not universal, German products are normally authenticated by measuring chamazulene and a-bisabolol content.

Gastrointestinal Effects

Historically, chamomile has been widely used as a digestive aid and carminative and in many gastrointestinal conditions, including the management of colic, indigestion, gastritis, diarrhea, and peptic ulcers. However, there is currently little scientific evidence to support its use in these conditions.

Diarrhea

One positive trial exists to support the use of a chamomile-based pectin product (Kamillosan) in the treatment of acute diarrhea. A double-blind, randomized control trial was conducted with 79 children aged 6 months to 5$\frac{1}{2}$ years who were diagnosed with acute non-complicated diarrhea. It found that children randomized to receive Diarrheosan (chamomile fluid extract plus apple pectin) had significantly reduced duration of diarrhea compared to those treated with a placebo.

Both groups received the same rehydration and diet. The results of this trial are limited, however, because it is difficult to establish which ingredient resulted in the beneficial effect of the product. Further research is required to determine if chamomile alone has any value in the treatment of acute non-complicated diarrhea.

Infantile Colic

There are currently two randomized controlled trials supporting the use of infusions (teas) that include chamomile in alleviating infantile colic. Because neither assessed the effect of chamomile alone, however, it is very difficult to determine the role of chamomile, if any, in the results described in the trials. Further research is necessary to assess the effect of chamomile on infantile colic.

One trial evaluated the effect of an herbal tea preparation on infantile colic in a prospective double-blind study involving 68 babies. The preparation contained extracts of *M. chamomilla*, vervain (*Verbena officinalis*), licorice (*Glycyrrhiza glabra*), fennel (*Foeniculum vulgare*), and lemon balm (*Melissa officinalis*). Parents were instructed to administer either 150 mL of the herbal tea or a placebo beverage at every colicky episode, for a week. The use of tea eliminated the colic in 19 (57%) of 33 infants, whereas the placebo was helpful in only 9 (26%) of 35 (p < 0.01). The mean colic score was significantly improved in tea-treated infants. No significant differences were noted in the number of night wakings in either group.

> *Further research is necessary to assess the effect of chamomile on infantile colic.*

In a second randomized, double-blind, placebo-controlled trial involving 88 babies, it was determined that a standardized herbal preparation (ColiMil) containing chamomile (71.1 mg/kg/day), fennel (65.7 mg/kg/day), and lemon balm (38.8 mg/kg/day) administered daily for 1 week reduced crying time among breastfed colicky infants compared with a placebo (p < 0.005).

Mouth and Gum Irritations

Three trials and a case report have studied the effects of a preparation containing German chamomile (Kamillosan) on conditions affecting the mouth or gums, with mixed results. Two of the trials looked specifically at the product's use as an oral rinse in the prevention and treatment of radiation- or chemotherapy-induced mucositis. The results of these two trials were contradictory. One randomized, placebo-controlled, double-blind trial (N=164) found chamomile mouthwash, in addition to cryotherapy, did not significantly reduce 5-fluorouracil (5-FU)-induced stomatitis (p = 0.32). This trial involved randomizing patients upon their first session of 5-FU. Patients received either chamomile (30 drops of extract in 100 mL) or a placebo mouthwash prior to their treatment and three times daily for 14 days. All patients also received oral cryotherapy (ice chips) for 30 minutes with each dose of 5-FU stomatitis, as graded by health-care providers and patients. A smaller, uncontrolled trial in a similar population of patients (N=96) found differing results: chamomile rinse was found to decrease stomatitis resulting from chemotherapy and radiation treatment. Finally, a double-blind German study found that chamomile extract had an astringent and cooling action in patients suffering from mouth or gum irritation.

There is no established mechanism of action to explain chamomile's use in the prevention and treatment of mouth or gum irritation. It is believed, however, that the sesquiterpene bisabolol constituents are responsible for chamomile's anti-inflammatory properties.

Other Uses

Insomnia and Anxiety

Despite the herb's reputation as a mild hypnotic, there are no human trials to support the use of chamomile as a sedative. The best scientific evidence to date for this indication comes from a study to determine the effects of chamomile tea on patients' hemodynamic parameters during ventricular catheterization procedures. Although the reserachers found virtually no change in their outcome of interest, they found that chamomile had a striking hypnotic effect. Ten of the 12 patients fell asleep after ingesting the tea and remained asleep throughout the catheterization procedure. Clearly this is an area where more research is needed.

There is in vitro evidence to support chamomile's use as a sedative. Apigenin, a chemical component of chamomile, was found to bind GABA receptors in vitro, which suggests a possible mechanism of action that may explain chamomile's reported sedative properties.

> *Despite the herb's reputation as a mild hypnotic, there are no human trials to support the use of chamomile as a sedative.*

Symptoms of the Common Cold

One randomized, placebo-controlled trial, with no mention of blinding, reported steam inhalation of German chamomile as resulting in a dose-dependent reduction in the severity of symptoms of the common cold. Sixty untreated outpatients with uncomplicated common colds were randomly assigned to one of four groups: a control group with a 35% alcoholic solution as the inhalation ingredient and three groups with increasing doses (13 mL, 26 mL, and 39 mL) of alcohol-based chamomile extract (Kneipp Kamillen-Konzentrat). Patients self-assessed the efficacy of the inhalation in alleviating their symptoms. The study found that upper and middle respiratory tract symptoms were relieved more than other cold symptoms. The onset of action was within 15 minutes, reaching a maximum effect at 30 to 120 minutes. More research in this area is needed. Steam inhalation is a widely accepted practice and could prove to be an effective and safe option for the symptomatic relief of cold symptoms.

Skin Irritations

Topical use of chamomile-based products for a variety of dermatological conditions is commonplace in Europe, especially Germany. One German study supports the use of Kamillosan, a proprietary product containing chamomile, specifically in the treatment of patients suffering from inflammatory dermatoses on their hands, forearms, and lower legs. In this comparative study, 161 patients who had initially been treated with 0.1% difluocortolone valerate were randomized to receive one of several treatments. Kamillosan was shown to be equally effective to 0.25% hydrocortisone and superior to 5% bufexamac and 0.75% fluocortin butyl ester.

While the exact mechanism of action is unknown, apigenin is implicated by its anti-inflammatory properties. Apigenin, a constituent of the essential oil of chamomile, was found to inhibit lipopolysaccharide (LPS)-induced IL-6 and/or TNF-alpha production, both in vitro and in rat models.

Wound Healing

One German randomized, placebo-controlled, double-blind trial (N=14) found chamomile extract to significantly decrease the size and healing time of weeping wounds. Patients included in the study had undergone dermabrasion of tattoos. Chamomile was found to have a statistically significant drying effect, which was thought to be the mechanism of action responsible for its beneficial effects in oozing wounds.

Adverse Effects
Skin Reactions

Several case reports of contact dermatitis and urticaria have been reported in humans. The majority of these reports are due to contact skin irritation after exposure to the fresh plant as opposed to ingestion of chamomile products. Allergic sensitivity is rare but possible. There is a documented case of a woman with recurrent facial dermatitis who tested positive for reactivity to German chamomile. She had been consuming chamomile tea frequently during the previous year. The consumption of the tea had immediately preceded at least some of the relapses of her facial eczema, sometimes accompanied by lip swelling. Upon total avoidance of chamomile tea for 4 months, she reported no further relapses.

Anaphylaxis

There is one documented case of fatal anaphylaxis (asphyxia, resulting in the death of a newborn the following day) during the administration of a chamomile-containing enema during labor. The enema contained glycerol and Kamillosan, and the 35-year-old woman had no previous history of allergic reaction. The case report analyzes the case and provides further information from immunological testing with chamomile components. The results highlight the potential hazard of allergenic proteins present in chamomile extracts. The authors suggest that chamomile-containing products should be appropriately labeled with such warnings.

Other cases of anaphylactic reactions have been reported, including a case of severe anaphylaxis after the ingestion of chamomile tea by an 8-year-old boy previously diagnosed

> *There have been several reports in the literature of suspected anaphylaxis associated with chamomile, but it is unclear whether German chamomile was the offending agent in many of these studies.*

with hay fever and bronchial asthma. The reaction occurred after his first exposure to chamomile tea, and further immunological testing suggested a type I IgE-mediated immunologic mechanism for the reaction. There have been several reports in the literature of suspected anaphylaxis associated with chamomile, but it is unclear whether German chamomile was the offending agent in many of these studies.

Conjunctivitis

Washing the eyes with chamomile tea is a folk remedy used to treat conjunctivitis and other ocular reactions. However, some cases of contact dermatitis following application have been reported. In one study, it was shown that conjunctivitis may be induced by washing the eyes with chamomile tea. It was determined that chamomile pollen was the allergen responsible for the reaction.

Cautions/Contraindications

Pregnancy and Lactation

German chamomile is commonly regarded as safe and is often used by pregnant women and lactating women for a variety of reasons, including topically for nipple care. Its reputation for safety is based largely on historical evidence, however. German chamomile's safety in pregnancy or lactation has not been established. German chamomile is historically believed to affect female menstrual cycles, as well as uterine stimulation, and to cause teratogenicity in animals when taken orally. Thus, it is not recommended for use in pregnancy. Other sources state that there are no specific contraindications for the use of chamomile in pregnancy or lactation. Clearly, more research is needed.

Sensitivity to Asteraceae

German chamomile is contraindicated in people with hypersensitivity to plants of the Asteraceae family (arnica, marigold, yarrow, ragweed, asters, chrysanthemums, echinacea), as cross-sensitivity is known to exist between members of this family (which is also known as Compositae). One study has shown a high degree of cross-reactivity between mugwort (*A. vulgaris*) and chamomile (*A. chamomila*). Twenty-four patients with asthma or rhinitis, sensitized primarily to *A. vulgaris*, were tested for sensitivity to chamomile via bronchial, conjunctival, and oral challenges. Sensitization to *A. vulgaris* seems to be a primary risk factor for adverse symptoms after ingesting chamomile infusions. Bronchial provocation tests also show chamomile pollen as a relevant inhalant allergen.

According to an English abstract, a study tested 30 adult patients suffering from atopic dermatitis with a mix of extracts from Asteraceae (or Compositae) plants, including chamomile (*Chamomilla recutita*). Among 9 Asteraceae-mix-sensitive patients, 5 were positive to chamomile. There appears to be a high risk for Asteraceae sensitivity among people with "extrinsic" atopic dermatitis. This is the first study to quantify such a relationship. Further research is needed.

Drug Interactions

Anticoagulants

A 70-year-old woman on warfarin therapy (4 mg 3 d/wk, 6 mg 4 d/wk) was admitted with a cough and difficulty sleeping, as well as bilateral pedal edema. She was diagnosed with an upper respiratory tract infection and sent home. Five days later, she returned with multiple internal hemorrhaging. She had been using 4 to 5 dollops a day of a chamomile-based cream on her legs to treat the edema. She had also been consuming 4 to 5 cups of chamomile tea to soothe her throat. German chamomile contains coumarin or coumarin derivatives, which have been shown in vitro to increase bleeding time. The potentiation of warfarin's pharmacologic activity has been identified as a potential risk. Patients taking German chamomile and warfarin concurrently should be educated about the potential for increased bleeding and should be closely monitored.

Drugs Metabolized by Cytochrome P450 CYP1A2 and CYP3A4

German chamomile extract has been shown in vitro to inhibit the cytochrome P450 system, especially CYP1A2 and CYP3A4. However, there is no documented evidence of this effect in humans. Patients taking German chamomile and other drugs metabolized by these cytochrome systems should be educated about the potential for a drug interaction and should be monitored closely by their health-care team.

Sedatives (Benzodiazepines)

Theoretically, the concurrent use of chamomile with conventional sedatives may result in an additive effect. There is in vitro evidence to support chamomile's use as a sedative. Apigenin, a chemical component of chamomile, was found to bind GABA receptors in vitro and is thus thought to be responsible for chamomile's sedative properties. It is theoretically possible that chamomile may potentiate the effects of other sedating drugs, especially those that share the same mechanism of action, such as benzodiazepines.

> *It is theoretically possible that chamomile may potentiate the effects of other sedating drugs, especially those that share the same mechanism of action, such as benzodiazepines.*

Selected References

Fidler P, Loprinzi C, O'Fallon J, et al. Prospective evaluation of a chamomile mouthwash for prevention of 5-FU-induced oral mucositis. Cancer 1996;77(3):522–25.

Saller R, Beschorner M, Hellenbrecht D, Buhring M. Dose-dependency of symptomatic relief of complaints by chamomile steam inhalation in patients with common cold. European Journal of Pharmacology 1990; 183:728–29.

Segal R, Pilote L. Warfarin interaction with *Matricaria chamomilla*. Canadian Medical Association Journal 2006;174(9):1281–82.

Dosage Regimens

Internal

- Dried flower heads: 2–4 g three times daily.
- Liquid extract (1:1 in 45% ethanol): 1–4 mL three times daily.
- Tincture (1:5 in 45% ethanol): 3–10 mL three times daily.

External

- Topical preparations are usually 3% to 10% chamomile by weight.

Infusion

- An infusion is the most popular dosage form. Since a large proportion of the medicinally active components are contained in the volatile oil, it is important to cover the container while making the infusion.

  Pour hot water (150 mL) over a heaped tablespoonful (approximately 3 g) of German chamomile flowers, cover, and after 5 to 10 minutes pass through a tea strainer. Unless otherwise prescribed for gastrointestinal complaints, a cup of the freshly prepared tea is drunk three or four times a day between meals. For inflammation of the mucous membranes of the mouth and throat, use the freshly prepared tea as a wash or gargle.

Children

- German chamomile is reputed to be very safe and is often used in children; however, there is no evidence to support or refute these claims. Further research is required before doses in children can be recommended.

Chaste Tree

Vitex agnus-castus L.

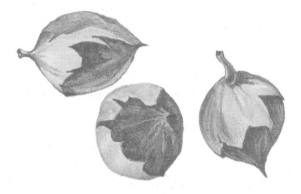

THUMBNAIL SKETCH

Common Uses
- Premenstrual syndrome and menopause symptoms
- Menstrual cycle irregularities
- Mastodynia (breast pain)
- Insufficient lactation and hyperprolactinemia (elevated prolactin levels)
- Acne resulting from a hormonal imbalance

Active Constituents
- The action of chaste tree appears to be determined by a number of different constituents. The iridoid agnuside is often used as a marker molecule to confirm authenticity.

Adverse Effects
- Nausea (rare)
- Headache
- Menstrual irregularities
- Diarrhea
- Dyspepsia
- Acne
- Pruritus

Cautions/Contraindications
- Pregnancy
- Children

Drug Interactions
- Oral contraceptives
- Hormone replacement therapy
- Interaction (theoretical) with dopamine antagonists, such as haloperidol and metoclopramide

Doses
- *Extract standardized for fruit content (9 g/100 mL):* 40 drops daily
- *Dried fruit:* 0.5–1 g three times daily
- *Tincture:* 0.2–0.4 mL (1:2) or 3–10 mL (1:5) daily

Note: Chaste tree may not have an immediate action. Treatment should be uninterrupted and last for several months for most indications.

Introduction

Family
- Verbenaceae

Synonyms
- Chasteberry
- Agnus-castus
- Monk's pepper

Medicinal Forms
- Dried fruit (berries)
- Standardized extract
- Tincture

Description
Chaste tree is a deciduous, aromatic shrub native to Mediterranean Europe, central Asia, and parts of India but now widely cultivated in subtropical regions. The chaste tree grows to 6 to 7 meters (20 to 25 feet) and has palm-shaped leaves. Small, lilac-like flowers grow in whorls on long spikes and produce purple, peppercorn-shaped berries.

Parts Used
The distinctive purple berries are the parts used medicinally.

Traditional Use
Chaste tree has been used since the time of Ancient Greece and Rome, where it played a part in religious ceremonies and medicinal practice. It was reputed to decrease libido in women and was used to "secure" chastity. Wives of Roman legionnaires spread the aromatic leaves of the chaste tree on their beds while their husbands were at war. The herb was included in monks' diets (hence the popular name "monk's pepper"), planted liberally in the grounds of many Catholic monasteries, and worn in clothing to promote celibacy. Chaste tree has long been considered of particular importance in women's health care, including symptoms of menopause, menstrual problems, breastfeeding problems, and infertility.

Current Medicinal Use
While more research is needed, a growing amount of scientific evidence supports the use of this herb in women's health issues. Chaste tree berry is primarily used for the unpleasant consequences of menses and menopause (premenstrual syndrome, mastodynia, dysmenorrhea) due to its amphoteric, or balancing, quality. It is considered one of the major galactagogues, or agents for increasing lactation in nursing mothers. Chaste tree berry may also be effective in managing cases of acne caused by hormonal imbalance and in promoting fertility.

Relevant Research

Preventative and Therapeutic Effects

Constituents
- Flavonoids: isovitexin, orientin, castican, chrysophanol D.
- Iridoids: aucubin, agnuside, eurostide.
- Volatile oil: a mixture of monoterpenes and sesquiterpenes, including cineol, limonene, and pinene.
- Essential fatty acids: linoleic acid.
- Miscellaneous: vitamin C, carotenes, castine (a bitter principle).

Note: An extract of the whole plant, rather than one constituent in particular, is considered medicinally active. The flavonoid agnuside is often used as a reference constituent as a measure of authenticity. Ketosteroids with a structure similar to sex hormones have been isolated from the leaves and flowers. The clinical relevance of this is unknown, since these plant parts are rarely used medicinally.

Women's Health Care

Chaste tree has been reported to be useful in the management of many female conditions, including premenstrual syndrome, mastodynia, premenstrual acne, menopause, insufficient lactation in nursing mothers, and ailments resulting from corpus luteum insufficiency.

Premenstrual Syndrome

Several clinical trials have reported that chaste tree may provide symptomatic relief for women suffering from premenstrual syndrome (PMS). Although most of the studies suggest that chaste tree may be helpful for PMS symptoms, most studies used an open-label design. Since the women knew they were receiving chaste tree, it is possible that the studies are simply reporting an expectancy, or placebo, effect. Thus, further trials using a randomized, double-blind design are needed to confirm the positive preliminary findings, which are discussed in more detail below.

One randomized, double-blind, placebo-controlled study involving 178 participants found that women ingesting chaste tree (extract Ze 440, 1 tablet daily for three menstrual cycles) had an improved rating of their irritability, mood alteration, anger, headache, and breast fullness compared to those in the placebo group. These findings confirmed those of an earlier multi-center, open-label trial involving 50 women of the same chaste tree extract. This study reported a significant reduction in PMS symptoms over the eight menstrual cycles that the women ingested chaste tree (Extract Ze 440) daily as assessed by the validated Moos Menstrual Distress Questionnaire. Similarly, a study of 36 women diagnosed with PMS found a generalized improvement in both physical and psychological symptoms at a dose of 40 drops of a proprietary brand of chaste tree tincture (Agnolyt) daily over 3 months.

> *Several clinical trials have reported that chaste tree may provide symptomatic relief for women suffering from premenstrual syndrome (PMS).*

Normalization in the luteal phase was also noted. This is supported by an uncontrolled observational study including 1,542 women with a mean age of 34.7 years diagnosed with PMS in which Agnolyt was shown to be useful. Results were based on patient and physician assessment. A majority of patients noted either complete relief or improvement in their symptoms. These favorable results were supported by the physician assessment (71% very good; 21% satisfactory). The dose given was 40 drops daily, with improvement seen after 25 days.

Two studies specifically looked at the effects of chaste tree among women with more severe types of PMS symptoms. One open-label, uncontrolled study investigated the treatment of moderate to severe PMS in 109 women treated with chaste tree tablets (4 mg dried ethanolic VAC BNO 1095 extract, 1 tablet daily) for three menstrual cycles. Comparison of before and after symptom assessment diaries showed that 68% of the women experienced a response after three menstrual cycles, and the authors concluded that this is a useful treatment for moderate to severe PMS, with good tolerability and safety.

Another study has suggested that chaste tree may be useful in treating premenstrual dysphoric disorder (a severe form of PMS). This double-blind trial involved 41 women randomized to receive either fluoxetine (a selective serotonin reuptake inhibitor used to treat premenstrual dysphoric disorder) or chaste tree extract for 2 months. The dose of treatment medication was 20 to 40 mg daily for both groups. The results showed that treatment with chaste tree extract decreased five mainly physical symptoms associated with premenstrual dysphoric disorder, compared with the seven mainly psychological symptoms that were relieved with fluoxetine treatment. The authors concluded that both treatments were well tolerated and appear to be promising in the management of premenstrual dysphoric disorder.

Other Menstrual Disorders

Many studies have indicated that chaste tree may prove useful in several menstrual situations: abnormal menstrual cycle, including normalization of menstrual flow in women suffering from irregular, frequent menstruation; heavy menstruation; pregnancies in cases of long-standing primary and secondary infertility; progesterone levels in women suffering from compromised corpus luteum function; and secondary amenorrhea (absence of menstruation after a woman has had her first period). However, most were observational studies that did not have control groups and did not blind the participants. More studies that are randomized and double-blinded are needed to confirm the preliminary positive findings discussed in detail below.

One study demonstrated in an uncontrolled observational study of 2,447 women presenting with a variety of menstrual disorders (including heavy menstruation, weak menstruation, irregular menstruation, and dysmenorrhea) that a chaste tree tincture (42 drops daily, mean duration of treatment of 153 days) was therapeutically effective. Both patients and physicians noted an appreciable improvement in symptoms. Instances of multiple diagnoses and concurrent drug use were noted but not controlled for. These favorable findings are supported by a multi-center trial in 1,571 women presenting with menstrual disorders. At a dose of 40 drops of Agnolyt daily, with a mean treatment time of 135 days, improvement was noted in 89.1% of cases.

A randomized, double-blind, placebo-controlled trial involving 97 women using another chaste tree product, Mastodynon (30 drops twice daily for three menstrual cycles), suggested that this product may decrease the intensity of pain experienced by women with cyclical mastalgia (breast pain). A significant difference between the chaste tree and the placebo group was noted after one and two menstrual cycles, but the results were not quite statistically significant after three cycles. Another placebo-controlled trial assessing Mastodynon demonstrated a 74.5% improvement, as determined by the use of a "pain scale," in 55 women suffering from severe mastopathy with cyclic mastalgia. There was no statistically significant change in prolactin or progesterone levels.

> *One study demonstrated in an uncontrolled observational study of 2,447 women presenting with a variety of menstrual disorders (including heavy menstruation, weak menstruation, irregular menstruation, and dysmenorrhea) that a chaste tree tincture (42 drops daily, mean duration of treatment of 153 days) was therapeutically effective.*

Lactation

Chaste tree is a galactagogue (i.e., it increases production of milk in nursing mothers). Two studies have supported this indication. In practice, the onset of action takes several weeks, but the increase in production is marked.

Hyperprolactinemia

In a randomized, double-blind, placebo-controlled trial in 52 women suffering luteal phase defects due to latent hyperprolactinemia (high levels of the hormone prolactin in blood), a commercial brand of chaste tree, Strotan, given as 20 mg daily, was shown to be beneficial. Latent hyperprolactinemia was evaluated by monitoring prolactin levels 15 and 30 minutes after an IV injection of 200 mcg of thyroxin-releasing hormone (TRH). After 3 months, it was noted in the test group that prolactin levels were decreased, shortened luteal phases normalized, and progesterone deficits eliminated when compared to the placebo group. With the exception of a luteal rise in 17 beta-estradiol in the test group, all other hormonal parameters were unchanged.

Mechanism of Action

It has been suggested that the mechanism of action of chaste tree is centrally mediated, rather than a direct hormone-like action. It has been hypothesized that by acting at the level of the pituitary, it promotes LH (luteinizing hormone) and inhibits FSH (follicle stimulating hormone) release. This consequently results in an increase in progesterone levels at the expense of estrogen. Many practitioners have noted that chaste tree appears more progesteronal than estrogenic in nature. However, a study demonstrated that chaste tree did not influence FSH or LH, either basal levels or when stimulated by addition of luteinizing hormone-releasing hormone (LHRH).

Latent hyperprolactinemia has long been known to accompany many of the unpleasant symptoms of premenstrual syndrome, particularly mastalgia. It has been hypothesized that the medicinal action of chaste tree is primarily due to its action on prolactin levels. In vitro and in vivo experiments have shown that components of chaste tree inhibit secretion of prolactin. Further, this action is antagonized with administration of a dopamine antagonist (haloperidol), suggesting that constituents present in chaste tree bind directly to central dopamine receptors. It has also been noted that chaste tree contains an agent or agents with affinity for both the D1 and D2 receptors. It appears that the action of chaste tree on prolactin levels is not due to any cytotoxic (cell damaging) effects.

> *It has been hypothesized that the medicinal action of chaste tree is primarily due to its action on prolactin levels.*

While this goes some way toward explaining the therapeutic properties of chaste tree, a complete pharmacology is yet to be elucidated, and it is unlikely that its medicinal action is solely due to its influence on the dopaminergic system. A recent animal study examining the effects of chaste tree on premenstrual syndrome, for example, has confirmed that two extracts from this plant interact with mu-opiate receptors, which decrease pain sensation when activated.

Other studies suggest that whether chaste tree exerts an antagonistic or agonistic action on prolactin levels may be dependent on both basal levels and drug dose. In a recent trial performed in 20 healthy male subjects, it was demonstrated that at low doses an antagonistic quality was predominant, the reverse being seen at higher doses. It was also noted that there was a "smoothing out" effect (a decrease in the extent and frequency of prolactin concentration peaks and troughs) independent of the dose given. The authors make the assumption that this specific extract of chaste tree contained both antagonistic and agonistic constituents, possibly acting at different sites. It was also noted that the initial level of prolactin concentration affected the action of the extract tested. The unblinded nature of this study and the small number of participants should be noted. In addition, male subjects were selected because they tend to have more stable prolactin levels than women.

Miscellaneous Effects

Numerous instances of pregnancy were reported in the trials discussed above, including in women with established infertility. One randomized, placebo-controlled, double-blind clinical trial involving 96 women suggested that chaste tree (Mastodynon, 30 drops twice daily for 3 months) may be beneficial for women with sterility due to secondary amenorrhea and luteal insufficiency.

A number of uncontrolled studies have suggested that chaste tree may prove useful in the management of acne vulgaris of a hormonal etiology.

It has also been reported that chaste tree, either alone or combined with other herbal medicines, may prove useful in the management of the unpleasant consequences of menopause, notably fluid retention, hot flashes, anxiety, and depression.

> *Chaste tree, either alone or combined with other herbal medicines, may prove useful in the management of the unpleasant consequences of menopause, notably fluid retention, hot flashes, anxiety, and depression.*

Adverse Effects

Adverse effects seem to be quite rare with chaste tree. Situations of dry mouth, disturbed sleep, tachycardia, nausea, allergic skin reaction, vomiting, a sensation of epigastric pressure, confusion, giddiness, acne, pruritus, alopecia, erythema, and headache have been noted in some studies. Changes in menses, including increased flow and changes in cycle, have also been noted. One instance of multiple follicular development was described in a patient undergoing unstimulated in vitro fertilization treatment upon introduction of a herbal medicine containing chaste tree. Although no similar situations are reported in the literature, the author of the original article suggests caution in this application.

Cautions/Contraindications

Chaste tree should not be used in children or during pregnancy. Although it is reputed to stimulate milk production, concerns have been raised regarding its use for this purpose, given the lack of conclusive information. The use of this herb should also be avoided in individuals with hormone-sensitive tumors.

Drug Interactions

It is advisable not to use chaste tree with oral contraceptives or hormone replacement therapy. Chaste tree should also be used with caution in individuals taking dopamine antagonists, such as haloperidol and metoclopramide.

Dosage Regimens

- Dried fruit: 0.5–1 g three times daily.
- Tincture: 0.2–0.4 mL (1:2) or 3–10 mL (1:5) daily.
- Standardized extract: Many of the clinical trials mentioned above have been carried out using a commercial brand of alcohol-based tincture standardized for fruit content (9 g/100 mL of tincture) called Agnolyt. The suggested daily dose is 40 drops daily.

Note: Many authors note that chaste tree does not have an immediate action. Treatment should be uninterrupted and last for several months when used for most of the above indications. In certain situations, the duration of treatment should be appreciably longer (e.g., 5 to 7 months for anovulatory cycles and infertility and up to 18 months for secondary amenorrhea of more than 2 years).

Selected References

Atmaca M, Kumru S, Tezcan E. Fluoxetine versus *Vitex agnus-castus* extract in the treatment of premenstrual dysphoric disorder. Human Psychopharmacology 2003;18: 191–95.

Berger D, Schaffner W, Schrader E, Meier B, Brattstrom A. Efficacy of *Vitex agnus-castus* L. extract Ze 440 in patients with pre-menstrual syndrome (PMS). Archives of Gynecology and Obstetrics 2000;264(3):150–53.

Prilepskaya VN, Ledina AV, Tagiyeva AV, Revazova FS. *Vitex agnus-castus*: Successful treatment of moderate to severe premenstrual syndrome. Maturitas 2006;55(1):S55–S63.

Schellenberg R. Treatment for the premenstrual syndrome with agnus-castus fruit extract: Prospective, randomised, placebo-controlled study. British Medical Journal 2001;322(7279): 134–37.

Cranberry

Vaccinium macrocarpon Ait.

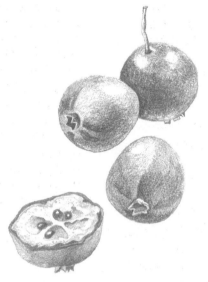

THUMBNAIL SKETCH

Common Uses
- Urinary tract infections (prevention)
- *H. Pylori* infection (suppression)

Active Constituents
- Fructose
- An unidentified large molecular weight compound

Adverse Effects
- None known

Cautions/Contraindications
- None known

Drug Interactions
- Warfarin

Doses
- *Cranberry juice:* 150–600 mL daily
- *Concentrated cranberry juice capsules:* 300–400 mg twice daily

Introduction

Family
- Ericaceae

Synonyms
- *Oxycoccus macrocarpus* Ait. Pursh

Medicinal Forms
- Juice
- Juice capsules

Description
Cranberry is a leathery-leaved evergreen bush with characteristic shiny red berries and pale pink flowers, native to the marshland of Northern Europe, Eastern Canada, and the eastern United States.

Parts Used
The ripe berries are the part of the plant used medicinally.

Traditional Use
Folk wisdom has long held that drinking cranberry juice will prevent urinary tract infections. Early clinical trials generally supported this claim; however, there were some negative findings and much controversy over the hypothesized mechanism of action. A recent large clinical trial aimed at ending the controversy found cranberry juice to be clinically effective in the prevention of urinary tract infections but has generated controversy of its own.

Current Medicinal Use
Cranberry is used primarily for the prevention of recurrent and uncomplicated urinary tract infections, though not as a treatment for acute infections.

Relevant Research

Preventative and Therapeutic Uses

Constituents
- Berries.
- Proanthocyanidins.
- Fructose.
- Flavonol glycosides: leptosine.
- Catechin.
- Triterpenoids.
- **Organic acids**: citric acid, malic acid, benzoic acid, quinic acid.
- **Miscellaneous**: vitamin C, unidentified large molecular weight molecule.

Urinary Tract Infections
Many early trials of the effectiveness of cranberry for the prevention or treatment of urinary tract infections involved small numbers of participants and were not blinded or controlled. Similar criticism may be made of relatively recent clinical trials that have suggested that cranberry juice may be useful for the prevention or treatment of urinary tract infections. Overall, there is significantly more evidence that cranberry may be useful for helping to prevent urinary tract infections than that it can help treat an active infection.

A 2008 systematic review evaluating the use of cranberry for prevention of urinary tract infections examined 10 studies that included a total of 1,049 participants. The authors of this review concluded that cranberry treatments are an effective method of preventing urinary tract infections in young women, that the evidence for this application in the elderly is inconclusive, and that the use of cranberry products in patients with neurogenic bladders is not effective. The four randomized controlled trials from this review that were selected for inclusion in the formal meta-analysis were chosen because they were of sufficient methodological quality and they all provided outcome data in a format that allowed it to be reanalyzed.

Two of the selected studies examined urinary tract infections in young women. One study randomized 150 women with active urinary tract infections caused by *Escherichia coli* to receive either 50 mL of cranberry-lingonon juice daily, 100 mL *Lactobacillus GG* drink 5 days a week, or no treatment for 6 consecutive months. The authors reported that the recurrence of the first urinary tract infection by 6 months was significantly lower in the cranberry treatment group (16%) than in the *Lactobacillus GG* drink (39%) or control group (36%).

A second study recruited 150 sexually active women with recurrent urinary tract infections and randomized them to receive either cranberry juice (250 mL three times daily) with placebo tablets, cranberry tablets (1:30 parts concentrated juice twice a day) with placebo juice, or placebo tablets and placebo juice. Results showed that both the cranberry products significantly decreased the incidence of urinary tract infections compared to the placebo group. This study also reported that cranberry tablets were more cost-efficient per year than cranberry juice when taken for preventative measures.

The third study included in the meta-analysis focused on the use of cranberry in the elderly, a population that often receives cranberry products in institutional settings because of this population's increased risk of acquiring urinary tract infections. This study examined the prevention of urinary tract infections in 376 hospitalized male and female elderly individuals, randomized to receive 300 mL of either cranberry juice or placebo juice for an average length of 18 days. Although this is the largest trial completed to date examining the use of cranberry products in an elderly population, the study was inconclusive because the number of urinary tract infections that arose was lower than

expected. The urinary tract infections that did arise were two times more common in the placebo group (14 of 189) than the cranberry treatment group (7 of 187).

> *Overall, there is significantly more evidence that cranberry may be useful for helping to prevent urinary tract infections than that it can help treat an active infection.*

The fourth study included in the meta-analysis examined the ability of cranberry products to prevent urinary tract infections in a group of 48 patients diagnosed with a neurogenic bladder condition resulting from spinal cord injuries who used intermittent catheterization. Participants were randomized to receive either 2 g cranberry capsules or placebo capsules once a day for 6 months. Urine samples collected monthly from these individuals showed no difference between the two groups, and the authors concluded that cranberry tablets are not effective for prevention of urinary tract infections in individuals with neurogenic bladders receiving intermittent catheterization.

Withdrawals for some of the studies identified in this review were high, ranging from 20% to 55%. Common reasons included moving away, gastrointestinal upset, taste, and inconvenience. Several patients also experienced symptoms of reflux after ingesting cranberry juice. Indication of urinary tract infection was determined through bacterial load in urine samples, which varied between studies.

Anti-adherence Properties
It was originally thought that cranberry juice acted by increasing urine acidity. Other studies, however, have challenged this theory. Currently, the most popular theory is that cranberry possesses "anti-adherence" properties, which prevent bacteria from attaching to the lining of the urinary tract. For example, two compounds have been

found in cranberry that inhibit the adhesion of *E. coli* to urinary tract cells. Fructose, found in all fruit juices, and another compound, found only in cranberry and blueberry juice, have been shown to inhibit *E. coli* fimbrial adhesions.

Anticancer Activity

In vitro screening tests have suggested that the proanthocyanidin fraction of cranberry has potential anticarcinogenic activity. However, a recent randomized controlled trial reported that consumption of 750 mL of cranberry juice every day for 2 weeks had no effect on antioxidant status or oxidative DNA damage. These findings suggest that previous in vitro potential may not translate into clinical application.

H. Pylori Infection

A double-blind, randomized controlled trial involving 189 subjects has suggested that cranberry juice can be used to suppress *H. pylori* infection, thereby decreasing the risk of ulcers. Subjects consumed either 500 mL of cranberry juice or a placebo juice daily for 90 days, and a significant decrease in the number of urea-positive breath test patients were seen in the treatment group by day 35. Urea breath tests detect emissions in the breath caused by the breakdown of urea by *H. pylori* bacteria.

Adverse Effects

None reported.

Cautions/Contraindications

None reported.

Drug Interactions

Several case reports have raised concern about possible interactions between cranberry and warfarin, a common blood-thinning drug. One review states that this concern stems from cranberry's proposed effect on liver metabolism of warfarin, but more studies are needed to confirm this interaction.

Dosage Regimens

Prevention of urinary tract infections
- Juice: 150–600 mL cranberry juice daily.
- Capsule: 300–400 mg concentrated cranberry juice capsules twice daily.

Note: Cranberry juice should not be used as a substitute for antibiotics in acute urinary tract infections.

Selected References

Jepson RG, Craig JC. Cranberries for preventing urinary tract infections [update of Cochrane Database Syst Rev 2004(2): CD001321:RMID:15106157]. Cochrane Database of Systematic Reviews 2008(1): CD001321.

Pham DQ, Pham, AQ. Interaction potential between cranberry juice and warfarin (review). American Journal of Health-System Pharmacy 2007;64(5):490–94.

Zhang L, Ma J, Pan K, Go VL, Chen J, You WC. Efficacy of cranberry juice on *Helicobacter pylori* infection: A double-blind, randomized placebo-controlled trial. Helicobacter 2005; 10(2):139–45.

Dandelion

Taraxacum officinale
G.H. Weber ex Wiggers

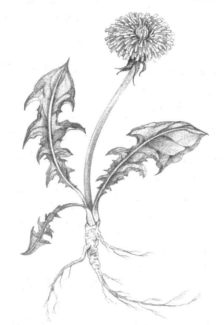

THUMBNAIL SKETCH

Common Uses
- *Root:* Liver (hepatobiliary) disorders, dyspepsia, loss of appetite
- *Leaves:* Water retention

Active Constituents
- Terpenes/terpenoids
- Bitter principle
- Phytosterols
- Inulin
- Minerals (potassium)

Adverse Effects
- Contact dermatitis (possible)

Cautions/Contraindications
- *Root:* Occlusion of bile ducts, paralytic ileus
- *Leaves:* Occlusion of bile ducts

Drug Interactions
- Leaf may potentiate the action of diuretics

Doses
- *Dried root (infusion or decoction):* 3–5 g three times daily
- *Root tincture (1:5 in 25% ethanol):* 5–10 mL three times daily
- *Dried leaf (infusion):* 4–10 g three times daily
- *Leaf liquid extract (1:1 in 25% alcohol):* 4–10 mL three times daily

Introduction

Family
- Asteraceae
  (also known as
  Compositae)

Synonyms
- Lion's tooth
- Fairy clock
- Wet-a-bed
- Pissenlit
- Dent-de-lion
- Irish daisy
- Puffball
- Swine's snout

Medicinal Forms
Leaf
- Dried leaf
- Infusion
- Tincture

Root
- Dried root
- Infusion
- Decoction
- Tincture

Description

Dandelion is a perennial herb native to Europe, now found throughout North America, that can grow to a height of 30 centimeters (12 inches). The oblong leaves grow in a rosette from a milky taproot, which sends up one or more leafless flower stems, each bearing a single yellow, multiple-petal flower. The name "dandelion" is a corruption of the Latin "dens leonis," or "lion's teeth," which derives from the appearance of the flower. A puffball tuft or cluster of "parachute" seeds follows the flower.

Parts Used

The leaf and root of the dandelion are used medicinally. The constituents of this plant, and arguably their medicinal action, change dramatically with the seasons. Generally speaking, the roots are best collected between June and August, when they are most bitter. Fresh dandelion leaves are commonly used in salads and sandwiches, the dried root is used as a coffee substitute, and the flowers are used in making dandelion wine and spirits.

Traditional Use

Members of the *Taraxacum* genus have been used by many cultures for their therapeutic properties. Dandelion is considered one of the primary herbs in the British herbal tradition, the roots being used for liver and digestive problems and the leaves for their diuretic properties in cases of edema. This latter action is demonstrated eloquently by the French name *pissenlit*. Dandelion has also been used in conditions as varied as fevers, boils, diarrhea, and hemorrhoids. In addition, it has been used in China and the Indian subcontinent for various conditions, including snake bites, abscesses, and appendicitis, as well as for its nutritional value.

Current Medicinal Use

Even though dandelion has a long history of medicinal use, very little scientific research has been conducted on the herb. Dandelion has both a choleretic (promoting production of bile) and a cholagogue (causing contraction of the bile duct, initiating the flow of stored bile) activity and is used to help the body detoxify. Since it is a digestive bitter, dandelion may help in cases of mild dyspepsia and indigestion. Dandelion leaf has mild diuretic properties.

Relevant Research

Preventative and Therapeutic Effects

Constituents

- Terpenoids (including the triterpenoids): taraxerol, taraxacin, lactucin, taraxasterol.

- Acids: chlorogenic acid, caffeic acid.

- Carbohydrates: fructose, glucose, inulin, sucrose. (During the summer, the fructose in the root is converted into inulin, to be reconverted back in the winter.)

- Vitamins and minerals: leaves are rich in potassium (297 mg/100 g), vitamin A (14,000 IU/100 g), vitamin C, vitamin B complex, zinc, manganese, copper.

- Phytosterols: sitosterol, stigmasterol, taraxasterol, campesterol. (The composition of the sterol portion found in the leaves undergoes extensive seasonal fluctuation.)

- Flavonoid glycosides: luteolin 7-glucoside, luteolin 7-diglucosides.

- Sesquiterpene lactones and taraxacoside: Many references are made to the bitter principle (also called taraxin) found primarily in dandelion root. This portion consists mainly of a mixture of sesquiterpene lactones and taraxacoside.

Effect on Liver Function

Dandelion root plays a major part in modern herbal practice, where it is considered to be safe for the management of many liver-related conditions. It is considered both a choleretic (promoting production of bile) and a cholagogue (causing contraction of the bile duct and initiating the flow of stored bile). These properties are firmly part of herbal tradition, but there are no clinical trials available to confirm or disconfirm this use. Studies have shown that administration of dandelion increased bile flow in dogs and rats and aided in the management of a variety of gallbladder conditions. In addition, a product in which dandelion is one of nine ingredients has been used to treat hepatitis. Given the importance of the liver as an organ of elimination within the herbal tradition, dandelion root is thought to be a useful and protective adjunctive therapy to chemotherapy.

> *Dandelion root plays a major part in modern herbal practice, where it is considered to be safe for the management of many liver-related conditions.*

Diuretic Action

One study demonstrated in rats and mice that dandelion possessed diuretic properties (promoted urination) when given in high doses. This study noted that an extract made from the leaves had a more pronounced diuretic action than the root. This appears to confirm the distinction between leaf and root noted by herbalists. The authors found that a 4% aqueous solution of dandelion leaf (15 mL/kg) had a diuretic effect comparable to furosemide at a dose of 80 mg/kg, and at a concentration of 8 mL/kg given for 30 days resulted in a marked weight loss.

In a more recent animal trial, no real diuretic effect was noted when an extract of *Taraxacum officinale* was administered to female wistar rats. Although no specifics of dose were given, the dandelion root was used in the preparation of the extract. Even though the diuretic action of dandelion has been shown in animal studies, the exact mechanism is as yet unknown. It appears that there may be numerous constituents playing a role in this function, including sesquiterpene lactones, found in the terpenoid portion, inulin, and potassium.

The high potassium content of dandelion leaf extract has been shown to offset the loss of potassium in the urine that can be responsible for the negative hepatic and circulatory effects of other diuretics. Herbalists also use this attribute when managing hypokalemia (abnormally low concentration of potassium ions in the circulating blood).

Miscellaneous Effects
Anti-inflammatory Effect
Some studies have suggested that oral and injected administration of dandelion extract can suppress induced inflammatory reactions in mice. For example, one study demonstrated that an ethanolic extract of dandelion suppressed in vitro production of the new blood vessels, which may contribute to inflammation, in a dose-dependent manner; directly decreased acute inflammation by decreasing permeability of blood vessels in mice; and decreased sensitivity to painful stimuli in mice.

Antimicrobial Effect
Extracts made from dandelion pollen have been shown to exert an antimicrobial action against *Proteus*, *Escherichia*, and *Salmonella* in vitro.

Digestion
Dandelion root is described as a digestive bitter and is often used in the treatment of dyspepsia and to stimulate the appetite.

Genitourinary
Investigators have hypothesized that the historical role of dandelion in the management of kidney stones could be due to the degradation of potential mucopolysaccharide foci by the saponins present in the plant. One animal study administering an extract of dandelion root to female rats found no significant differences between the incidence of kidney stones in the treatment group and the control group.

Hypoglycemia
A hypoglycemic action was noted in rabbits following esophageal administration. The fall in blood sugar was pronounced at high doses, and it has been suggested that dandelion could be acting in a similar fashion to conventional sulphonylurea hypoglycemics used to manage type 2 diabetes. Other trials have found contradictory results.

Adverse Effects
Contact dermatitis has been noted after frequent exposure to the fresh herb. This is unlikely to be clinically important because most herbal products are made from the dried material. Even when given as a large part of the diet (32%) for a prolonged period of time (209 days), dandelion root was not shown to have carcinogenic potential in rats.

Cautions/Contraindictions
Leaf: Dandelion leaf should be used with caution in cases of occlusion of the bile ducts.

Root: Dandelion root should be used with caution in cases of occlusion of the bile ducts and/or gallbladder, empyema, and paralytic ileus. Possible cross-reactivity has been noted between different members of the Asteraceae/Compositae (Sunflower) family, including dandelion, in sensitive individuals. Historical and anecdotal evidence suggests avoidance of excessive doses during pregnancy or lactation, but no evidence has been published to support this claim.

> *Because dandelion is considered a weed by many gardeners, it is very often heavily sprayed with a variety of herbicides and pesticides. Thus, people should be cautioned against collecting this herb from gardens, by roadsides, or from crop fields.*

Note: Because dandelion is considered a weed by many gardeners, it is very often heavily sprayed with a variety of herbicides and pesticides. Thus, people should be cautioned against collecting this herb from gardens, by roadsides, or from crop fields. It has also been noted that *Taraxacum officinale* growing in urban areas may contain enough heavy metals (lead, zinc, and copper) to be potentially harmful if taken orally.

Drug Interactions

No specific interactions between this plant and any pharmaceutical preparations could be found. One study suggests caution in using any herbal diuretic with conventional diuretics.

Dosage Regimens

- Dried root (infusion or decoction): 3–5 g three times daily.
- Root tincture (1:5 in 25% ethanol): 5–10 mL three times daily.
- Dried leaf (infusion): 4–10 g three times daily.
- Leaf liquid extract (1:1 in 25% alcohol): 4–10 mL three times daily.

Selected References

Houghton P. Bearberry, dandelion and celery. Pharmaceutical Journal 1995;255:272–73.

Jeon HJ, Kang HJ, Jung HJ, Kang YS, Lim CJ, Kim Y, Park EH. Anti-inflammatory activity of *Taraxacum officinale*. Journal of Ethnopharmacology 2008;115:82–88.

Devil's Claw

Harpagophytum procumbens DC.

Common Uses
- Inflammation of joints (including osteoarthritis, rheumatoid arthritis, and gout)
- Indigestion and dyspepsia (stomach pain)

Active Constituents
- Iridoid glycosides (harpaside, harpagoside)

Adverse Effects
- Digestive upset (mild)

Cautions/Contraindications
- Peptic ulcer (active)

Drug Interactions
- None

Doses
For digestive indications:
- *Dried tuber in decoction:* 500 mg three times daily
- *Tincture (1:5 in 25% ethanol):* 1 mL three times daily

For other indications:
- *Dried tuber in decoction:* 1.5–2.5 g three times daily
- *Liquid extract (1:1 in 25% ethanol):* 1–2 mL three times daily
- *Dried tuber:* 100–250 mg three times daily

Introduction

Family
- Pedaliaceae

Synonyms
- Harpagophytum
- Grapple plant
- Wood spider

Medicinal Forms
- Dried tuber
- Decoction
- Tincture
- Liquid extract

Description

Devil's claw is native to southern and eastern Africa, notably the veldt of the Transvaal region. It is a trailing herbaceous perennial, growing to 1.5 meters (5 feet) in length, with lobed leaves whose brilliant "devil" red to purple flowers and woody, barbed, claw-like fruit are responsible for its descriptive name. The plant produces tubers that are harvested as herbs.

Parts Used

The secondary storage root or tuber is the part principally used medicinally when dried.

Traditional Uses

Decoctions of dried roots have long been taken as a tea or tonic by the indigenous peoples of Africa for a variety of digestive and rheumatic conditions. After devil's claw was introduced to European herbal medicine by G.H. Mehnert, this herb became so popular that by 1976 it was estimated that 30,000 arthritic patients in the United Kingdom alone were using it.

Current Medicinal Use

Devil's claw is primarily used in the management of inflammatory joint diseases, such as osteoarthritis, rheumatoid arthritis, and gout. Since devil's claw is considered a bitter tonic, it may be of help in the management of various gastrointestinal complaints, including dyspepsia and digestive upsets.

Relevant Research

Preventative and Therapeutic Effects

Constituents
- Iridoid glycosides: harpagide, harpagoside, procumbide.
- Phenolic acids: chlorogenic acid, cinnamic acid.
- Flavonoids: kaempferol, luteolin.

Note: Harpagoside, which appears to be the constituent of most interest, is primarily found in the secondary tubers. The flowers, stem, and ripe fruit appear to be devoid of this agent.

Musculoskeletal Effects

Devil's claw has been reputed to have anti-inflammatory and antirheumatic properties. It is commonly used in the management of inflammatory joint diseases, such as osteoarthritis, rheumatoid arthritis, and gout. The authors of a 2006 review concluded that there is clinical evidence that devil's claw may be beneficial for the treatment of pain and improvement of mobility in a variety of musculoskeletal conditions. They also argue that the evidence indicates that devil's claw is effective as an anti-inflammatory and analgesic preparation, particularly in the relief of arthritic conditions. However, most of the research has been done in animals, making it difficult to determine devil's claw's clinical effects in humans.

> *The evidence indicates that devil's claw is effective as an anti-inflammatory and analgesic preparation, particularly in the relief of arthritic conditions.*

Osteoarthritis

Devil's claw is a popular herbal remedy for the treatment of osteoarthritis. A 2004 systematic review examined five randomized controlled trials that assessed devil's claw for osteoarthritis and came to an overall conclusion that a component of devil's claw, harpargoside, is more effective than a placebo and as effective, if not more effective, than conventional drugs, such as phenylbutazone or diacerhein. A 2007 review reached a similar conclusion, based on a review of five clinical trials.

Low Back Pain

A Cochrane Collaboration review of herbal medicine for low back pain identified three high-quality trials and concluded that devil's claw seemed to reduce pain more than a placebo. A 2007 review reached a similar conclusion, based on a review of six clinical trials. Details of the key trials from the Cochrane review are described below.

A randomized, placebo-controlled, double-blind, 4-week study of 118 patients presenting with low back pain found that treatment with devil's claw was not significantly better than treament with a placebo in two out of three outcome measures. The primary outcome measure was the amount of a specific opiod analgesic (Tramadol) taken by patients in the last 3 weeks of the study. Secondary outcome measures included relief according to the Arhus Low Back Pain Index and the number of patients pain-free at the study's conclusion.

While the number of patients pain-free at the conclusion of the trial was significantly higher in the treatment group than in the placebo group, there was no significant difference between the groups with respect to the Arhus Low Back Pain Index or the amount of analgesic ingested. This study has been criticized because the consumption of analgesic could not be equated with the subjective experience of pain.

A second randomized, controlled, 4-week study of 183 patients found that daily doses standardized to 50 mg or 100 mg harpagoside (WS 1531) may be equally effective as bed rest, paracetamol (acetaminophen), or non-steroidal anti-inflammatory drugs (NSAIDs), with fewer side effects.

A pilot double-blind, 6-week study of 88 patients reported that daily doses standardized to 60 mg harpagoside (Doloteffin) demonstrated equivalent efficacy as daily doses of 12.5 mg rofecoxib, an NSAID. A 1-year follow-up after this pilot study again suggested comparable efficacy between the rofecoxib and harpagoside groups and confirmed high tolerance of devil's claw extracts.

Two additional trials not included in the Cochrane review — one an open-label trial with 130 patients, the other a double-blind pilot study with 197 patients — also suggest that devil's claw may be beneficial in the management of the symptoms of low back pain.

Anti-inflammatory Effect

Many authors have suggested that devil's claw can exert an anti-inflammatory action. Aqueous extracts of devil's claw were shown to possess anti-inflammatory activity when injected into both rats and mice. However, the anti-inflammatory properties appeared to be abolished after oral administration or after an acid treatment.

One animal study reported that an aqueous extract of devil's claw may possess an anti-inflammatory action comparable to that of phenylbutazone. Extracts of devil's claw were shown, however, to possess no appreciable action in reducing rat hind paw edema induced by either carragennan or *Mycobacterium butyricum* when compared to standard NSAID agents. Even at doses far higher (100 times) than the "standard recommended dose" of devil's claw, no inflammatory action was seen nor any inhibitory action on prostaglandin synthetase action noted.

In an attempt to demonstrate a possible mechanism of anti-inflammatory action, one study found that 500 mg of devil's claw, standardized to 3% total glucoiridoids per unit dose, had no influence on eicosanoid production in humans. There was also no statistically significant difference in blood clotting times between the two groups.

Digestive Effects

Devil's claw has been classified as a "bitter tonic" useful in the management of various gastrointestinal complaints, including dyspepsia and digestive upsets due to poor gallbladder or pancreatic function. An in vitro study has indicated that the iridoid components of devil's claw, harpagoside and harpagide, affect the contractile response of guinea pig ileum. The authors infer that this could be a result of an action on the mechanism that controls influx of calcium into the cells.

> Devil's claw has been classified as a "bitter tonic" useful in the management of various gastrointestinal complaints, including dyspepsia and digestive upsets due to poor gallbladder or pancreatic function.

Miscellaneous Effects

Cardiovascular Protection

Crude methanolic extracts of *Harpagophytum procumbens* exert a dose-dependent protective effect on experimental ventricular arrhyth-mias (abnormal rapid heart rhythms that originate in the lower chambers of the heart) induced by various means in both rat and isolated rabbit hearts. Some authors have suggested that this action is in part due to an inhibition of calcium influx into the myocardial cells (muscle cells of the heart) because it was shown to be protective against arrhythmias induced by digitalis. This action appears to be the result of a synergistic interplay of constituents rather than solely the harpagoside. Also noted was a positive inotropic effect (increased force or energy of muscular contractions) at low doses and a negative inotropic effect (decreased force or energy of muscular contractions) at higher doses.

Antimicrobial Effects

Extracts made from the secondary roots of devil's claw exerted weak antifungal action against various fungi.

Adverse Effects

A "slight digestive upset" was reported by two patients participating in one study. One individual in another study reported morning frontal throbbing headache, tinnitus (ringing in the ears), severe anorexia, and loss of appetite, but no attempt appears to have been made to determine whether these effects were due to the devil's claw product being investigated.

Cautions/Contraindications

Given the action of devil's claw as a classic bitter, it may theoretically increase gastric acid secretion. This fact has led to a caution on its use in cases of active peptic ulcer disease. Historically, the use of devil's claw has been contraindicated in pregnancy due to its alleged abortifacient action (i.e., it has the potential to cause abortion). Although this situation could be due to a simple mistranslation, it is still a valid point of concern until more information is known.

Drug Interactions

No interactions between this herb and any pharmaceutical preparations could be found. Given the influence mentioned above in animal studies of *Harpagophytum procumbens* on cardiac muscle, its use in high doses may interact with cardiac and hypo- or hypertension therapy.

Selected References

Gagnier JJ, Chrubasik S, Manheimer E. *Harpagophytum procumbens* for osteoarthritis and low back pain: A systematic review BMC. Complementary and Alternative Medicine 2004;4:13.

Gagnier JJ, Tulder MW, Berman B, Bombardier C. Herbal medicine for low back pain: A Cochrane review. Spine 2007;32(1):82–92.

Grant L, McBean DE, Fyfe L, Warnock M. A review of the biological and potential therapeutic actions of *Harpagophytum procumbens*. Phytotherapy Research 2007;21:199–209.

Dosage Regimens

For digestive indications:

- Dried tuber in decoction: 500 mg three times daily.
- Tincture (1:5 in 25% ethanol): 1 mL three times daily.

For other indications:

- Dried tuber in decoction: 1.5–2.5 g three times daily.
- Liquid extract (1:1 in 25% ethanol): 1–2 mL three times daily.
- Dried tuber: 100–250 mg three times daily.

Note: Many of the clinical trials have used a dose range of 400–500 mg of dried herb three times daily. While many products are standardized for harpagoside content, it would be prudent to use whole-plant extracts until the importance of this constituent is verified.

Dong Quai
Angelica sinensis (Oliv.) Diels

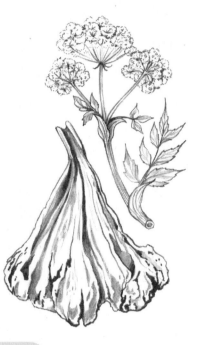

THUMBNAIL SKETCH

Common Uses
- Women's health care (including the unpleasant consequences of menopause, dysmenorrhea, and amenorrhea)
- "Blood tonic" (dependent on a suitable diagnosis in traditional Chinese medicine)

Active Constituents
- Components of both the alcohol and aqueous soluble portions have been shown to possess therapeutic properties

Adverse Effects
- Diarrhea and phototoxic skin reaction (rare)

Cautions/Contraindications
- Pregnancy, hypermenorrhea (heavy periods), hemorrhagic (bleeding) disease, history of spontaneous abortion

Drug Interactions
- No examples of drug interactions found, but caution is recommended in cases of concomitant administration with oral anticoagulants

Doses
- *Raw herb:* 3–10 g (or equivalent) daily

Introduction

Family
- Apiaceae (also known as Umbelliferae)

Synonyms
- Chinese angelica
- Tang kuei
- Dang gui
- Female ginseng
- Female tonic
- Woman's herb
- Toki
- Tangwi
- *A. polymorpha* Maxim. Var. *sinensis* Oliv.

Medicinal Forms
- Fresh root (steamed or fried in vinegar)
- Dried root (as a soup)

Description

Dong quai is a fragrant perennial plant, growing to 2 meters (6 feet) tall, with large green leaves, hollow stems, and clusters of white flowers. It is native to southwestern China and Japan, where it is now cultivated extensively.

Similar plants are often used in place of *Angelica sinensis*, including *Angelica acutiloba* (Siebold & Zucc.); Kitag (Korean or Japanese dong quai); *Ligusticum glaucescens* Franch (wild chin quai); and *Levisticum officinale* Koch (European dong quai). While these plants do possess therapeutically useful qualities, they are considered by most to be inferior to *Angelica sinensis*.

Parts Used

The root, with its distinctive aroma and bittersweet, pungent taste, is the part used medicinally. The larger roots are more prized than the smaller ones. As a general rule, the larger the root, the sweeter the taste and the better the quality.

Traditional Use

Dong quai is arguably one of the oldest and most established therapeutic agents used in the traditional Chinese medicine (TCM) healing model. It is considered to be a tonic that can strengthen and invigorate the whole individual or specific organ groups. While dong quai exerts its tonifying action on many sites, it is classically considered to be one of the major "blood tonics," often used to "build the blood." Even though it has numerous applications, it was considered to be of particular importance in the management of female conditions, such as menopause and dysmenorrhea (pain during menstruation). It is in the realm of women's health care that most people will encounter the use of dong quai in the Western world.

Another member of the same genus, *Angelica archangelica* L. (Angelica), shares some of the same constituents and actions as dong quai, but it is used primarily as a digestive tonic, especially in cases of indigestion and flatulence. *Angelica archangelica* L. is also used extensively in the liquor industry, as a flavoring in liqueurs, such as benedictine and chartreuse.

Current Medicinal Use

Until more conclusive scientific research has been conducted, it is best to use dong quai as intended in traditional Chinese medicine. In the hands of an appropriately trained practitioner, dong quai may be useful in the management of menstrual and menopause conditions, as well as some cardiovascular conditions.

Relevant Research

Preventative and Therapeutic Effects

Constituents

- **Volatile oils:** ligustilide, n-butylidene phthalide, n-valerophernone-O-carboxylic acid.

- **Furanocoumarins:** psoralen, bergapten, archangelicin.

- **Organic acids:** ferulic acid, succinic acid, myristic acid.

- **Miscellaneous:** vitamin A, vitamin E, various members of the vitamin B group, polysaccharides (including-AR-4E-2), angelica immunostimulating polysaccharide (AIP).

Cardiovascular Effects

Traditional Use

Within the traditional Chinese medicine model, dong quai is prescribed for conditions of "blood deficiency," a situation that often presents with a variety of symptoms, including pale lips and tongue, dull or pale face with sallow complexion, depression and fatigue, poor memory, oligomenorrhea (infrequent periods), and amenorrhea (absence of menstrual period in a woman of reproductive age). While many of these symptoms may be equated with the Western concepts of anemia and cardiovascular disease, it is important to realize that conditions diagnosed following a TCM tradition cannot be directly equated with a conventional medical diagnosis.

Cardiac Activity

Several experimental studies suggest that extracts of *Angelica sinensis* exert an inhibitory action on cardiac muscle contraction. Both aqueous and alcoholic extracts of *Angelica sinensis* have been shown to antagonize arrhythmias (abnormal heart beat) induced by a number of agents (including epinephrine, strophanthin, digitalis, atropine, and datura flower) in both in vivo and in vitro models. A quinidine-like action (prolonged atrial refractory period, lowered cardiac excitability) was demonstrated in anesthetized dogs given an ether extract of *Angelica sinensis* root. In addition, a 2% fluid extract of *Angelica sinensis* has been shown to markedly increase blood flow to and from the heart and decrease oxygen consumption of the heart muscles in the isolated hearts of guinea pigs.

Vascular Action

It has been demonstrated that *Angelica sinensis* exerts a predominately hypotensive effect in vivo. This drop in blood pressure appears to be rapid and short-lived. It was thought that this action was in part due to a decreased cardiac output, but this has been shown not to be the case. It is more likely due to a vasodilatory action resulting from muscarinic and histaminic receptor stimulation. Early investigations suggested that the hypotensive action was solely due to the non-volatile components, and the volatile constituents were thought to have a stimulating action. This has since been shown not to be the case.

> *A 2% fluid extract of* Angelica sinensis *has been shown to markedly increase blood flow to and from the heart and decrease oxygen consumption of the heart muscles in the isolated hearts of guinea pigs.*

Antithrombotic Action

In vitro experiments have demonstrated that aqueous extracts of *Angelica sinensis* could suppress platelet aggregation induced by ADP and collagen. The agent thought to be predominantly responsible for this action is ferulic acid. It has been postulated that the decrease in platelet aggregation could be due to inhibition of cyclo-oxygenase and thromboxane A2, resulting in a subsequent decrease in the production of bioactive eicosonoids. Osthole, extracted from a related species (*Angelica pubescens* Maxim.), has also shown to decrease platelet aggregation by inhibiting thromboxane B2. It has also been postulated that the antithrombotic action could be due to a decrease in fibrinogen levels and blood viscosity. This influence on the blood's coagulating system is far from certain, with some suggesting that an effect cannot be demonstrated.

Antilipidemic Effect

Angelica sinensis root added to the feed (5% w/w) of albino rats and rabbits with experimental hyperlipidemia exerted a demonstrable antilipidemic effect. While the exact mechanism is unknown, it does not appear to be due to an effect on cholesterol absorption.

Women's Health

Traditional Use

Dong quai is considered useful in the management of a variety of women's conditions, including abnormal, suppressed, or difficult menstruation, dysmenorrhea (pain during menstruation), dysfunctional uterine bleeding (see contraindications), premenstrual syndrome (PMS), preparation for conception, recovery after birthing, and unpleasant consequences of menopause. As mentioned above, many of these conditions are diagnosed and treated using models outside of the conventional medical model.

Menstrual Problems

Although dong quai has a long history of use in traditional Chinese medicine for treating problems associated with menstruation, little scientific research of its use in specific Western diagnoses has been conducted, which makes it difficult to recommend it for any specific condition.

A common Chinese patent formula containing *Angelica sinensis* root (Xiao Yao Powder) was seen to decrease symptoms of PMS in 10 women. A randomized, placebo-controlled trial involving 49 women found that a phytoestrogen combination containing 60 mg soy isoflavones, 100 mg dong quai, and 50 mg black cohosh significantly decreased the frequency of menstrual migraine attacks, as well as significantly decreasing the frequency of all migraines, the severity of headaches, and the doses of triptans and analgesics, compared to the placebo group, when ingested for 24 weeks. The clinical contributions of the dong quai in this product cannot be determined from this study.

In addition, dong quai root has been shown to have an action on uterine tissue in various animal models. It appears that this effect depends on the extract used. The volatile oil fraction causes direct muscular relaxation, completely abolishing contractions in a dose-dependent fashion. The active constituent appears to be ligustilide. The volatile oil antagonizes excitation caused by either histamine or epinephrine, while the non-volatile fractions have an opposite action resulting in strong uterine contractions. The alcoholic extract has a more pronounced effect than the aqueous one. When administered parenterally, there is no difference between the fractions, and they all cause excitation.

Pressure within the uterus was shown to influence the action of dong quai on rabbit uterine fistula. When the existing pressure was elevated, contraction became slower and more rhythmic. It has been suggested that this action is responsible for dong quai's effectiveness in the treatment of dysmenorrhea (uterine pain during menstruation).

Menopause

Although dong quai has been used by traditional Chinese medicine practitioners to treat a subset of women suffering with menopausal symptoms, attempts to quantify its effects in women with the Western diagnosis of menopausal symptoms have been largely unsuccessful. For example, in a double-blind, randomized, placebo-controlled, 24-week trial, 71 postmenopausal women who had follicle-stimulating hormone levels of less than 30 mIU/mL with hot flashes were administered dong quai extract standardized to 0.5 mg/kg ferulic acid, and it was found that dong quai alone was no more helpful than a placebo in relieving menopausal symptoms. No statistically significant differences were observed in endometrial thickness, vaginal maturation, and menopausal symptoms. A product containing dong quai (Angelica-Paeonia Powder) was shown to

> *Although dong quai has been used by traditional Chinese medicine practitioners to treat a subset of women suffering with menopausal symptoms, attempts to quantify its effects in women with the Western diagnosis of menopausal symptoms have been largely unsuccessful.*

alleviate symptoms commonly seen with menopause in 43 cases. Specific details of this trial were not available at the time of preparing this monograph. In addition, a trial of a botanical formula containing dong quai (and *Arctium lappa* L., Asteraceae, *Glycyrrhiza glabra* L., Fabaceae, *Leonurus cardiaca* L., Lamiaceae, and *Dioscorea villosa* L., Dioscoreaceae) conducted at the National College of Naturopathic Medicine found that symptoms of menopause were decreased when compared to a placebo group. As was correctly noted by the authors, given the small sample number (13), no definite conclusions can be made. No conclusions can be drawn for dong quai in particular from this investigation since the other herbal ingredients in the botanical formula have demonstrable therapeutic actions in their own rights.

The many positive actions of dong quai on the female reproductive system have long been considered to result from phytoestrogenic properties. This assumption is now being questioned because many of the actions of this herb are probably not estrogen-dependent. Studies in mice have found dong quai to be devoid of estrogenic action. Conversely, both aqueous and petroleum ether extracts, when given intraperitoneally and subcutaneously, are reported to have an estrogen-like action.

As has been demonstrated, the evidence supporting the therapeutic usefulness of *Angelica sinensis* comes predominantly from the Asian medical model and there is a distinct lack of quality clinical information. It should also be noted that what little evidence there is from a conventional Western standpoint normally involves products in which dong quai is only one of many ingredients. More research is required before the traditional uses of dong quai can be supported by evidence from a biomedical paradigm.

Miscellaneous Effects

Antimicrobial Effects

An aqueous decoction of dong quai has been shown to exert a weak antimicrobial action against a variety of bacteria, including *E. coli*, *Salmonella typhi*, and *Shigella dysenteriae*.

Metabolic Effect

When added to the feed of rats (5% to 6% of diet), *Angelica sinensis* was shown to reduce or prevent testicular disease resulting from vitamin E deficiency.

Central Nervous System

Parenteral administration of tang kuei essential oil from Japan has been shown to exert tranquilizing, hypnotic, and anesthetic actions in a variety of animal models.

Analgesic Action

Dong quai is used within TCM for various conditions associated with pain primarily due to a TCM diagnosis of "blood stagnation." This analgesic action appears to depend on the quality and origin of the pain.

Adverse Effects

Even though tang kuei extract from Japan accelerated the death of mice that had been given carbon tetrachloride, in practice adverse effects caused by *Angelica sinensis* appear to be very rare. The LD_{50} of dong quai administered intravenously to mice was 100.6 g/kg.

Diarrhea is possible because of dong quai's relaxant action on the smooth muscle of the digestive tract. This appears more likely if the individual has a "weak" digestive system already.

> *In practice adverse effects caused by* Angelica sinensis *appear to be very rare. The* LD_{50} *of dong quai administered intravenously to mice was 100.6 g/kg.*

Concerns have been raised regarding the presence of furancoumarins (psoralen and bergapten) in *Angelica sinensis* and the subsequent increased possibility of a photosensitization, resulting in a dermatitis-like skin reaction. Examples of phototoxic reactions have been noted when high doses of psoralens from other plants (e.g., celery) have been administered in conjunction with UV light.

There is one report of a case in which a 35-year-old man in Singapore experienced gynecomastia (enlarged breast tissue) after self-medicating with dong quai (dose not available, product labeled 100% dang gui root powder) for 1 month. His hormone levels were reported to be normal, and his symptoms resolved completely within 3 months after discontinuing dong quai.

It has been noted that parenteral administration of the volatile oil results in severe pain, nausea, hot flushes, and chills. These reactions are usually self-limiting. In addition, it has been reported that the intravenous injection of the volatile components of the plant may cause kidney failure. A case of anaphylactic shock resulting from the injection of a product containing angelica has also been noted.

Cautions/Contraindications

Given its action on uterine smooth muscle, dong quai should not be used during the first trimester of pregnancy or in individuals with a history of spontaneous abortion. Given the lack of information, many suggest that consumption of dong quai should be avoided at any stage of pregnancy, except when used by an appropriately trained health-care provider. There are three unpublished case reports of rashes in infants who were being breastfed by women ingesting dong quai. The rashes were reported as resolved when dong quai was discontinued. Specific details of these cases are not available.

Practitioners of traditional Chinese medicine advise that "tonic" herbs, such as dong quai, should not be used during acute illness (e.g., the flu and colds). In addition, dong quai should be avoided in cases of hemorrhagic disease and hypermenorrhea.

Drug Interactions

Plant medicines rich in coumarins may interfere with concomitant anticoagulant therapy. There is one case report in the literature that describes a 46-year-old African-American woman diagnosed with atrial fibrillation and stabilized on warfarin who experienced a greater than twofold increase in international normalized ratio (INR) after taking dong quai (Nature's Way, one 565 mg tablet once or twice daily) concurrently for 4 weeks. The patient's INR returned to acceptable levels 1 month after discontinuing the dong quai.

Dosage Regimens
• Raw herb: 3–10 g (or equivalent) daily.

Note: Although dong quai is available in liquid extract and tincture preparations, there is little reliable information available on proper dosages.

Selected References

Hirata JD, Swiersz LM, Zell B, Small R, Ettinger B. Does dong quai have estrogenic effects in postmenopausal women? A double-blind, placebo-controlled trial. Fertility and Sterility 1997;68(6):981–86.

Page RL, 2nd, Lawrence JD. Potentiation of warfarin by dong quai. Pharmacotherapy 1999;19(7):870–76.

Echinacea

E. angustifolia DC., E. purpurea (L.) Moench, E. pallida (Nutt.) Nutt.

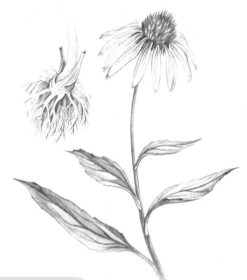

THUMBNAIL SKETCH

Common Uses

Internal
- Colds, flus (supportive)
- Upper respiratory tract and lower urinary tract infections

External
- Skin abrasions and ulcerations

Active Constituents
- Polysaccharides
- Glycoproteins
- Alkamides
- Caffeic acid derivatives (such as echinacoside, cichoric acid, and cynarin)

Adverse Effects
- Rare allergic reactions manifesting as asthma attacks, anaphylaxis, or urticaria

Cautions/Contraindications

Internal
- Progressive systemic diseases (e.g., tuberculosis, multiple sclerosis)
- Autoimmune conditions (e.g., diabetes mellitus, lupus, rheumatoid arthritis)
- HIV/AIDS (use controversial)

External
- None known

Drug Interactions
- Opposes effects of immunosuppressants (theoretical)

Doses

Internal
- *Dried herb:* 1 g three times daily
- *Hydroalcoholic tincture (1:5 in 45% ethanol):* 2–5 mL three times daily
- *Liquid extract (1:1 in 45% ethanol):* 0.5–1.0 mL three times daily
- *Expressed juice (E. purpurea):* 6–9 mL daily in divided doses

External
- Semi-solid preparations should contain at least 15% expressed juice (E. purpurea)

Introduction

Family
- Asteraceae
  (also known as
  Compositae or
  Sunflower family)

Synonyms
- Purple coneflower
- Purple Kansas
  coneflower
- Black Simpson
- Red sunflower
- Comb flower
- Cock up hat
- Missouri snakeroot
- Kansas snakeroot
- Indian head

Medicinal Forms
Root
- Dried root
- Tincture
- Liquid extract

Aerial Parts
- Expressed juice
  (liquid or semi-
  solid)

Description

There are nine echinacea species indigenous to the North American Midwest, from Saskatchewan to Texas, but only three species of this perennial are collected or cultivated as medicinal herbs. *Echinacea angustifolia* is the smallest of these plants, growing to only 0.5 meter (18 inches). Although commercial cultivation of *Echinacea angustifolia* has been initiated, much of the medicinal supply is still wild-harvested. The tap root of *Echinacea angustifolia* can reach 1 to 1.5 meters (3 to 5 feet) in length. *Echinacea pallida* is larger, growing to approximately 1 meter (40 inches) in height. *Echinacea purpurea*, the most common purple cone flower, can grow from 0.5 to 1.5 meters (18 inches to 5 feet) tall. The entire medicinal supply of this third species is cultivated. Each species features several spreading, soft purple flower rays and a conical disk composed of numerous purple, tubular florets, from which the name "purple coneflower" derives. The genus name may derive from the Greek *echinos* for "sea urchin" or "hedgehog," after its bristly leaves and cone.

Echinacea angustifolia is the favored species in North America and is often the only species listed in North American reference texts. It has been argued that it is largely the favorite simply because of familiarity — it is native to North America, and knowledge about this species has been handed down through generations of herbalists and Native Peoples healers. However, *E. angustifolia* is largely still harvested from wild sources, which raises concerns about both the sustainability and quality of the supply. Limited efforts are currently under way to cultivate *E. angustifolia* for medicinal purposes.

In contrast, *Echinacea purpurea* is the species that is most commonly commercially cultivated. In addition, the vast majority of both pharmacological and clinical studies have been conducted with *E. purpurea*, primarily with the commercial product Echinacin, which is the expressed juice of the aerial parts of the plant, with alcohol added as a preservative. Echinacin was used in the creation of the Commission E monograph in Germany.

Parts Used

The roots are primarily used medicinally; however, there is evidence that the aerial parts of *E. purpurea* also have some medicinal action.

Traditional Use

Echinacea species were used extensively as medicinal herbs by native North American tribes, reportedly to treat a variety of ailments, including mouth sores, toothaches, colds, sore throats, burns, and snake bites. Its use for snake bites gave rise to several common names, such as "Missouri snakeroot" and "Kansas snakeroot."

H.F.C. Meyer, a German physician working in Nebraska, is credited with introducing echinacea to the medical profession when he began selling a patent formula containing a root extract of *E. angustifolia* in the 1870s. In 1887, Meyer brought echinacea to the attention of John King, a well-known Eclectic physician, and John Uri Lloyd, a prominent pharmacist and manufacturer, who undertook a number of trials of the product and then began marketing echinacea products as anti-infective agents. By 1915, echinacea products were available from many other pharmaceutical companies, including Merck, Wyeth, and Parke Davis. Although the Eclectics embraced the use of echinacea, it was widely criticized by the "regular" medical establishment of the time, who argued that there was no scientific evidence to support its use. However, from 1916 to 1950, *E. angustifolia* and *E. pallida* roots were listed as official drugs in the National Formulary of the United States.

To meet the growing European demand for echinacea, a German company, Madaus AHG, attempted to import *E. angustifolia* seeds from the United States. The species imported, however, was subsequently demonstrated to be *E. purpurea*. The majority of European research on echinacea in the past 50 years was conducted using the Madaus product Echinacin, which is made from the expressed juices of the aerial parts of *E. purpurea* combined with 22% ethanol as a preservative.

Current Medicinal Use

Several hundred articles and a number of books have been written about echinacea, and a large proportion of the literature was originally published in German. Echinacea has been shown to have immunological activity. While the results from clinical trials are sometimes conflicting, there is a growing body of information to show that it may be useful in treating colds, flus, and infections of the upper respiratory tract and lower urinary tract when administered internally. This herb also has anti-inflammatory activity and is administered externally to manage skin abrasions and ulcerations.

Relevant Research

Preventative and Therapeutic Effects

Constituents

Although the three species are often considered interchangeable clinically, their chemical constituents differ. One study found no characteristic chemical differences between the aerial parts of the three species; however, the alkylamides in the roots did differ significantly. *E. angustifolia* may be distinguished from *E. purpurea* because the former contains isobutylamides, echinacoside, and cynarin, and the latter contains distinctive polyacetylenes and polyenes. Echinacoside — the chemical for which many echinacea products are standardized — has been found in both *E. angustifolia* and *E. pallida* but not *E. purpurea*. However, cynarine, a quinic acid derivative, has been detected only in *E. angustifolia* and may be useful for discriminating between it and the other two species. In addition, echinacein, the isobutylamide generally thought to cause the "tingling of the tongue" associated with echinacea products, has been identified only as a constituent of *E. angustifolia*.

E. angustifolia

- **Carbohydrates:** sucrose, pentosans, fructose.
- **Polysaccharides:** inulin storage (fructans), hetero-polysaccharides (structural).
- **Phenolic compounds:** caffeic acid derivatives, echinacoside, 3-malonylglucoside cynarin (roots only), chlorogenic, isochlorogenic acid (leaves and stems).

- **Flavonoids:** a variety including luteolin, kaempferol, and quercetin derivatives, rutoside.
- **Fatty acids:** linoleic, oleic, cerotic, and palmitic acids.
- **Polyacetylenes:** a variety of polyynes and polyenes.
- **Alkylamides:** echinacein and a variety of others, including pyrrolidides, piperidides, isobutylamides (pattern of alkylamides differs from *E. purpurea*).
- **Alkaloids:** tussilagine, isotussilagine (pyrrolizidines that do not contain 1,2-unsaturated necine ring system necessary to confer liver toxicity).
- **Miscellaneous:** betaine hydrochloride, phytosterols, n-triacontanol, behenic acid ethyl ester.

E. purpurea

- **Carbohydrates:** fructose.
- **Polysaccharides:** a variety of hetero-polysaccharides (structural), including arabinogalactan, xyloglucans.
- **Phenolic compounds:** caffeic acid derivatives, chicoric acid, caftaric acid and derivatives (mainly aerial parts).
- **Flavonoids:** several, including a variety of kaempferol, quercetin, and rutin derivatives, rutoside.
- **Fatty acids:** linoleic, oleic, cerotic and palmitic acids.
- **Polyacetylenes:** a varitey of polyynes and polyenes.
- **Alkylamides:** echinacein and a variety of isobutylamides (pattern of alkylamides differs from *E. angustifolia*).
- **Alkaloids:** tussilagine, isotussilagine (pyrrolizidines that do not contain 1,2-unsaturated necine ring system necessary to confer liver toxicity).
- **Miscellaneous:** glycine betaine, cyanidins, glycoproteins.

E. pallida

The polyacetylenes of *E. pallida* are very susceptible to oxidation; thus, the chemical composition of the roots depends on storage conditions.

- **Carbohydrates:** sucrose, petosans.
- **Polysaccharides:** inulin storage (fructans), hetero-polysaccharides (structural).
- **Phenolic compounds:** caffeic acid derivatives, echinacoside, des-rhamnosyl-verascoside, 6-0–caffcoyl-echinacoside (roots only), caftaric acid and derivatives (mainly aerial parts), chlorogenic and isochlorogenic acid (leaves and stems).
- **Flavonoids:** a variety including luteolin, kaempferol and quercetin derivatives, rutoside
- **Fatty acids:** linoleic, oleic, cerotic, and palmitic acids.
- **Polyacetylenes:** a variety of polyynes and polyenes, keto alkynes and keto alkenes.
- **Alkylamides:** traces.
- **Miscellaneous:** betaine hydrochloride, cyanidins.

Immunological Activity

The immunostimulatory action of echinacea appears to depend on the synergistic action of several constituents. Although several different compounds have been shown to possess immunological activity, echinacea's effects on the immune system cannot be attributed to any single compound. Most of the scientific research has been conducted with isolated fractions of *E. purpurea* (often a polysaccharide extract) and *E. angustifolia*. Very little research has reported on *E. pallida*.

Upper Respiratory Tract Infections (Including the Common Cold)

There have been a number of systematic reviews assessing the efficacy of using echinacea to treat cold symptoms. The two most recent and high-quality reviews are described below. All these reviews concluded that echinacea may have a positive effect when used to treat the common cold, although more detailed studies are needed to confirm this use, and one challenge for all the reviews is the wide range of different echinacea products available, including those made from different species, different parts of the plant, and different extraction processes.

A 2008 systematic review of randomized controlled trials compared echinacea treatment with no treatment, a placebo, or other active treatment in the management of the common cold. The authors identified 14 treatment trials that included 1,126 participants enrolled in trials because they were already experiencing cold symptoms and another 1,910 participants enrolled in trials who were instructed to start self-treatment if they experienced cold symptoms during the trial period. Of the trials that compared echinacea treatment with a placebo, nine comparisons showed significantly positive results for the echinacea group, two identified a positive trend in favor of echinacea, and six reported insignificant results (i.e., no difference between echinacea and placebo).

> *Most importantly, it is necessary to determine which specific extracts of echinacea are associated with positive clinical effects in humans.*

These trials used a wide variety of echinacea products, including pressed juice from aerial parts of *E. purpurea* and tinctures or extracts of *E. purpurea*, *E. angustifolia*, and *E. pallida*. Trials using combination products were not included in this review. The authors concluded that both the pressed juice and extracts of *E. purpurea* may have positive effects when used to treat cold symptoms in adults in the first day or two after the onset of a cold. There was not sufficient evidence to confirm the use of other forms of echinacea, but this was largely due to the fact that these were the only forms tested in more than one clinical trial to date.

A second review conducted in 2007 identified seven randomized placebo-controlled trials, four positive and three negative, that met their inclusion criteria for a meta-analysis investigating the use of echinacea to treat the common cold. The authors chose to include trials of products containing echinacea in which the trials evaluated the duration or incidence of cold symptoms. The authors reported that products containing echinacea decreased the duration of cold symptoms by 1.4 days compared to a placebo. This review has been critiqued for selecting studies with methodological flaws, including small studies with inadequate blinding, and overlooking negative effects presented in trials.

Although some of these preliminary results appear promising, further research is required to confirm the efficacy of echinacea in the management of acute upper respiratory tract infections or the common cold. Most importantly, it is necessary to determine which specific extracts of echinacea are associated with positive clinical effects in humans.

Prevention of Upper Respiratory Tract Infections (Including the Common Cold)

A review was completed in 2008 that assessed the efficacy of echinacea products for the prevention of upper respiratory tract infections. The authors chose to include only trials that used echinacea as a monotherapy (single therapeutic agent) compared to a placebo, with no other active prevention strategy. They also excluded trials in which participants were artificially exposed to rhinovirus. This review identified two randomized, placebo-controlled clinical trials with a total of three echinacea treatment groups and 411 healthy volunteers. Participants were administered either 4 mL pressed echinacea juice, *Echinacea purpurea* root extract, or *Echinacea angustifolia* root extract, which were compared with the placebo for either 8 or 12 weeks. Neither of these trials found a statistically significant decrease in the incidence of upper respiratory tract infections in the participants treated with echinacea compared to the placebo. The authors did note a slight decrease in the number of participants that experienced one or more episodes of a cold in the treatment groups, and they concluded that this small potential effect may become more evident in larger trials.

> *Overall, current evidence from clinical trials suggests that prophylactic ingestion of echinacea is unlikely to result in a clinically significant reduction of the incidence, severity, or duration of the common cold.*

A review conducted in 2007, including a total of 731 participants, identified nine randomized controlled trials, five negative and four positive, investigating the use of echinacea for preventing upper respiratory tract infection. These included one trial that used echinacea in combination with other supplements and also included three trials in which participants were artificially exposed to rhinovirus. A meta-analysis of these trials determined that participants in the echinacea treatment group had a decrease of 65% in the chance of experiencing an upper respiratory infection compared to control or a placebo; however, when participants were exposed to rhinovirus, there was a decrease of only 35%. The authors of this review postulated that this decreased benefit may be a result of heterogeneity in echinacea's ability to defend against certain viruses and concluded that echinacea appears to be effective in prevention of upper respiratory tract infections. These authors have been criticized for their methods of rating articles and selective weighing of articles for their meta-analysis.

One additional negative double-blind, randomized, placebo-controlled trial investigating echinacea for prevention of colds has been published since these reviews were completed. This trial randomized hospital workers to receive either 3 capsules of *E. purpurea* (300 mg each, part of plant not specified) or a placebo (parsley) daily for 8 weeks during the winter. A total of 28 participants in the echinacea group and 30 participants in the placebo group completed the study, and the authors reported that 5 fewer sick days (9 vs. 14) were needed in the echinacea treatment group over this period of 8 weeks. They concluded that this was not a statistically significant result and that echinacea was ineffective in decreasing the incidence of upper respiratory tract infections in this study.

Overall, current evidence from clinical trials suggests that prophylactic ingestion of echinacea is unlikely to result in a clinically significant reduction of the incidence, severity, or duration of the common cold. Larger — and more costly — clinical trials are necessary to confirm these findings. The expense may be worthwhile, given the popularity of this herb in preventing colds and flus.

Complex Action

Research teams have demonstrated that extracts of *E. purpurea* increase phagocytosis significantly in vitro and in vivo; increase proliferation of phagocytes in spleen and bone marrow; stimulate migration of granulocytes to the peripheral blood; stimulate macrophages to excrete tumor necrosis factor (TNF); stimulate macrophages to secrete interleukin-1 (IL-1) and interleukin-6 (IL-6); stimulate monocytes to produce IL-1, IL-6, and TNF; stimulate macrophages to produce interferon-B2; independently and directly activate macrophages to cytotoxicity; increase properdin levels; and increase the number of PMN and activate the adherence of PMN to the endothelial cells.

In addition, studies revealed that *E. purpurea* extracts appear to have no direct action on T lymphocytes, no induction of lymphokine (MAF) production, no significant stimulation of B cell proliferation, and no enhancement of specific immune responses (antibody production). Studies with *E. angustifolia* extracts have demonstrated a statistically significant increase in the phagocytic activity of peritoneal macrophages in mice.

One study demonstrated that many of the effects of *E. purpurea* extracts previously noted in vitro or in animal models were also found when an extract was given to human test subjects. Effects demonstrated in humans include activating the adherence of PMN to endothelial cells, increasing phagocytosis, migration of granulocytes from bone marrow into the peripheral blood, increasing production of IL-6, and decreasing the suppression of immune system markers that normally occur with exercise.

> *The pharmacology of this herb and its many constituents is complex, emphasizing the need for additional research in determining echinacea's mode of action.*

In contrast to earlier studies, a double-blind, placebo-controlled crossover study (N=20) of the nonspecific immune response after the oral ingestion for 14 days of the freshly expressed juice of *E. purpurea* (dose not specified), identical in composition to the commercially available German product Esberitox, reported that echinacea did not enhance phagocytic activity of polymorphonuclear leukocytes, nor that of monocytes, when compared with the placebo. In addition, in this study the echinacea dose did not influence the production of TNF-alpha, nor that of interleukin 1-beta. Unexpectedly, the echinacea did decrease serum ferritin concentration.

Clearly, the pharmacology of this herb and its many constituents is complex, emphasizing the need for additional research in determining echinacea's mode of action. Given that the majority of studies discussed above were completed with defined-composition extracts, it is difficult to extrapolate the results of these studies to consumption of the varied commercially available preparations of echinacea species in clinical settings.

Anti-Inflammatory Activity

Several small studies support echinacea's historical use as an anti-inflammatory agent. In one clinical study, patients with chronic inflammation (9 due to viral infections, 14 due to bacterial infections) were administered injections of Echinacin (1 ampoule intermuscularly once daily for 7 days). There was an increase in the total lymphocyte count, with a decreased percentage of T4 cells. Similar results were obtained in another study of patients suffering from contact eczema (N=4), neurodermatitis (N=6), herpes simplex (N=8), and *Candida* infection (N=10). Echinacin was applied topically daily for 7 days. After 7 days, the proportion of T helper cells was decreased, but an overall lymphocytosis was observed.

A pilot study assessing the use of oral *Echinacea purpurea* extract to treat low-grade autoimmune idiopathic uveitis (an inflammation of one or more layers in the eye) enrolled 51 participants who ingested either 150 mg echinacea twice daily, accompanied by conventional steroid therapy, or steroid therapy alone for 9 months (blinding and randomization not described in the report). The authors reported that participants taking echinacea experienced shorter treatment periods and concluded that echinacea may be a safe and effective treatment for treating this form of inflammatory uveitis.

Antibacterial and Antiviral Activity

Echinacea has been shown to have only very weak activity as an antiviral, antibacterial, or antifungal agent. Several extracts of *E. angustifolia* (echinacoside and an alcoholic extract) have shown limited inhibitory activity against *Staphylococcus aureus*, *Escherichia coli*, *Pseudomonas aeruginosa*, and *Trichomonas vaginalis* in vitro. Several compounds isolated from *E. purpurea* were also shown to have weak activity against *E. coli* and *Pseudomonas aeruginosa*. Echinacea does not appear to be clinically useful as an antibiotic.

Several teams of researchers have noted the antiviral activity of echinacea. Echinacin (*E. purpurea*) was reported to have some activity in mice against encephalomyocarditis virus (EMC virus) and vesicular stomatitis virus (VSV). In addition, extracts of *E. purpurea* were found to have some activity against influenza, herpes, VSV, and poliovirus in vitro. Extracts of *E. pallida* have also been reported to exhibit some inhibition of VSV. Given that the antiviral activity observed requires the presence of 0-2-diethylamino ethyl dextran (DEAE) (in vivo) and did not develop in the presence of hyaluronidase (in vitro), an "interferon-like" mechanism of action without the induction of interferon has been hypothesized.

> *Echinacea does not appear to be clinically useful as an antibiotic.*

Miscellaneous Effects

Anticancer

Echinacin (*E. purpurea*) was given at 60 mg/m2 intermuscularly daily on days 3 to 10 and then twice weekly as part of an immunotherapy protocol for 15 outpatients with metastasizing, far-advanced colorectal cancers. The protocol included cyclophosphamide (LDCY) 300 mg/m2 every 28 days and thymostimulin 30 mg/m2 on days 3 to 10 and then twice weekly. Stimulation of the phagocytic activity of peripheral blood leukocytes was noted 14 days after the low-dose cyclophosphamide and attributed to the effect of the Echinacin. Mean survival time was 4 months, and two patients survived more than 8 months. Given the advanced stage of the disease in these patients, comparison of these survival times with others reported in the literature was not possible. A randomized, placebo-controlled trial is needed to assess the effects of this protocol on survival. A second study has suggested that components of echinacea may have the potential to promote anticancer activity.

Radiation Protection

One study in irradiated rats suggests that *Echinacea purpurea* promoted the effective functioning of the vitamin E redox system by mobilizing the body's stores of liposoluble vitamin A, carotene, and vitamin E. The relevance of this for humans is not clear.

Chemotherapy-Induced Leukopenia Prevention

There is one open prospective study with matched historical controls of 15 patients with advanced gastric cancer undergoing palliative chemotherapy who were injected (IV) with 2 mg of the polysaccharide fraction isolated from *Echinacea purpurea* (EPS-EPO VIIa) for 10 days, beginning 3 days before chemotherapy. The results of this pilot study suggest that this extract of echinacea, administered IV, might be effective in reducing chemotherapy-induced leukopenia. This evidence is promising and suggests that further research in this area may be warranted.

Skin Photodamage Protection

One study suggests that echinacea species have a dose-dependent protective effect on the free radical-induced degradation of type III collagen. The authors suggest that echinacea products may be useful in the prevention and treatment of photodamage of the skin. Further research is needed to confirm these preliminary findings.

Recurrent Genital Herpes

There is one randomized, double-blind, placebo-controlled crossover trial designed to assess whether an extract of echinacea (*Echinacea purpurea*, Echinaforce brand) could influence the clinical course of recurrent genital herpes. Fifty patients took 800 mg of echinacea twice daily for 6 months; however, no statistically significant benefit could be detected when the echinacea and placebo groups were compared (outcomes included frequency and severity of genital herpes recurrences).

Snake Bites

Historically, echinacea species were used for the treatment of snake bites and were reported to reduce the spread of venom. Scientific investigation of this phenomenon occurred primarily in the 1950s and centered on the effect of echinacea on hyaluronidase. All these studies were conducted with the German product Echinacin, which is made from the expressed juices of the aerial parts of *E. purpurea*, combined with 22% ethanol as a preservative. Echinacin has been shown to inhibit hyaluronidase production in vitro and in vivo. One study suggested that 0.04 mL of Echinacin was equivalent to 1 mg of cortisone, using a modified spreading test in rats. It has been hypothesized that in addition to a direct effect on hyaluronidase production, Echinacin may also stimulate changes in fibroblasts, resulting in an indirect effect on the hyaluronic acid-hyaluronidase system.

Comparative Studies

One study found that the ethanolic root extracts of all three species caused a 20% to 30% increase in phagocytosis in vitro and in vivo, with *E. purpurea* appearing slightly (non-significantly) more active than the other two species. Another trial found that *E. purpurea* was significantly more active in vitro than the other species. However, this trial has been criticized because the researchers used only 30% alcohol to make the extracts of each of the species and the tinctures of *E. angustifolia* used clinically are usually made with 80% alcohol. The different alcohol concentrations would likely result in the extraction of different compounds from the plant material. The sources of the three species were not reported.

Adverse Effects

While many reviews, including that of the German Commission E, indicate that there are no known toxic effects, several case reports and one clinical study identify possible adverse effects that may be associated with the use of echinacea. In addition, individuals with allergies to the sunflower family (Asteraceae, or Compositae) may theoretically experience mild allergic symptoms when ingesting echinacea.

Clinical Studies

One human study has suggested that consumption of standardized 1,000 mg *E. purpurea* for 10 days alters gastrointestinal flora and may increase the chance of diarrhea and inflammatory bowel disease after long-term use. Further studies are needed to determine if this is indeed a risk.

One case of echinacea-associated anaphylaxis has been reported in a 37-year-old woman who ingested 5 mL (approximately double the manufacturer's recommended amount) of an echinacea tincture containing *E. angustifolia* whole plant and *E. purpurea* root. The patient experienced an immediate burning of the mouth and throat, followed within a few minutes by tightness in the chest, generalized urticaria, and diarrhea. Her symptoms resolved completely during 2 hours of observation in the emergency department, with no need for further treatment (the patient self-medicated with 75 mg promethazine orally prior to being transported to the hospital).

> *As with most herbal adverse event reports, little or no attempt has been made to determine the quality of the echinacea products to rule out potential adulterants that may be the cause of the patients' symptoms.*

At least 26 cases suggestive of possible immunoglobulin E-mediated hypersensitivity (4 anaphylaxis, 12 acute asthma, 10 urticaria/angioedema) associated with echinacea have been reported to the Australian adverse drug reactions reporting system. In addition, there is a case report of recurrent erythema nodosum that was temporally associated with the use of echinacea. However, as with most herbal adverse event reports, little or no attempt has been made to determine the quality of the echinacea products to rule out potential adulterants that may be the cause of the patients' symptoms.

One case of echinacea-induced severe acute hepatitis has also been reported. The 45-year-old male patient had started taking echinacea root tablets at a daily dosage of 1,500 mg after he had caught a cold to help his immune system. After about 2 weeks of echinacea ingestion, he started experiencing fatigue and jaundice and was admitted to the hospital. One month after discontinuation of echinacea, the man's symptoms had resolved and his laboratory tests were normalized.

Animal Studies

Using the Lorke method on mice, LD50 values of less than 2,500 and 5,000 mg/kg have been found for a polysaccharide mixture from the aerial parts of E. purpurea and from a cell culture of E. purpurea respectively. The animals died not from the echinacea, but from the hyperosmolar solution injected in such large amounts. E. purpurea cell cultures have also been tested for possible gene toxicity in human lymphocyte cultures and found to have no significant toxic effects in short- or long-term experiments. No hepatotoxic effects have been found, or are expected, with the pyrrolizidine alkaloids in echinacea species because they do not contain the 1,2-unsaturated necine ring system.

Finally, some concern has been raised given the reported in vitro stimulation of the secretion of TNF and the potential role of TNF in cachexia and endotoxic shock. However, it has been argued that an increase in the secretion of TNF has been demonstrated only by using purified polysaccharides derived from E. purpurea cells cultured in vitro and that these polysaccharides are not present in most commercial products. More recent evidence questions whether echinacea affects TNF at all.

In the past, Echinacea purpurea roots have been adulterated with Parthenium integrifolium L., Asteraceae (Missouri snakeroot), which may have caused other adverse effects.

Cautions/Contraindications

External

None known.

Internal

Echinacea should be used with caution by patients with progressive systemic diseases (e.g., tuberculosis, leucoses, multiple sclerosis) or autoimmune conditions (e.g., diabetes mellitus, lupus, rheumatoid arthritis). Use of echinacea is also controversial in HIV/AIDS. However, it has been argued that these contraindications are not necessary. A few studies argue that no clinical evidence exists to support these claims and cites historical evidence that echinacea has actually been used to treat tuberculosis and leukemia.

> *Echinacea should be used with caution by patients with progressive systemic diseases (e.g., tuberculosis, leucoses, multiple sclerosis) or autoimmune conditions (e.g., diabetes mellitus, lupus, rheumatoid arthritis).*

There is currently very little research investigating the safety of echinacea use by women who are pregnant. One prospective controlled cohort study conducted by the Motherisk Program at the Hospital for Sick Children in Toronto (N=206) concluded that gestational use of echinacea and echinacea products does not appear to be associated with increased risk for major malformation. Additional research in this area is required to confirm these findings.

Dosage Regimens

Echinacea has widely been reported to lose its ability to stimulate the immune system if taken continuously for extended periods of time, but there appears to be little scientific evidence to clearly support or confirm this claim. It has been argued that oral doses of echinacea have never been shown to lose their effectiveness; recent clinical trials have demonstrated continued effects from echinacea at 8 weeks or more. This opinion is supported by Kerry Bone. Another study reviews the literature and recommends that echinacea products be taken cyclically: 10 to 14 days on, with a 3-day rest period. The German Commission E monograph suggests that echinacea should not be taken continuously (internally or externally) for more than 8 weeks.

Internal
- Dried herb: 1 g three times daily.
- Hydroalcoholic tincture (1:5 in 45% ethanol): 2–5 mL three times daily.
- Liquid extract (1:1 in 45% ethanol): 0.5–1.0 mL three times daily.
- Expressed juice (*E. purpurea*): 6–9 mL daily in divided doses.

External
- Semi-solid preparations should contain at least 15% expressed juice (*E. Purpurea*).

Note: Commercially available products are sometimes standardized for cichoric acid, polysaccharide, or alkamide content. These compounds are believed to have clinical activity. Some products are standardized for echinacoside content, which is a method of demonstrating authenticity (for *E. angustifolia*) rather than a measure of therapeutic potency.

Drug Interactions

None are reported by the German Commission E; however, echinacea's effects theoretically oppose the action of immunosuppressants.

Selected References

Linde K, Barrett B, Bauer R, Melchart D, Woelkart K. Echinacea for preventing and treating the common cold. Cochrane Database of Systematic Reviews 2008 (3).

Shah SA, Sander S, White MC, Rinaldi M, Coleman CI. Evaluation of echinacea for the prevention and treatment of the common cold: A meta-analysis. Lancet Infectious Disease 2007;7:473–80.

Elder

Sambucus nigra L.

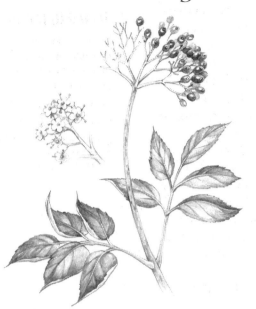

Common Uses
- *Internal:* Respiratory tract ailments (especially with fever and phlegm colds, flu, sinusitis, hay fever, and bronchitis), diuretic (urinary) ailments
- *External:* Eczema, boils, dermatitis

Active Constituents
- Flavonoids
- Triterpenes
- Essential oils
- Sterols
- Phenolic acids

Adverse Effects
- None noted with berries or flowers of American or European elder

Cautions/Contraindications
- Pregnancy and breastfeeding
- Autoimmune conditions (caution)
- Drug interactions
- Antidiabetic medications (theoretical)

Doses
Internal
- *Dried flowers:* 3–5 g three times daily
- *Liquid extract (1:1 in 25% ethanol):* 3–5 mL three times daily
- *Tincture (1:5 in 25% ethanol):* 10–25 mL three times daily

External
- Elder flowers can also be used externally in the form of poultices, ointments, and salves

Introduction

Family
- Caprifoliaceae

Synonyms
- Sambucus
- Black elder
- Common elder
- Pipe tree
- Bore tree
- Bour tree
- Hylder
- Hylantree
- Eldrum
- Hollunder
- Sureau
- Sweet elder (canadensis)
- Rob elder (canadensis)
- Elderberry (canadensis)
- S. nigra L. ssp. canadensis (L.) R. Bolli

Medicinal Forms
- Internal
- Dried flowers infusion
- Liquid extract
- Tincture
- External
- Poultices
- Salves
- Ointments

Description

Both the *Sambucus nigra* L. (European elder) and *S. nigra* L. ssp. *canadensis* (L.) R. Bolli (American elder) tree are used medicinally. They share similar indications and appearance, except that the European elder is slightly larger, growing up to 10 meters (33 feet) in height as compared to 4 meters (22 feet) for its North American cousin. *S. nigra* L. ssp. *canadensis* (L.) R. Bolli is native to the eastern United States and Canada, while *Sambucus nigra* L. is commonplace throughout the hedgerows of the United Kingdom and Europe. Both species can now be found throughout North America. The tree blooms with yellow-white flowers in late spring, and the berries turn from dark red to black.

Parts Used

While the flowers are the part most commonly used medicinally, most parts, notably the leaves and berries, are considered to have therapeutic properties.

Traditional Use

Known as Mother Nature's medicine chest, elder has traditionally been used to treat a wide variety of ailments, including coughs, colds, allergies, and arthritis. Elder is also rich in folklore, believed to be a good charm and used to drive away robbers and kill snakes. In rural England, it was considered a grave offence to damage any part of the tree, since it was thought to be inhabited by the Elder Mother and intrinsically linked to Mother Earth. Elderberries are also used as food in making elderberry pie and wine. Another species, red elderberry (*Sambucus racemosa*), has long been used by the Haida, Saanich, and Cowichan peoples of British Columbia in the treatment of many conditions, ranging from women's health to uses similar to those for *Sambucus nigra* L. and *S. nigra* L. ssp. *canadensis* (L.) R. Bolli.

Current Medicinal Use

Based on traditional evidence, elder flowers are used in the treatment of many respiratory conditions where there is fever and/or phlegm (colds, flu, hay fever, sinusitis, recurrent ear infections, bronchitis, croup) and ailments of the urinary system. Ointments, lotions, and salves made from elder flowers are used to treat various skin conditions and irritations (eczema, dermatitis, urticaria).

Relevant Research

Preventative and Therapeutic Effects

Constituents
Based on investigations of European elder only.

Flowers
- **Flavonoids:** quercetin, kaempferol, isoquercetin, rutin, astragalin.
- **Triterpenes:** ursolic acid, amyrin, 30 hydroxyursolic acid.
- **Essential oil:** fatty acids, alkanes.
- **Phenolic acids:** chlorogenic acid, p-coumaric acid, caffeic acid.
- **Miscellaneous:** mucilage, tannins, potassium, pectin, proteins (plastocynin).

Leaf
- Similar to above, with cyanogenic glucosides (sambunigrin) also present.

Berries
- Fruit acids, tannins, anthocyanin pigments, pectin, traces of essential oil.

Bark
- Phytohemagglutins, lectin, triterpenoids, cyanogenic glucosides.

Component Effects
Preparations made from various parts of the plant are suggested to be useful in the management of many conditions. Different parts are used for different indications.

Flowers
Elder flowers are used — alone or in combination with other herbal remedies, such as peppermint — in the treatment of many respiratory conditions where there is fever and/or phlegm, including colds, flu, hay fever, sinusitis, recurrent ear infections, bronchitis, and croup. Gargles made from the flower are used to ease sore and irritated throats. Preparations of elder flower are particularly popular in pediatric cases.

The flowers have also been used for many conditions of the genitourinary tract, such as cystitis and renal stones. Generally, elder may be indicated in situations where diuresis is required.

In addition, ointments, lotions, and salves made from elder flowers are used to treat various skin conditions, including eczema, dermatitis, urticaria, and generally irritated skin.

Berries
The berries are considered useful as an antirheumatic (anti-arthritis) and laxative. Liquid extracts made from the berries are now commonly used in monodiets, juice fasts, and detoxification protocols.

Flu
In a 2007 review, two double-blind, randomized controlled trials were found in which elder was used to treat viral infections associated with flu symptoms. Both showed positive results when participants ingested Sambucol (a syrup that contains 38% standardized elder extract along with raspberry extract, glucose, citric acid, and honey) for 3 days. Children were given 30 mL daily and adults ingested 60 mL daily of the elder treatment or a placebo. In the first trial, of the 27 patients who completed the study, 25 had laboratory confirmation of influenza A or B infection, and all were experiencing typical early flu symptoms. Elder supplementation resulted in a significant improvement in symptoms, including fever, and led to recovery in 2 days on average, which was at least 4 days earlier than those in the control group. Clinically significant improvement in flu symptoms was observed in 14 of 15 subjects in the treatment group 2 days after their first dose, with complete symptom recovery in 13 of 15 subjects in the elder group after 3 days. However, in the placebo group, only

4 of the 12 participants recovered completely within 3 days of their first dose and only 5 of the 12 subjects in the placebo group had recovered after 5 days.

In the second trial, patients experiencing early flu symptoms received 15 mL of Sambucol or placebo syrup four times daily for 5 days. Symptoms were reported to be relieved 4 days sooner than in the control group, and the use of rescue medication was significantly reduced in the elder group. It also took the placebo group 7 to 8 days to reach the same level of subjective improvement that the patients in the treatment group reached in 3 to 4 days.

Since the product tested in both trials contained other ingredients, such as raspberry extract, glucose, citric acid, and honey, it is impossible to attribute the effect of the treatment entirely to the elder. Further research appears warranted.

Cholesterol-Lowering Effects

Current research suggests that intake of elderberry juice may not result in changed blood cholesterol levels and may not affect low-density lipoprotein (LDL) stability. A randomized, placebo-controlled pilot study with 6 subjects originally reported a reduction of plasma cholesterol concentrations after 2 weeks and an increase in the resistance to oxidation of LDL after 3 weeks of taking elderberry juice. However, when the same authors conducted a full-scale randomized, placebo-controlled trial, they found no significant differences in the outcomes of the placebo and the treatment group. The full-scale study included 34 participants who

> *Current research suggests that intake of elderberry juice may not result in changed blood cholesterol levels and may not affect low-density lipoprotein (LDL) stability.*

took either 400 mg capsules of spray-dried powder containing 10% anthocyanes three times daily (which is equivalent to 5 mL elderberry juice) or a placebo for 2 weeks, and a subgroup of 14 subjects who continued for an additional week to test for resistance to oxidation of LDL. All participants were instructed to follow a diet containing 35% fat. The authors suggest that elderberry at higher, or "nutritionally relevant," doses may be effective at lowering cholesterol. One criticism of this study is that the participants were young volunteers, and whether they had high LDL cholesterol levels was not disclosed.

> *Elder may be able to stimulate insulin secretion and sugar metabolism. More research is needed to explore its use in humans diagnosed with diabetes.*

Diabetes

Although elder flower is traditionally recommended in folk medicine for use in symptoms associated with diabetes, no studies in humans have yet been published to support its efficacy. However, in a controlled in vitro study, aqueous extract of elder flower significantly increased glucose (sugar) uptake, glucose oxidation, and sugar synthesis in rats' abdominal muscle. Elder may be able to stimulate insulin secretion and sugar metabolism. More research is needed to explore its use in humans diagnosed with diabetes.

Miscellaneous Effects

Pharmacological findings provide preliminary explanations for some of elder's indications. Extracts of *Sambucus nigra* L. have been shown to exert a diuretic effect in rats, primarily as a result of the flavonoid and potassium content. This may explain its use in disorders of the genitourinary tract. As well, a methanolic extract of the branch tips of red elderberry has been shown to exhibit activity against bovine (cow) respiratory syncytial virus. Red elderberry has also been shown to have some other antiviral activity, as well as antibacterial and antifungal activity. While the extracts of various species of *Sambucus* have been used as diagnostic tools (e.g., as an indication of immunocompetence), no human clinical trials could be found to substantiate the above indications.

With respect to elder's antiviral activity, although studies in humans are needed to support its protective effects in HIV infection, six case studies reported that taking a combination of thymus extract and elderberry extract resulted in a diminished viral burden in patients with HIV. A combination product of elder flower extract with *Hypericum perforatum* (St. John's wort) and *Saponaria officinalis* (soapwort) was also found to stop the replication of herpes virus-1 in a test tube study.

Other miscellaneous actions of elder have also been reported. For example, taking an elder extract has been shown to have mild anti-inflammatory properties in rats, and lectins (sugar-binding proteins) extracted from European elder have been shown to possess antispasmodic properties in vitro. In test tube studies, elderberry extract has been able to fight oxidative stress via inhibition of LDL oxidation and binding to free radicals. This may make elder a potentially valuable therapeutic role in cardiovascular disease, cancer, neurodegenerative disease, peripheral vascular disease, autoimmune diseases, and multiple sclerosis. Because elderberry may also improve endothelial cell (a type of cell that makes up blood vessels) function, its use may prevent some vascular diseases.

Adverse Effects

The flowers and ripe seeds appear to be free from adverse effects and are considered in the United States as GRAS (generally regarded as safe). Substances found in other parts of the plant, notably the cyanogenic glycosides, have the potential to cause gastrointestinal distress, including nausea, diarrhea, and vomiting. One authority cautions that the seeds of *Sambucus racemosa* may cause irritation to the mucous membranes. Although the lectins have been shown to have the potential to cause birth defects in pregnant mice, the doses administered were far above those possible in normal practice.

Cautions/Contraindications

Caution has been recommended against use in pregnancy and during breastfeeding, as well as against long-term use, because there is a lack of toxicity data and the safety of elder taken during pregnancy has not yet been established.

Because elderberry might have stimulating effects on the immune system, its use may worsen the symptoms of autoimmune diseases by stimulating disease activity. Therefore, patients with autoimmune diseases, such as multiple sclerosis, systemic lupus erythematosus, rheumatoid arthritis, or others, are advised to avoid taking elderberry.

Drug Interactions

No drug interactions have been recorded. However, elder may be able to lower blood sugar levels and thus may have additive effects when used with antidiabetic medications that also lower sugar levels.

Dosage Regimens
Internal (General)
- Liquid extract of dried flowers (1:1 in 25% ethanol): 3–5 mL three times daily.
- Tincture of dried flowers (1:5 in 25% ethanol): 10–25 mL three times daily.
- Tea made from 3–5 g of the dried flowers steeped in 250 mL boiling water for 10 to 15 minutes, taken three times daily.

External
- Elder flowers can also be used externally in the form of poultices, ointments, and salves.

Note: Even though parts from the whole plant have been used historically, medicinal use should be limited to the flowers and ripe berries (which are usually boiled). Elder flowers are also often taken in the form of cordials and for nutritious rather than medicinal reasons.

Selected References

Guo R, Pittler MH, Ernst E. Complementary medicine for treating or preventing influenza or influenza-like illness. The American Journal of Medicine 2007;120(11):923–29.

Murkovic M, Abuja PM, Bergmann AR, Zirngast A, Adam U, Winklhofer-Roob BM, et al. Effects of elderberry juice on fasting and postprandial serum lipids and low-density lipoprotein oxidation in healthy volunteers: A randomized, double-blind, placebo-controlled study. European Journal of Clinical Nutrition 2004 Feb;58(2):244–49.

Evening Primrose

Oenothera biennis L.

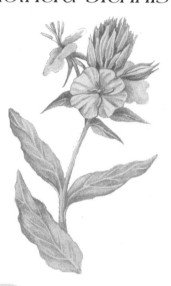

Common Uses

- Atopic eczema
- Diabetic neuropathy
- Women's health care (including premenstrual syndrome, mastalgia, and endometriosis)
- Rheumatoid arthritis
- Multiple sclerosis
- Sjögren's syndrome
- Psychiatric conditions (schizophrenia, hyperactivity in children, dementia)
- Alcoholism
- Obesity

Active Constituents

- Fixed oil (containing gamma-linolenic acid and linoleic acid)

Cautions/Contraindications

- Mania
- Epilepsy

Drug Interactions

- None documented, but concerns have been raised regarding use with phenothiazines, non-steroidal anti-inflammatory drugs (NSAIDs), corticosteroids, anticoagulants, beta-adrenergic antagonists, and some anticancer drugs

Doses

- *Adults:* 2–8 g seed oil daily in divided doses with food
- *Children:* 2–6 g seed oil daily in divided doses with food

Introduction

Family
- Onagraceae

Synonyms
- Tree primrose
- Sundrop
- King's cure-all

Medicinal Forms
- Seed oil (capsules or liquid form)

Description

Evening primrose is a biennial standing 1 to 3 meters (3 to 6 feet) in height. The stem rises from a fibrous taproot, with a flat, basal rosette of leaves. The plant blooms in early summer, producing large yellow flowers. The capsular pods that form after the individual blooms die contain brown seeds rich in fixed oil. Evening primrose is actually not a primrose (Primulaceae family) at all but a member of the fuchsia (Onagraceae) family. Its name arises from the fact that the flowers open in the evening to allow pollination by insects, especially moths. While *Oenothera biennis* L. is native to North America, it is now naturalized throughout Western Europe, brought there accidentally as sea trade increased between the two continents.

Parts Used

While the root and whole plant of evening primrose have been used in the past, the fixed oil from the seeds is now the primary form used therapeutically.

Traditional Use

Evening primrose has been used for both medical and culinary purposes in the past. The root was used as a vegetable because of its pungent flavor, and the whole plant was indicated in the management of many conditions, including gastrointestinal disorders, asthmatic coughs, neuralgia, and whooping cough. These numerous indications gave rise to the plant being commonly referred to as the king's cure-all.

Evening primrose oil was one the first nutritional and botanical supplements to gain popularity in the renaissance of alternative medicine. The popularity of evening primrose oil supplements is such that a survey of complementary medicine use in Australia in 1993 showed that more than 12% of all women supplemented with this product.

Current Medicinal Use

As a source of preformed gamma-linolenic acid, evening primrose oil may be of use in a number of conditions, especially those with an inflammatory component. Evidence from clinical trials of the efficacy of evening primrose for specific conditions is usually not complete and is often conflicting. Despite this, it is commonly used in women's health care and for treating atopic eczema. No matter what the reason for taking evening primrose oil, it needs to be taken for a prolonged period of time (over 6 months) for best results.

Relevant Research

Preventative and Therapeutic Effects

Constituents

Given that the fixed oil of evening primrose oil is the part used medicinally, this analysis of the plant's constituents is limited to the seeds.

Approximately 14% fixed oil, comprising approximately:

- *Cis*-linoleic acid (70%)
- *Cis*-gamma-linolenic acid (9%)
- Oleic acid
- Palmitic acid
- Stearic acid

Essential Fatty Acids

To understand the suggested pharmacology of evening primrose oil, it is necessary to review some basic points regarding essential fatty acid (EFA) biochemistry and nomenclature. By definition, an essential fatty acid is one that the body cannot make. There are two basic types, omega 3 (derived from alpha-linolenic acid) and omega 6 (derived from linoleic acid). These essential fatty acids are polyunsaturated (they contain more than one double bond). A particular fatty acid is named by determining the position of the first double bond from the methyl end of the carbon-carbon backbone of the molecule. For example, an omega 3 fatty acid contains a double bond between the third and fourth carbon atom. The essential fatty acids have a *cis* rather than a *trans* configuration, and the omega 3 and omega 6 series are not interchangeable.

Both alpha-linolenic and linoleic acid can be modified via desaturation or elongation reactions. While neither alpha-linolenic nor linoleic acid have any direct biological effect, their metabolites have pronounced physiological properties. The enzymatic mechanism by which these changes occur is very similar, if not identical, in both the omega 3 and omega 6 series. The physiological action of EFAs occurs in one of two primary ways. EFAs play a role in the physical properties of cell membranes, influencing their flexibility and fluidity, and thus they affect membrane-based receptors and systems. EFAs also act as precursors of biologically active eicasonoids such as prostaglandins and leukotrienes.

In the omega 6 series, *cis*-linoleic acid (LA) is converted to gamma-linolenic acid (GLA), which in turn is converted to dihomogamma-linolenic acid (DGLA). The rate-limiting step for this process is the desaturation of LA to GLA by the enzyme delta-6 desaturase. The DGLA can then be metabolized further to form arachadonic acid (AA) by delta-5 desaturase. DGLA can also be acted upon by cyclo-oxygenase to form prostaglandin E1 (PGE1). PGE1 is generally seen as beneficial, preventing inflammation and platelet aggregation, decreasing blood pressure, and regulating the immune system. On the other hand, arachidonic acid gives rise to harmful pro-inflammatory mediators. While it may be assumed that any increase in GLA would lead to a later increase in both the anti-inflammatory and inflammatory moieties, this does not appear to be the case. Administration of large amounts of GLA increases DGLA levels but not AA levels. It is thought that the beneficial metabolites of DGLA, including PGE1, play a role in limiting the release of arachidonic acid from its phospholipid stores. Also, while the conversion of GLA to DGLA is rapid, the activity of delta-5 desaturase is quite slow.

Since the body can manufacture GLA, it should not theoretically be considered an essential fatty acid. In practice, this may not be the case due to the inefficiency of the rate-limiting enzyme mentioned above, delta-6 desaturase. This enzyme system appears to be compromised in many situations, including aging, diabetes, excessive consumption of alcohol, viral infections, and atopic eczema.

A deficiency in certain nutritional cofactors (e.g., zinc, pyridoxine, and magnesium) can also lead to a decreased activity of this enzyme system. The existence of a decreased rate of delta-6 desaturation in atopic individuals is not universally accepted.

The therapeutic rationale for the use of evening primrose oil is that, since it is rich in GLA, it bypasses the rate-limiting delta-6 desaturase stage.

Dermatological Conditions

Atopic Eczema and Dermatitis

The fact that delta-6 desaturation may be slower in atopic individuals has led to the suggestion that oral administration of evening primrose oil could be beneficial in the management of atopic eczema. A number of clinical studies support this claim, showing that evening primrose oil significantly improved symptoms, including itching, inflammation, and dryness. The evidence is not universally positive, with a number of studies showing that evening primrose was not superior to a placebo in the management of this condition. Consequently, the use of evening primrose oil orally in the management of atopic eczema in North America remains controversial. In contrast, evening primrose oil is considered suitable in the management of atopic eczema in many countries, including the United Kingdom, Germany, Australia, and New Zealand.

Several explanations for the failure of evening primrose oil in some studies have been suggested. First, omega 3 EFAs (deep-sea fish oil) may be as important as omega 6, implying that combination products containing both may be more beneficial. In some cases of atopy, other desaturation steps apart from the delta-6 stage could be involved. Finally, not all cases of atopic eczema are due to disorders of fatty acid metabolism.

There are no clinical trials of the oral use of evening primrose oil for eczema or dermatitis; however, in a survey of 100 children with atopic dermatitis, 13% of children who had evening primrose oil supplemented into their diet felt that it had helped their skin.

Evening primrose oil is considered suitable in the management of atopic eczema in many countries, including the United Kingdom, Germany, Australia, and New Zealand.

Examples of the multiple studies of topical preparations containing evening primrose oil are described below. Topical application of a cream containing 12.5% evening primrose oil given to 20 volunteers with dry skin significantly increased sebum content without changing transepidermal water loss. While the volunteers had an atopic disposition, they did not show symptoms of frank atopic dermatitis. Evening primrose oil, when applied topically, did not prevent steroid-induced thinning of the skin caused by the twice daily application of 0.1% betamethasone valerate.

When a cream made up of 20% evening primrose oil was applied to 155 participants, 137 of whom had atopic dermatitis, there was significantly less reddening, scaling, drying, itching, and hardening of the skin. Topical treatment with a cream containing evening primrose oil as a main ingredient (amount was not disclosed) in 37 children with atopic dermatitis, aged 6 months to 12 years old, resulted in significantly decreased dryness and itchiness of the skin compared to the control group of 39 children.

Psoriasis

The supplementation of evening primrose oil and marine oil (i.e., omega 6 and omega 3) have proven unsuccessful in the management of psoriasis.

Scleroderma

Patients treated with evening primrose oil showed decreased hand pain, more healed ulcers, improved skin texture, and less dilated capillaries in the face, hands, or mouth. Incidents of Raynaud's phenomenon associated with scleroderma also decreased with evening primrose oil treatment. A combination treatment of fish oil and evening primrose oil did not show a significant improvement in symptoms over the control group, but another study points out that this may have been because the therapeutic effects of the placebo (sunflower oil) and additional supplementation (lithium) could have interfered with the action of treatment.

> *Patients treated with evening primrose oil showed decreased hand pain, more healed ulcers, improved skin texture, and less dilated capillaries in the face, hands, or mouth.*

Asthma

Oral administration of evening primrose oil appears not to be effective in the management of various forms of asthma.

Diabetic Neuropathy

The ratio of linoleic and linolenic acid to their respective metabolites has been found to be elevated in diabetes. In diabetic patients, both delta-6 and delta-5 desaturase enzymes may be impaired. This impairment of normal fatty acid metabolism and subsequent production of physiological moieties may play an important role in the development of diabetic neuropathy. By administering preformed gamma-linolenic acid, as in evening primrose oil, this imbalance may be corrected. The discovery that evening primrose oil may correct deficient nitric oxide in the nerve ischemia seen in diabetes implies that evening primrose's action may be more complex than was originally proposed. The role played by cyclo-oxygenase activity in the neuroactivity of evening primrose oil appears to be an important factor to consider. A latency period noted in a recent animal study has led to the suggestion that the action of evening primrose

oil may be mediated by metabolically generated compounds rather than by one existing in the oil itself.

A beneficial role for the use of evening primrose oil in the correction of the neurovascular disorders seen in diabetics has been demonstrated in a number of animal studies. Administration of 4 g of evening primrose oil (360 mg gamma-linolenic acid) daily for 6 months to 22 diabetic patients suffering from diabetic neuropathy caused an improvement (objective and subjective) when compared to a placebo. Glycosylated hemoglobin levels were not influenced by evening primrose oil supplementation. These positive findings were confirmed in a later double-blinded, multi-center trial with 11 patients suffering from "mild diabetic neuropathy." The dose of evening primrose oil was higher than in the previous study (6 g daily equivalent to 480 mg of gamma-linolenic acid) and the trial was carried out over 1 year. The response to evening primrose oil appeared more pronounced in those with lower starting glycosylated hemoglobin levels, suggesting satisfactory blood sugar control.

However, another small study in children had inconclusive results. In that double-blind, placebo-controlled study, 11 children with insulin-dependent diabetes were given either 2 capsules of seed oil (each containing 45 mg of gamma-linolenic acid) or a placebo once daily for 4 months, then 4 capsules of evening primrose oil for another 4 months. The results were inconclusive as to whether evening primrose oil supplementation provides a protective effect on diabetic vascular complications.

> *A beneficial role for the use of evening primrose oil in the correction of the neurovascular disorders seen in diabetics has been demonstrated in a number of animal studies.*

It appears that the gamma-linolenic acid content of a supplement does not determine its efficacy in managing diabetic neuropathy. In a recent animal study, evening primrose oil supplementation was shown to outperform a number of other products rich in GLA (borage oil, black currant oil, and "fungal" oil).

Women's Health Care
Premenstrual Syndrome (PMS)

A number of studies have indicated that evening primrose oil may be of use in the management of premenstrual syndrome. The benefits are seen only following prolonged administration of 4 to 6 months. A proposed mechanism of action is that the PGE1 generated could influence the actions of prolactin, which is thought to play a role in the presentation of this syndrome. Women with premenstrual syndrome may also have difficulty in converting linoleic acid into gamma-linolenic acid. However, one review of the available literature concluded that evening primrose oil offered no benefit and argued that most of the information comes from low-quality, open studies and that the well-controlled studies were "small and modest" in design. The above comments about the need for prolonged administration could play a part in these negative findings.

> *A number of studies have indicated that evening primrose oil may be of use in the management of premenstrual syndrome.*

Mastalgia (Breast Pain)

Although it has been suggested that evening primrose oil is beneficial in the management of both cyclical and non-cyclical mastalgia (breast pain), most of the recent trials have not been positive. For example, while one study suggested it was as effective as bromocriptine, another suggested its effect to be only slightly greater than a placebo. One randomized, placebo-controlled, double-blind study of 120 women reported that ingestion of 3 g of evening primrose oil daily for 6 months did not offer a clear benefit over ingestion of control oils (corn oil and corn oil with wheat germ).

Another double-blind, placebo-controlled, parallel group, multi-center study of 555 women found that treatment with 2 g of evening primrose oil twice daily for at least 4 months did not result in a substantial difference over placebo fatty acids (coconut oil). An open label, non-randomized, comparative study of topical non-steroidal anti-inflammatory gel versus evening primrose oil found that the herbal supplementation reduced pain in the breast, but less significantly than did the drug treatment. A limitation was that the study lasted only 3 months, and it may take at least this amount of time for dietary supplements to produce their maximal effect.

The potential advantage of evening primrose oil over other more conventional therapies appears to be the lack of adverse effects. The suggested mechanism of action is via prolactin modulation. As with the case of premenstrual syndrome, benefits are only noted after prolonged use, usually 4 to 6 months.

Endometriosis

A combination product containing both gamma-linolenic acid and the omega 3 fatty acid eicosapentaenoic acid (Scotia HGA) was shown in a placebo-controlled trial to decrease the symptoms of endometriosis in 90% of cases.

Menopause Symptoms

While evening primrose oil is often used in the management of menopause, it appears to offer no benefit over a placebo in treating associated hot flashes and sweating. Most studies used combination products, making it difficult to identify any specific effects of evening primrose oil. For example, in one open-label, multi-center, randomized, group comparative efficacy and safety trial, 1,080

> *While evening primrose oil is often used in the management of menopause, it appears to offer no benefit over a placebo in treating associated hot flashes and sweating.*

women with menopausal symptoms received either 1 (N=562) or 2 capsules (N=518) daily for 6 months. Each capsule contained isoflavones (60 mg), primrose oil (440 mg), and vitamin E (10 mg).

The Blatt-Kupperman scale was used to monitor changes in menopausal complaints, including hot flashes, nervousness, insomnia, melancholy, dizziness, fatigue, muscle pain or soreness, headache, increased heartbeat, skin tingling or numbness, and other unpleasant abnormal sensations. A significant reduction in the Blatt-Kupperman scores were noted at the end of the trial; however, these findings were comparable for both treatment groups. Since everyone knew they were taking a supplement, it is possible that the changes were due to the placebo effect. Another study reported that daily ingestion of Efacal (a supplement containing 1 g calcium, 4 g evening primrose oil, and 440 mg marine fish oil) for 12 months by 42 postmenopausal women was not associated with significant increases in bone mineral density.

Inflammatory and Autoimmune Conditions

Rheumatoid Arthritis

Various in vitro and in vivo trials have demonstrated that prostaglandin E1 has anti-inflammatory properties. Since it has been suggested that evening primrose oil may increase the levels of this moiety, it may be therapeutically useful in the management of this condition. In a review of the relevant clinical trials, the authors conclude that the studies varied in both design and quality and that the evidence supporting its use in the management of this condition is not conclu-

sive. Any benefits appeared to be subjective rather than objective. Short-term administration appears to provide no clinical benefits, with relief being noted after 6 months in some studies. Since two of the clinical trials were of limited duration, this has been given as a possible explanation for their lack of positive results.

In a double-blind, placebo-controlled, 9-month trial of 38 patients suffering from psoriatic arthritis, a combination product containing evening primrose oil and fish oil (Efamol Marine) was seen to offer no therapeutic benefits.

Multiple Sclerosis

An association between multiple sclerosis and levels of linoleic acid has been noted. There is some evidence to suggest that evening primrose oil may be beneficial in reducing the severity, duration of relapses, and progression of the disease. The patients most likely to respond appear to be those with a recent diagnosis and less severe symptoms. The mode of action proposed is that the linoleic acid may be modifying an immune response and that the most benefit may be obtained by combining the therapy with a low animal fat, high polyunsaturated fat diet. The need to use the more expensive evening primrose oil rather than linoleic acid has been questioned.

Sjögren's Syndrome

Abnormalities in fatty acid metabolism have been noted in Sjögren's syndrome (a disorder in which a person's immune cells attack and kill their own tear- and saliva-producing cells). Supplementation with evening primrose oil has been shown to stimulate tearing and ease the drowsiness often present with this condition. However, a more recent randomized, double-blind, placebo-controlled trial reported that daily ingestion of 800 mg or 1,600 mg GLA (extracted from evening primrose oil) for 6 months by 90 patients with primary Sjögren's syndrome had no effect on fatigue compared to the placebo.

Cardiovascular Conditions

Essential fatty acids are known to play an important role in maintaining good cardiovascular health. Problems with essential fatty acid metabolism or inadequate intake are known to increase cholesterol, platelet aggregation, and blood pressure. Combination products of omega 3 and omega 6 oils may be useful in the management of various cardiovascular conditions. Both human and animal studies suggest that evening primrose oil can decrease blood pressure and inhibit platelet aggregation.

In a double-blind study, evening primrose oil supplementation was shown to result in symptomatic relief of patients suffering from Raynaud's phenomenon (a blood circulation disorder), but no changes in the objective measures were noted.

> *Essential fatty acids are known to play an important role in maintaining good cardiovascular health.*

Psychiatric Conditions
Attention Deficit Hyperactivity Disorder (ADHD)

Abnormalities in essential fatty acid metabolism have been noted in cases of children with hyperactivity disorder, behavioral problems, and learning difficulties, and the requirements for essential fatty acids and the incidence of hyperactivity are higher in boys than in girls. One review of clinical trials concluded that there are conflicting results for the therapeutic effects of evening primrose oil in children with attention deficit hyperactivity disorder. For example, two studies found treatment with evening primrose oil was linked to a decrease in inattention but not in hyperactivity.

The first was a randomized, double-blind, placebo-controlled crossover study in which 31 children (4 girls and 27 boys) with marked inattention and overactivity received 3 capsules twice daily of evening primrose oil (Efamol, each capsule containing 360 mg of linoleic acid and 45 mg of gamma-linoleic acid). The second was a randomized, placebo-controlled, double-blind study that involved 41 children (32 completed the trial) aged 8 to 12 years with both specific learning difficulties and above-average ADHD ratings (however, they were not officially diagnosed with ADHD or any other psychiatric disorder). The children in the treatment group were given either 8 capsules daily of evening primrose supplementation (480 mg docosahexaenoic acid, 186 mg eicosapentaenoic acid, 42 mg arachidonic acid, 96 mg gamma-linolenic acid, 864 mg *cis*-linoleic acid, and 8 mg thyme oil) or a placebo (olive oil) for 12 weeks.

In addition, a randomized, placebo-controlled, double-blind study that analyzed data from 104 children (of the 201 who enrolled in the trial) aged 7 to 12 years reported that administering a supplement containing evening primrose and fish oil for 15 weeks significantly improved parental — but not teacher — perceptions of hyperactivity and inattention.

Two other studies concluded that evening primrose oil had no significant effects on the behavior of children with this condition. The first of these negative studies was a randomized, placebo-controlled, double-blind study in which 50 children in the active treatment group were given a combination product containing fish oil and evening primrose oil supplementation (480 mg docosahexaenoic acid, 80 mg eicosapentaenoic acid, 40 mg arachidonic acid, 96 mg gamma-linolenic acid, and 24 mg alpha-tocopheryl acetate) for 4 months. The other study looked at 18 boys with ADHD who were given 4,000 mg evening primrose capsules.

Another placebo-controlled, double-blind study not included in the review involved hyperkinetic children aged 5 to 15. In this study, those who were given evening primrose oil supplementation did not exhibit

> *Abnormalities in essential fatty acid metabolism have been noted in cases of children with hyperactivity disorder, behavioral problems, and learning difficulties.*

improved behavioral patterns or changes in blood fatty acid composition compared to the placebo group. It is important to note that the placebo used in this case was safflower oil, a substance rich in essential fatty acids.

Another review of open-label case studies suggests, however, that supplementation with evening primrose oil may prove beneficial in treating hyperactivity. Clearly, more research is needed to clarify the role of evening primrose oil in the management of symptoms of attention deficit hyperactivity disorder.

Developmental Coordination Disorder (DCD)

One randomized, controlled, parallel (followed by one-way crossover) trial studied whether fatty acid supplementation (essential fatty acids from fish oil and evening primrose oil containing 558 mg EPA and 174 mg DHA delivered daily) affects behavioral and learning difficulties. A total of 117 children aged 5 to 12 years diagnosed with developmental coordination disorder in accordance with the *Diagnostic and Statistical Manual of Mental Disorders, 4th edition (DSM-IV)* were given either treatment or a placebo (olive oil) for 3 months, after which the placebo group was also given the fatty acid supplementation. Significant motor function improvement from baseline scores was seen in both the treatment and the placebo groups. However, only the treatment group showed favorable significant differences in reading and spelling, as well as in a wide range of ADHD-related symptoms.

When the fish oil and evening primrose oil supplementation was later given to the children in the placebo group, these children showed improvements comparable to those of the first group that received this treatment. The children in the first treatment group continued the supplementation in the second open-label part of the trial and maintained or improved on their earlier progress.

Dementia

Supplementation with evening primrose oil may prove beneficial in the management of various kinds of dementia, including Alzheimer's disease and those that are caused by aging.

Schizophrenia

While the exact pathophysiology of schizophrenia has yet to be determined, it has been suggested that abnormal essential fatty acid metabolism may be implicated. Decreased levels of linoleic acid in plasma phospholipids have been noted in schizophrenics. It has been suggested that they may have difficulty in producing PGE1, which may play a role in decreasing excessive central dopaminergic function, which is thought to play a role in the pathogenesis of the disease. Clinical research to date (placebo-controlled trials, open observational trials, and reported case histories) has produced contradictory results. In a group of psychiatric patients suffering from tardive dyskinesia induced by neuroleptics, evening primrose oil was reported to cause a "marginally significant" improvement. When four cofactors needed in essential fatty acid metabolism (zinc, pyridoxine, niacin, and vitamin C) were added to the treatment, this improvement, including enhancement of memory and alleviation of schizophrenic symptoms, was increased.

Miscellaneous Effects
Gastrointestinal Disorders

Evening primrose oil has been shown to "significantly improve stool consistency" in ulcerative colitis when compared to both a fish oil supplement and a placebo. No difference in the other symptoms (stool frequency, rectal bleeding, disease relapse, sigmoidoscopic appearance, or rectal histology) was seen. In a double-blind, placebo-controlled crossover trial, supplementation with evening primrose oil also produced some relief in women suffering from irritable bowel syndrome exacerbated premenstrually.

Postviral Fatigue Syndrome

Supplements containing evening primrose have been demonstrated to be effective in the management of postviral syndrome (aka chronic fatigue syndrome and myalgic encephalomyelitis) in both placebo-controlled trials and in clinical practice. In a double-blind, placebo-controlled trial of 63 adults with clear cases of postviral syndrome taking a combination product of evening primrose oil and fish oil (Efamol Marine), a pronounced improvement in symptoms (fatigue, muscle pain, dizziness, and poor concentration and memory) was noted. This study was carried out on volunteers with a clear viral cause to their condition. However, when a new study team attempted to replicate this 1990 study, their results contrasted sharply with the results of the original study. Although the patients' symptoms generally improved with time, the improvement was not statistically significant and there was no difference between the treatment and the placebo groups.

> *Supplements containing evening primrose have been demonstrated to be effective in the management of postviral syndrome (aka chronic fatigue syndrome and myalgic encephalomyelitis).*

Alcoholism

Alcohol is known to have multiple effects on the metabolism of essential fatty acids, causing depletion of linoleic acid stores, inhibiting the conversion of linoleic acid to gamma-linolenic acid, and stimulating the conversion of dihomogamma-linolenic acid to arachidonic acid. While alcohol initially increases PGE1 synthesis, long-term consumption causes a marked drop. Abrupt ending of alcohol consumption also causes a rapid fall in PGE1 levels. It has been hypothesized that administration of preformed gamma-linolenic acid may play a role in preventing alcohol toxicity and the development of alcohol addiction.

Human trials have shown that the administration of evening primrose oil decreases the need for tranquilizer use during the withdrawal phase and promotes the normalization of elevated liver enzymes. While long-term administration does not decrease the rate of relapse, it does appear to appreciably improve recovery of memory and visual-motor coordination. Animal studies have demonstrated that administration of evening primrose oil may decrease the damaging effect on the brain and decrease the potential of alcohol to cause birth defects in animals.

Renal (Kidney) Disease

Diets enriched with evening primrose oil have been shown to decrease the nephrotoxic (kidney-damaging) effect of cyclosporine in rats. Evidence from animal trials also suggests that evening primrose oil supplementation may prove beneficial in the treatment of urolithiasis.

Cancer

In vitro studies have shown that gamma-linolenic acid has antineoplastic properties. The clinical relevance of this has yet to be determined. An open-label trial with historical matched controls was conducted to assess the effects of adding 2.8 g GLA daily to tamoxifen therapy (20 mg daily) for 6 weeks in 30 patients with endocrine-sensitive breast cancer (20 stage I to stage II, 14 locally advanced, and 4 metastatic). Overall, the addition of GLA seemed to result in a significantly faster clinical response and a greater reduction in estrogen receptor expression. Additional research in this area is recommended.

Obesity

Evening primrose oil has been suggested to be useful in the management of obesity. Clinical studies on humans have reported mixed results. It is important to note that some authors suggest that not enough vigorous clinical trials exist to justify many of the uses suggested for evening primrose oil.

Adverse Effects

Evening primrose oil appears to be extremely safe. Adverse effects in humans are very rare and are limited to headache, nausea, and diarrhea. Evening primrose oil has been shown in animal studies to have no carcinogenic properties. At normal therapeutic doses (less than 4 g daily), it is unlikely that evening primrose oil would be harmful if taken in pregnancy; however, the composition of breast milk can be manipulated by supplementing the maternal diet with evening primrose oil.

Cautions/Contraindications

Evening primrose oil should not be used by individuals diagnosed with mania, because it may theoretically worsen the symptoms. Evening primrose oil should also be used with caution in patients suffering from epilepsy (see drug interactions).

Historically, evening primrose oil has been used by midwives to speed up cervical ripening in an effort to shorten labor. However, a recent open-label retrospective trial suggested that oral administration of evening primrose oil from the 37th week of pregnancy until birth does not shorten pregnancy or decrease the length of labor and may be associated with an increased incidence of prolonged rupture of membranes, increase of oxytocin, arrest of descent, and extraction of vacuum. Additional research is needed before evening primrose oil can be recommended in pregnancy.

Drug Interactions

No reports of interactions between evening primrose oil and conventional medication could be found. A possible increase in epileptic attacks has been suggested in schizophrenics taking phenothiazines who are also treated with evening primrose oil. The clinical likelihood of this occurring in practice has been questioned. A theoretical interaction between gamma-linolenic acid and both non-steroidal anti-inflammatory drugs and corticosteroids has been suggested. Whether this interaction would be synergistic or antagonistic depends on whether the GLA is acting as a precursor of PGE1 formation or if it modifies membrane composition.

The therapeutic action of a product containing GLA, such as evening primrose oil, may be decreased with patients taking beta blockers. This is due to the fact that cyclic AMP concentrations are in part mediated by beta adrenergic receptors, as well as the action of PGE1. Evening primrose oil should be used with caution in patients taking conventional anticoagulant therapy.

The cell death effect of anticancer drugs (paclitaxel and vinorelbine) may increase when given with products containing unsaturated fatty acids, such as evening primrose oil. The mechanism for this effect is not known, although it is possible that GLA increases the cell growth inhibition of anticancer drugs by promoting cell death signaling pathways.

Both omega 3 and omega 6 essential fatty acids are therapeutically important. Consequently, supplements combining both are becoming increasingly popular in practice.

Dosage Regimens

- Adults: 2–8 g seed oil daily.
- Children: 2–6 g seed oil daily in children suffering from atopic eczema.

Note: Evening primrose oil is usually taken in divided doses. Most evening primrose oil supplements contain 8% gamma-linolenic acid (GLA). Other nutritional supplements exist that may contain more GLA, such as borage (*Borago officinalis* L., Boraginaceae) oil, black currant (*Ribes nigrum* L., Grossulariaceae) oil, and algal sources. These sources of GLA are generally considered less biologically active than that from evening primrose oil. The vast majority of clinical evidence exists for evening primrose oil supplements. It is important to remember that both omega 3 and omega 6 essential fatty acids are therapeutically important. Consequently, supplements combining both are becoming increasingly popular in practice.

Selected References

Keen H, Payan J, Allawi J, Walker J, Jamal GA, Weir AI, et al. Treatment of diabetic neuropathy with gamma-linolenic acid. Diabetes Care 1993;16(1):8–15.

Morse PF, Horrobin DF, et al. Meta-analysis of placebo-controlled studies of the efficacy of Epogam in the treatment of atopic eczema: Relationship between plasma essential fatty acid changes and clinical response. British Journal of Dermatology 1989;121:75–90.

Richardson AJ, Montgomery P. The Oxford-Durham study: A randomised controlled trial of fatty acid supplementation in children with developmental coordination disorder. Pediatrics 2005;115:1360–66.

Stevens L, Zhang W, Peck L, Kuczek T, Grevstad N, Mahon A, et al. EFA supplementation in children with inattention, hyperactivity and other disruptive behaviors. Lipids 2003; 38:1007–21.

Feverfew

Tanacetum parthenium (L.) Schultz-Bip.

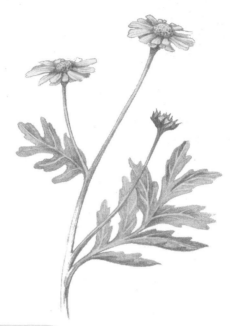

THUMBNAIL SKETCH

Common Uses
- Migraines (prophylactic treatment)
- Inflammatory joint disease

Active Constituents
- Sesquiterpene lactones (notably parthenolide)

Adverse Effects
- Mouth ulceration and gastrointestinal upset
- Postfeverfew syndrome (including nervousness, tension, fatigue, and joint ache)

Cautions/Contraindications
- Pregnancy and breastfeeding
- Children under 2 years of age

Drug Interactions
- Anticoagulant or antiplatelet therapy, such as warfarin or ASA (theoretical)
- Anticancer therapy, such as sulindac (theoretical)

Doses
- *Dried leaf preparation (Tanacetum parthenium (L.) Schultz Bip. containing at least 0.2% parthenolide)*: 125 mg daily
- *Dried aerial parts*: 50–200 mg daily
- *Tincture (1:5 in 25% ethanol)*: 5–20 drops daily

Note: For optimal results in the management of recurrent migraines, it is advisable to take feverfew continuously for a minimum of 4 to 6 weeks.

Introduction

Family
- Asteraceae (also known as Compositae)

Synonyms
- Featherfew
- Featherfoil
- Motherherb
- Flirtwort
- Midsummer daisy
- Pyrethrum
- Febrifuge plant
- Altamisa
- *Chrysanthemum parthenium* (L.) Bernh.
- *Leucanthemum parthenium* (L.) Gren & Godron
- *Pyrethrum parthenium* L.

Medicinal Forms
- Dried aerial parts
- Tincture

Description

Feverfew is an herbaceous perennial native to most of Europe, especially the Balkans, but now naturalized throughout the Americas, Europe, and the rest of the world. It stands 15 to 60 centimeters (6 to 24 inches) in height, with several flowers on a common stalk. The flowers may be as large as 2 centimeters (1 inch) with a yellow central disc and a single layer of outer white florets. The flowers have a strong odor, and the bitter-tasting leaves have a feather-like appearance. There have been numerous incidents in the past of other members of the Asteraceae family, such as German chamomile and tansy, being sold erroneously as feverfew. Confusion has also occurred because numerous Latin binomials have been applied to the plant.

Parts Used

The parts used medicinally are the aerial parts, especially the leaves.

Traditional Use

Feverfew has been used medicinally for a variety of indications dating back to Ancient Greece, and it use was been documented in many of the *materia medica* written in the Middle Ages. Feverfew was particularly popular in the management of fever — hence its name — headache, migraine, women's health care (threatened miscarriage, labor difficulties, menstrual irregularities), toothache, gastric upset, and insect bites. The bitter dried powder could be taken orally, mixed with either honey or wine, or used topically by adding the herb to baths.

Current Medicinal Use

While not conclusive, results from a number of clinical trials show that feverfew extracts standardized for parthenolide content may be effective in preventing migraines. Claims for its activity in managing arthritic conditions have not been substantiated.

Relevant Research

Preventative and Therapeutic Effects

Constituents
- Sesquiterpene lactones: germacranolides (including parthenolide, artemorin, chrysanthemonin), eudesmanolides (including santamarin, reynosin, magnolialide), guaianolides (including chrysartemin A, partholide, chrysanthemolide).
- Others: volatile oils (mainly monoterpene and sesquiterpene derivatives), pyrethrin, various flavonoids.

Note: Qualitative and quantitative differences exist between different chemical races of feverfew. For example, specimens rich in santamarin and reynosin have no parthenolide, and specimens rich in parthenolide have little or no reynosin or santamarin.

Pharmacological Actions

Extracts of feverfew appear to influence production of physiologically active eicasonoids. While feverfew suppresses prostaglandin production, it inhibits neither cyclo-oxygenase nor thromboxane A2 synthesis. Unlike the constituents of classic non-steroidal anti-inflammatory drugs (NSAIDs), constituents found in feverfew appear to inhibit cellular phospholipases, hence preventing the release of arachidonic acid and subsequent inflammation.

An additional action could be an inhibition of the activating factors of protein kinase C. Compounds present in feverfew may also exert an inhibitory action directly on the prostaglandin synthetase enzyme system, preventing the production of prostaglandins from arachidonic acid. It has been suggested that non-sesquiterpene lactones may also play a part in this inhibition of the production of eicasonoids.

Extracts of feverfew have been shown to exert an antisecretory and anti-aggregatory effect on blood platelets and polymorphonuclear leucocytes (white blood cells). With respect to human platelet activity, there appears to be little difference between a crude chloroform feverfew extract and parthenolide. Feverfew extract has been shown to decrease deposition of platelets on collagen substrates, leading some to suggest it be used as an antithrombotic drug. This inhibition of secretory and aggregatory activity appears to be due to an action on cellular sulphydryl groups. In addition, feverfew has been reported to inhibit release of serotonin by platelets and vitamin B_{12}-binding protein from polymorphonuclear leucocytes (white blood cells). Feverfew extract has also been shown to protect rabbit aortas against perfusion injury.

Feverfew extracts also appear to inhibit the release of enzymes from polymorphonuclear leucocytes. This action appears more pronounced than that seen with conventional non-steroidal anti-inflammatory drugs, such as indomethacin. This action could be responsible for feverfew's reputed effectiveness in the management of various arthritides and certain skin conditions, such as psoriasis. In addition, an extract of feverfew has been shown to inhibit histamine release from rat peritoneal mast cells stimulated by anti-IgE in a dose-dependent manner. The mode of action responsible for this anti-histaminic property is different from that of either quercetin or sodium chromoglycate.

A cytotoxic action for both a crude extract of feverfew and parthenolide has been demonstrated in in vitro studies. These compounds were found to inhibit cell growth in a variety of experiments with different types of cell lines. Intracellular thiols and calcium equilibrium may be partly responsible for parthenolide's ability to cause cell death. In non-human studies, parthenolide has also been shown to inhibit the anti-cell death transcription factor nuclear factor kappa B (NF-kB).

Numerous mechanisms of action for feverfew and some of its constituents have been identified in in vitro studies, but the relevance of these mechanisms to the use of feverfew leaf as a migraine prophylactic in humans is not at all clear. While most interest has been focused on the sesquiterpene lactones, notably parthenolide, it is possible that other constituents also exert a biological action. The possibility of a synergy between constituents has also been suggested.

Effect on Migraine

Three systematic reviews have concluded that the available studies indicate that feverfew may be more effective than a placebo in preventing migraines. While the results are encouraging, the efficacy of feverfew for migraine prevention has not been established beyond a reasonable doubt and rigorous studies are needed in future.

Research into this use was initiated primarily by a group of migraine sufferers in the late 1970s who used feverfew "successfully" in the treatment of their conditions. The public demand led to two documented clinical trials in the 1980s. Following a survey of migraine sufferers in which it appeared that feverfew may be beneficial, a placebo-controlled trial was performed with 17 selected volunteers who had consumed an average of 2.44 fresh feverfew leaves daily for at least 3 months and had a history of migraines, common or classic, for 2 years with no more than eight attacks per month. One group of 8 received "freeze-dried" feverfew (50 mg daily), and a second group of 9 received a placebo. Assessment was made by using diary cards scoring the visual symptoms, nausea, and headache (including times of onset and relief and of any additional treatment taken) according to a predetermined scale. The group given the feverfew product reported no change in condition, while the group given the placebo noted both an increased frequency of attacks (3.43 attacks/month as compared to 1.22/month before) and increased severity of headache, nausea, and vomiting over six periods of 4 months. The abrupt withdrawal of feverfew in two of the patients led to the recurrence of some symptoms. However, the observations and conclusions drawn from this study have been questioned because of the poor methodology.

The efficacy of feverfew in the preventative management of migraines was evaluated in a randomized, double-blind, placebo-controlled, crossover trial in 1988 with 76 selected volunteers who had suffered from migraines, classic or common, for 2 years or more, with at least one attack per month. Following a 1-month single-blind placebo run-in, the volunteers were given either 1 capsule of feverfew daily (mean weight 82 mg, equivalent to 2.19 mmol parthenolide) or a placebo. The treatment was continued for 4 months, and patients were then transferred to the other option. Conventional migraine medications were stopped at the

beginning of the trial. A symptom diary was used to record number and duration of individual attacks, severity of headache, and any associated symptoms. In addition, the overall impression of the patients was assessed by use of a visual analog scale and the selection of a predefined "descriptive" to describe the change in headache (much worse, worse, same, better, much better). Patients were assessed every 2 months during the double-blind portion of the study. Following treatment with feverfew, an improvement was noted in the number and severity of attacks, degree of vomiting, and general improvement (on the visual analog scale). There was no alteration in the duration of individual attacks.

> *Three systematic reviews have concluded that the available studies indicate that feverfew may be more effective than a placebo in preventing migraines.*

A recent well-designed, randomized, double-blind, placebo-controlled crossover trial of feverfew did not find such promising results. For this trial, 50 patients who had suffered from migraines since their youth and continued to suffer from at least one migraine, classic or common, at least once per month and had never taken feverfew in the past were selected. The patients involved suffered serious migraines that were not receptive to conventional medication. While all migraine-related medications were stopped at the start of the trial, volunteers were permitted to treat any attacks acutely using conventional symptomatic drugs. After a 1-month placebo phase, patients were treated with either a dried alcoholic extract of feverfew leaves containing 0.5 mg of parthenolide or a placebo. After 4 months, the patients were crossed over to the opposing group. The severity of the migraine attacks was recorded according to a predetermined scale and the number of headaches during months 2 to 4 recorded. There was no significant difference in the number of migraines experienced between the groups. Of the group of 44 volunteers that completed the study, 7 in the feverfew group reported "using considerably fewer antimigraine preparations."

This study has been criticized on a number of points. The investigators noted that, unlike the previous studies, the individuals selected had never used feverfew before. The feverfew product used an alcoholic extract rather than dried feverfew leaves. While extracts used were standardized for parthenolide, other necessary active moities could be absent. Concerns about the use of acute migraine drugs during the trial, and their effect on the assessment of the severity of the attacks, have also been raised. In addition, the appropriateness of the criteria used by the investigators to measure changes in symptoms — the International Headache Society's scale — has been questioned.

Two studies sought to investigate a dose response of a new feverfew extract (MIG-99) and found conflicting results. Both studies were randomized, multi-center, double-blind, and placebo-controlled. In the first trial, over a 4-week period, three doses of feverfew (2.08 mg, 6.25 mg, and 18.75 mg) given three times daily were compared with a placebo in 147 patients suffering from migraines with and without aura. In this study, feverfew extract MIG-99 failed to show a significant migraine prevention effect in general and a dose-response relationship was not observed. Feverfew was shown to be effective in only 49 patients with at least four attacks during the 28-day baseline period, and in these patients, the 6.25 mg dose (three times daily) was found most effective. In the second trial, over a 4-week period, feverfew (6.25 mg) given three times daily was compared with placebo in 170 patients experiencing migraines with and without aura. Although improvements were seen in both groups, the results showed that feverfew treatment was significantly more efficacious than treatment with the control.

> *While the vast majority of feverfew users take feverfew to prevent future migraines from happening, incidents of its proving useful in treating the symptoms of acute migraines have been documented.*

Three additional studies included feverfew as a main ingredient in a combination product. The first was a 3-month randomized, double-blind, placebo-controlled trial of 49 women, in which a daily dose of riboflavin (400 mg), magnesium (300 mg), and feverfew (100 mg) was found to offer comparable effects in migraine prevention to the placebo treatment of 25 mg riboflavin daily. However, there was a notable reduction in the mean number of migraines in both groups. A higher placebo response was reported than in any other placebo trials of migraine prevention, which suggests that 25 mg riboflavin may actually have therapeutic properties.

The second study was an open-label study that looked at the effectiveness of a sublingual combination product made of feverfew and ginger (GelStat Migraine) in 29 participants who experienced at least 15 migraines a month. It found that 59% of subjects were satisfied with this therapy and 41% preferred GelStat Migraine or felt it was equal to their pre-study medication.

The final trial was a 12-week prospective, open-label study that looked at the effectiveness of taking 2 capsules daily of Mig-RL (150 mg each of feverfew and *Spondilla alba* per capsule) in 12 patients diagnosed with migraine without aura. In the 10 patients who completed the trial, it was found that the treatment reduced migraine frequency and pain intensity.

While the vast majority of feverfew users take feverfew to prevent future migraines from happening, incidents of its proving useful in treating the symptoms of acute migraines have been documented. However, there are no research studies investigating its use to treat migraines.

Effect on Arthritis

While feverfew has been used in the management of various arthritic conditions, this claim is not supported by clinical research. In a double-blind, placebo-controlled study of 41 female patients suffering from rheumatoid arthritis, dried feverfew (70–86 mg, equivalent to 2–3 (µmol of parthenolide) taken once a day for 6 weeks was shown to offer no benefits over placebo. Patients were permitted to continue their conventional non-steroidal treatment throughout the study. Concerns were noted that the dose used might have been too low. The authors suggested that these findings did not exclude a benefit in the management of osteoarthritis or soft tissue damage.

Effect on Inflammatory Acne

Although feverfew's anti-inflammatory properties suggest that this herb would be beneficial in inflammatory skin disorders, its parthenolide component is a known skin sensitizer, so it is generally contraindicated for topical use. To solve this problem, a parthenolide-free extract of feverfew was developed (feverfew PFE™). The goal of developing this product was to eliminate the risk of skin sensitization, but along with it came the surprising discovery that the compound showed strong immunomodulatory activity. An open-label study that enlisted 25 patients with mild inflammatory acne found that 45 days of treatment with 1% feverfew PFE™ (Aveeno Daily Moisturizer Ultracalming) improved mild inflammatory acne. The patients used two daily applications of the moisturizer on their face. Further research is needed to investigate this use of feverfew.

Miscellaneous Effects

Although there has yet to be a study published on humans, research using mice and human cells has shown that feverfew may protect against ultraviolet B (UVB)-induced skin cancer.

Parthenolide has been shown to possess antimicrobial properties against a variety of gram-positive bacteria, fungi, and viruses. A weaker action has been noted against some gram-negative pathogens. The clinical relevance of this is unknown.

Feverfew's anti-inflammatory effects might be beneficial in atopic dermatitis, as well as cystic fibrosis. However, there has been a lack of studies in humans to verify its benefits.

A systemic review of herbal products for menopause found a lack of evidence to support the use of feverfew for menopausal symptoms.

> *Although there has yet to be a study published on humans, research using mice and human cells has shown that feverfew may protect against ultraviolet B (UVB)-induced skin cancer.*

Adverse Effects

Adverse effects are considered to be generally rare, primarily presenting as mouth sores and gastrointestinal upset. Mouth sores presented in 12% and swelling of the lips in 7% of patients in one British clinical trial. Mouth sores are due to a systemic rather than a direct irritant action; thus, putting feverfew into capsules does not decrease its presentation. Feverfew products may also cause inflammation of the mucous membranes of the mouth and throat, resulting in swelling of the lips and tongue and a loss of taste, which is likely to be reduced when the feverfew is taken as a tablet or capsule. These adverse effects present usually within the first week but may occur at any time in the first 2 months of treatment.

> *Another study described a group of symptoms, including nervousness, tension, fatigue, and joint aches, which was associated with withdrawal of feverfew products. The name "postfeverfew syndrome" was coined to describe this finding.*

One study that looked at the safety of using feverfew in patients with cancer reported fever, nausea, diarrhea, indigestion, chills, fatigue, and blurred vision. However, the fever was more likely related to a simultaneous viral illness. The blurred vision was in a known diabetic patient, and this symptom did not improve even after feverfew treatment was stopped.

Another study described a group of symptoms, including nervousness, tension, fatigue, and joint aches, which was associated with withdrawal of feverfew products. The name "postfeverfew syndrome" was coined to describe this finding. No other reference to this syndrome could be found.

Allergic reactions to feverfew have also been reported. Numerous examples of contact dermatitis have been noted in individuals handling the fresh feverfew plant. It is probable that parthenolide is the sensitizing component. There have been two case reports of contact dermatitis that worsened after using a moisturizer containing feverfew. Using diagnostic tests, both patients were confirmed to be allergic to parthenolide. An appreciable cross-sensitivity between feverfew and other plants containing these constituents has also been seen.

In a comparative study between a group of 30 migraine sufferers who had been taking a variety of feverfew products (leaves, capsules, or tablets of feverfew for at least 11 months) and a non-user control group, no significant genetic mutations were noted, suggesting feverfew may be safe for long-term use. However, additional research is needed to confirm this preliminary finding.

Cautions/Contraindications

Feverfew is considered an emmenagogue (an agent that may promote or increase menstrual flow) and abortifacient (an agent that may induce abortions); consequently, its use is contraindicated in pregnancy. Feverfew should not be given to children under 2 years of age. Feverfew products should not be taken for more than 4 months without consulting a physician. This caution is due to the lack of long-term information regarding toxicity. Feverfew should not be taken by people with known hypersensitivity to other members of the daisy (Asteraceae) family.

Drug Interactions

No documented instances of drug interactions occurring with feverfew in humans were found for this review. However, it has been suggested that the effect of feverfew may be reduced when it is taken concurrently with non-steroidal anti-inflammatory drugs (NSAIDs) or corticosteroids. Theoretically, feverfew may potentiate the action of anticoagulants and antiplatelet drugs, such as warfarin or ASA. Finally, in vitro studies suggest that feverfew may enhance the anticancer effects of sulindac.

Comparison of Dosage Forms

A very detailed review article discusses many concerns related to the practical use of feverfew preparations. Many of the statements made by manufacturers regarding the superiority of a particular product (freeze-dried or certain extracts) cannot be substantiated. The quality, with regard to parthenolide content, of commercial feverfew products has also been questioned. Investigation of commercially available feverfew products found that many did not contain the parthenolide content considered necessary for therapeutic efficacy. In addition, the parthenolide content of the dried feverfew leaf has been shown to decrease appreciably over time. This led to questions regarding effective shelf life and the need for more specific storage conditions.

Many factors, such as the season in which the feverfew is harvested and the growing conditions, can effect the sesquiterpene lactone content. To further complicate matters, the bioactivity (ability to inhibit the release of serotonin from bovine blood platelets) appears to vary within and between samples. This variance can be independent of the geographical source of the sample of *T. parthenium*.

The same review also noted that "there is no scientific evidence supporting either the superiority of the wild traditional feverfew or ineffectiveness of non-traditional or cultivated variants." In comparing capsule versus tablet formulations, it was stated that, "While there is no fundamental reason to reject tablets per se, it should be noted that their effectiveness would be dependent upon satisfactory disintegration/dissolution characteristics."

> *Many of the statements made by manufacturers regarding the superiority of a particular product (freeze-dried or certain extracts) cannot be substantiated.*

A 2004 study reported that the actual amount of parthenolide in Canadian commercial feverfew preparations varied from less than 8.4% to 446.3% of the amount claimed on the label. This meant that the daily delivered parthenolide could be as low as less than 2 mcg or as high as 5.639 mg. Keeping this in mind, studies that tested for the effects of parthenolide using commercially available feverfew products may have inadvertently reported inaccurate dose-response relationships.

Dosage Regimens

- Dried leaf preparation (*Tanacetum parthenium* containing at least 0.2% parthenolide): 125 mg daily.

Although it has been argued that administration should be limited to standardized extracts, other dosage forms seen in clinical practice include:

- Dried aerial parts: 50–200 mg s daily.
- Tincture (1:5 in 25% ethanol): 5–20 drops daily.

Note: For optimal results in the management of recurrent migraines, it is advisable to take feverfew continuously for a minimum of 4 to 6 weeks.

Selected References

Pittler MH, Ernst E. Feverfew for preventing migraine. Cochrane Database of Systematic Reviews 2004;1.

Vogler BK, Pittler MH, Ernst E. Feverfew as a preventive treatment for migraine: A systematic review. Cephalalgia 1998;18(10):704–8.

Garlic

Allium sativum L.

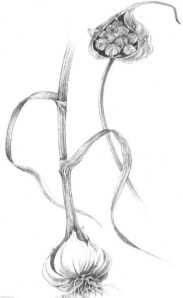

Common Uses
- Cardiovascular (protective effects, including decreased cholesterol levels, decreased blood pressure, decreased platelet aggregation)
- Antimicrobial
- Cancer (protection against cancer, especially stomach and colon cancer)
- Antifatigue
- Common cold (prevention and recovery)

Active Constituents
- Sulfur-containing products (including alliin, allicin, diallyl disulfide, and ajoene)

Adverse Effects
- Heartburn, flatulence, and gastro-intestinal upset (usually only at doses greater than 4 cloves daily)
- Contact dermatitis (if the skin is exposed to raw garlic for an extensive period of time)
- Postoperative bleeding

Cautions/Contraindications
- Pregnancy and breastfeeding
- Surgery (discontinue prior to surgery)
- Organ transplants (caution should be exercised after organ transplants)
- Pemphigus

Drug Interactions
- Anticoagulants (e.g., warfarin)
- Antithrombotic (ASA, aspirin)
- Antidiabetic therapy (possibly)
- Highly active antiretroviral therapy (HAART) used in treating HIV and AIDs, most notably ritonavir and saquinavir

Doses
- *Fresh garlic:* 3–30 g (1–8 cloves) daily
- *Dried cloves:* 2–5 g of fresh air-dried daily
- *Dried powder:* 400–1,200 mg of fully dried powder daily
- *Garlic oil:* 2–5 mg daily
- *Allicin:* 2–5 mg daily

Introduction

Family
- Liliaceae

Synonyms
- Russian penicillin (allicin)

Medicinal Forms
- Fresh cloves
- Oil
- Powder

Description
Garlic is a perennial growing from 30 centimeters to 1 meter (1 to 3 feet) tall, with pale pink or green-white flowers and a bulb composed of a cluster of cloves. Native to central Asia, garlic is now cultivated widely for culinary and medicinal purposes.

Parts Used
The garlic bulb is the part of the plant used medicinally. When intact, it is odorless; however, crushing the cells brings the enzyme alliinase into contact with the sulfur-containing compound alliin, converting it to allicin, which produces the characteristic garlic odor. Allicin is relatively unstable and is converted to a variety of other active sulfur-containing compounds. Some people argue that the potency of a garlic product can be determined by its ability to produce allicin, which in turn yields many of the other active components. Some commercial products are now standardized for their allicin yield.

Traditional Use
Garlic has been used medicinally since approximately 3000 BC. The Latin name, *Allium*, is derived from the Celtic word for pungent, hot, and burning, properties common to all the Allium species. The species name, *sativum*, means "cultivated" or "planted," referring to the fact that garlic is no longer found in the wild. It was one of the earliest cultivated crops and continues to be extensively grown for both medicinal and culinary purposes.

Garlic has been described as an aphrodisiac, as well as a treatment for a large variety of other conditions, including colds, coughs, high blood pressure, hypertension, diarrhea, rheumatism, and snake bites. In addition, garlic oil has been used to "expel" roundworms and was generally considered to be a good antiseptic. Traditionally, garlic was used to treat diabetes in Norway and Central Europe. It was considered a heart and arthritis remedy in Ayurvedic (traditional Indian) medicine, in which it was also sometimes used for fatigue, parasitic disease, digestive disorder, and leprosy. In traditional Chinese medicine (TCM), garlic was used in controlling dysentery and as an antiparasitic, antifebrile, and stomachic.

Over the past 100 years, more than 1,300 papers have reported on the chemical constituents, mechanisms of action, and clinical applications of garlic, making it one of the most extensively researched medicinal plants. A review from 1985 provides an excellent account of many of these.

Current Medicinal Use

A growing amount of evidence now shows that the sulfur-containing constituents have medicinal properties, including antimicrobial, cardioprotective, and potentially anticancer actions. Garlic is primarily used to decrease high cholesterol and blood pressure. When taken as either a supplement or part of the diet, garlic has been associated with a decrease in some types of cancer, such as colorecectal cancer.

Medicinal Forms

It has been estimated that when crushed or chopped, 1 g of fresh garlic will release 3.7 mg of allicin, which appears to be the precursor for many of the major active constituents of garlic. Dried garlic contains no allicin, but it does contain both alliin and alliinase, and thus theoretically should be able to produce allicin. Allinase is inactivated by acids, so the conversion to allicin does not occur in the stomach. It has been suggested that dried garlic is most effective if it is ingested as an enteric-coated formulation so it is released in the alkaline environment of the intestine. In the intestine, the conversion to allicin occurs rapidly, and allicin is quickly combined with cysteine to produce 5-allylmercaptocysteine, which prevents the distinctly odored allicin from being absorbed into the bloodstream. Thus, this form of garlic is relatively odorless and most likely still effective. Odorless garlic products may be also prepared by coarsely chopping, peeling, and rapidly freeze-drying the cloves before powdering so there is little opportunity for enzymatic conversion of the odorless alliin to the odoriferous allicin and related breakdown products.

Oil-based products are less likely to be efficacious because allicin is unstable in an oil base. Similarly, in aqueous products, allicin suffers substantial degradation. A 1992 German study investigating the allicin content of 18 German garlic products found that only 5 had an allicin yield equivalent to the 4 g of fresh garlic (or more) that the German Commission E considers necessary for therapeutic activity.

Relevant Research

Preventative and Therapeutic Effects

Constituents

- **Enzymes:** alliinase, peroxidase, myrosinase, (manganese, copper, zinc) superoxide dismutase.

- **Sulfur-containing compounds:** alliin (S-allyl cysteine sulfoxide); allicin (diallyl thiosulfinate), which is formed when the enzyme alliinase acts on alliin when the garlic clove is crushed; allyl methanethiosulfinate; diallyl disulfide (breakdown product of allicin); diallyl trisulfide; allyl methyl trisulfide; S-allyl-mercaptocysteine; ajoene ($C_9H_{14}S_3O$), formed by combining allicin and diallyl disulfide, which is considered unstable and may rearrange to a variety of polysulfides; 2-vinyl-4H-1,3-dithiin; 2-vinyl-4H-1,2-dithiin; S-allylcysteine; allixin.

- **Miscellaneous:** neutral lipids (predominant), phospholipids, glycolipids; essential amino acids (of particular importance are those containing sulfur, for example, cysteine and methionine, as well as arginine); anthocyanins; quercetin and its flavone aglycone analogs; kaempferol glycosides; scordinins (biologically active thioglycosides); tellurium compounds.

Note: The biological action of garlic is generally thought to be due to its organic sulfur compounds, specifically those containing the allyl $CH_2=CH-CH_2$ group. It has been estimated that 1 g of fresh garlic will release 3.7 mg of allicin when crushed or chopped.

Cardiovascular Effects

A systematic review including 45 randomized controlled trials and 73 additional studies reporting adverse effects concluded that the trials "suggest possible small short-term benefits of garlic on some lipid and antiplatelet factors, and insignificant effects on blood pressure. Conclusions regarding clinical significance are limited by the marginal quality and short duration of many trials and by the unpredictable release and inadequate definition of active constituents in study preparations."

Cholesterol Levels

The ability of garlic to decrease triglycerides and low-density lipoprotein (LDL) cholesterol in the blood has been documented by numerous studies. However, studies reporting no lipid- or cholesterol-lowering effect have also been published. Studies during the past 25 years have reported that the ingestion of garlic can decrease blood cholesterol, sometimes by as much as 20%. However, the study designs, doses, forms (raw or powder), study populations, and blinding mechanisms (the smell of garlic makes it very difficult to conducted blinded studies) vary widely, making it difficult to reach firm conclusions regarding the efficacy of garlic for this indication.

For example, one study severely criticized both the quality of commercial garlic products and the methodological quality of the 13 controlled trials they reviewed. They concluded that while experiments with fresh garlic are consistent in showing that garlic lowers cholesterol levels, the doses required to achieve this effect are extremely high (a minimum of 7 cloves daily). In addition, it appeared that the effects of garlic ingestion lasted only a few hours. In response to this finding, several manufacturers began producing dehydrated garlic preparations (water accounts for up to 60% of the bulk of garlic) that are standardized for alliin content.

Other reviews of double-blind controlled studies have concluded that ingestion of garlic significantly decreases lipid and cholesterol levels. A 1993 meta-analysis of five placebo-controlled, randomized trials, which assessed the effect of garlic on total blood cholesterol in individuals with cholesterol levels greater than 5.17 mmol/L (200 mg/dL), concluded that the oral ingestion of the equivalent of $^1/_2$ to 1 clove of raw garlic daily significantly decreased blood cholesterol levels by approximately 9%. The study suggests that these effects are possible with relatively low doses of garlic. However, problems with the low quality of the trials included in the analysis continue to be of concern.

A 1994 meta-analysis of 16 trials with a combined total of 952 subjects found an overall 12% reduction in total blood cholesterol in those taking garlic compared to those taking a placebo. This effect was apparent after approximately 1 month and persisted approximately 6 months after the therapy was discontinued. Garlic powders were also reported to reduce triglyceride levels by an average of 13%. However, the authors cautioned that more than half the trials reviewed were of poor quality.

> *The ability of garlic to decrease triglycerides and low-density lipoprotein (LDL) cholesterol in the blood has been documented by numerous studies.*

A 2000 meta-analysis of 13 randomized, placebo-controlled studies concluded that although garlic appears to be superior to a placebo in reducing total cholesterol levels, the size of the effect is modest and the clinical use of garlic in the management of hypercholesterolemia (high levels of cholesterol in the blood) remains debatable. An updated 2002 meta-analysis included three additional trials in which the effect of garlic was found to be even less, while four double-blind, randomized controlled trials (encompassing the results of 3,670 participants) published after this updated meta-analysis all reported no changes in lipid levels for hypercholesterolemic patients.

Two randomized controlled trials suggest that garlic may decrease total blood cholesterol and increase HDL (high-density lipoprotein) cholesterol in patients diagnosed with type 2 diabetes.

In one of the few studies comparing garlic to standard lipid-lowering products, garlic was compared in a double-blind clinical trial with bezafibrate in 98 patients. There was no significant difference in the outcome measures between the two groups — both groups had significant reductions in triglyceride, total cholesterol, and LDL levels, as well as increased HDL levels.

Several mechanisms of action have been postulated to explain garlic's effects on cholesterol levels, including increased bile acid excretion, reduced 3-hydroxy-3-methylglutaryl coenzyme A reductase activity, and inhibition of squalene epoxidase, the final enzyme in the synthetic pathway of cholesterol by tellurium compounds found in garlic bulbs. All of these mechanisms decrease the hepatic (liver) production of cholesterol. It appears that components of garlic (e.g., allicin, diallyl disulfide, allyl mercaptan, and the vinyl-dithiins) may all play a role in interfering with cholesterol biosynthesis although via a variety of different mechanisms.

In addition, it is suggested that components of garlic may decrease the activity of lipogenic enzymes (e.g., glucose-6-phosphate dehydrogenase, malic dehydrogenase, and 4a-methyl oxidase), which leads to a decrease in fatty acid synthesis. Another hypothesis is that components of garlic may exert cardioprotective effects by decreasing the levels of glycosaminoglycans (GAGs). The amount of GAGs has been shown to be proportional to the susceptibility of different species to cholesterol-induced athersclerosis. GAGs are able to bind to plasma lipoproteins and thus have been implicated in lipid accumulation in developing lesions. A more recent idea is that the reduction in platelet aggregation by aged garlic extract is due to its ability to inhibit calcium mobilization within cells, either by binding with it or by changing the chemical messengers inside platelets. It has also been proposed that sulfur components of garlic may be metabolized to release hydrogen sulfide, which has cardioprotective properties inside the body.

One study presents findings that suggest the hypothesis that garlic decreases the susceptibility of isolated LDL to oxidation may not be correct. Based on the results of animal experiments, one comprehensive review concluded that only raw cloves or garlic that has been boiled for 20 minutes or less have blood lipid–lowering properties. Of interest is that, in several studies, there is an initial rise in cholesterol, triglycerides, LDL, and VLDL (very low-density lipoprotein) blood levels during the first few months of garlic ingestion. Researchers have postulated that this initial increase could be due to the garlic causing tissue lipids to move into circulation.

Blood Pressure

Although several trials have demonstrated garlic's ability to decrease blood pressure, others have not been able to show such an effect. A 1994 meta-analysis that reviewed eight randomized controlled trials of at least 4 weeks in duration (all of which used Kwai garlic powder) concluded that there is currently insufficient evidence to routinely recommend garlic use in patients with hypertension. Of the eight studies reviewed, only three were conducted in hypertensive subjects and only seven compared garlic to a placebo. Overall, three showed a significant reduction in systolic blood pressure and four showed a significant decrease in diastolic blood pressure. A 2006 review identified three additional studies on the effects of garlic on blood pressure since 1993 and not yet mentioned above — two of which showed a reduction, while one did not. One of the positive studies had no control group, but the other two studies were randomized and controlled.

For example, a double-blind, placebo-controlled study of 42 patients getting 300 mg three times daily of standardized garlic powder in tablet form found no effects on blood pressure. In contrast, a double-blind, placebo-controlled crossover study of 41 men (total blood cholesterol 220–290 mg/dL) taking 7.2 g of aged garlic or a placebo daily for 4 to 6 months reported a 5.5% decrease in systolic blood pressure and a slight reduction in diastolic blood pressure in the group taking garlic. In addition, a study of 47 patients with mild hypertension (mean diastolic blood pressure 102 mmHg) who took 600 mg dried garlic powder (Kwai) daily or a placebo for 12 weeks reported that the supine diastolic blood pressure in the group taking the garlic was significantly lower at 8 weeks and 12 weeks than that of those in the control group.

The ability of garlic to decrease blood pressure may be due to its ability to inhibit adenosine deaminase, the enzyme that degrades adenosine to inosine, enhancing the physiological effects of adenosine on the heart.

> *Although several trials have demonstrated garlic's ability to decrease blood pressure, others have not been able to show such an effect.*

Platelet Aggregation (Blood Clotting)

The anti–blood clotting effects of garlic have been extensively studied, and an excellent review of the inhibition of platelet aggregation by a variety of components of garlic is available. It is important to note that, at dietary levels, platelet function does not appear to be impaired by garlic.

A review of 13 trials, most rated as poor in quality, concluded that although fresh garlic reliably decreases platelet aggregation, it does so only at very high doses (more than 7 cloves per day) and the effects appear to last for only a few hours. Other studies have found decreased platelet aggregation at significantly lower doses. For example, one double-blind, placebo-controlled crossover study of 10 individuals randomized to receive either 900 mg (1.3% alliin) daily or a placebo found no significant effects at 6 hours. At 7 and 14 days, however, those taking the garlic had decreased platelet aggregation caused by adenosine diphosphate (ADP) and decreased platelet aggregability in response to collagen. In contrast, another clinical study of daily consumption of 600 mg garlic powder in tablet form (equal to 1.7 g of cloves) for 4 weeks found no inhibitory effects of platelet aggregation.

Another randomized, double-blind, placebo-controlled study of 34 healthy volunteers taking between 2.4 and 7.2 g of aged garlic extract daily reported that only at the highest supplementation level (7.2 g daily) did garlic show a slight increase in the threshold of adenosine diphosphate (ADP)-induced aggregation and reduced adhesion to von Willebrand factor. Platelet adhesion to collagen was inhibited only at higher levels of supplementation, but adherence to fibrinogen was potently inhibited at all levels of supplementation. These findings are similar to those of an earlier study.

It has been suggested that garlic causes a slow buildup of active constituents, making higher single doses necessary to achieve inhibition of platelet aggregation, but lower doses of garlic may have anticoagulant effects in long-term administration.

Garlic has been shown to inhibit platelet aggregation induced by epinephrine, adenosine diphosphate, and collagen. Both alliin and allicin have been shown to inhibit collagen-induced platelet aggregation; however, allicin is approximately 15 times more active. In vitro studies indicate that platelet cAMP (cyclic adenosine monophosphate), cyclo-oxygenase, and thromboxane synthetase activity are not affected by either of these constituents of garlic. It should be noted that the antithrombotic (anti-blood clotting) effects of allicin are destroyed above 56°C (133°F) and at a pH greater than 8.5.

> *A review of 13 trials, most rated as poor in quality, concluded that although fresh garlic reliably decreases platelet aggregation, it does so only at very high doses (more than 7 cloves per day) and the effects appear to last for only a few hours.*

Several studies have noted decreased or complete lack of the antithrombotic action of garlic after it has been exposed to heat. The exact antithrombotic mechanism of action is unknown; however, raw garlic has been shown to irreversibly inhibit cyclo-oxygenase activity in a dose-dependent manner and to decrease thromboxane B2 levels. Thus, other constituents of garlic must play a role in this effect.

Although allicin is considered one of the most potent anti-aggregation constituents in garlic, it is not found in the blood stream after oral ingestion of garlic. Shortly after it is absorbed into the blood stream, it is converted to allyl mercaptan. Allicin may also be converted to ajoene, which has been identified as an active antithrombotic agent. However, ajoene is often not present in commercial garlic pills or powders of steamed garlic distillates. Ajoene has been shown to inhibit platelet aggregation traditionally induced by a variety of stimulatory agents, including collagen, ADP, epinephrine, arachidonic acid, platelet-activating factor, and thrombin. This activity is increased by prostacyclin (PGI2), forskolin, indomethacin, and dipyridamole.

Several mechanisms have been postulated for the antithrombotic activity of ajoene. It is thought, for example, to inhibit the exposure of fibrinogen receptors on platelet membranes. Other researchers have suggested that it may interact with a purified blood protein, which in turn may play an important role in the activation of platelets.

Additional components of garlic (e.g., diallyl disulfide and methyl allyl trisulfide) have also been implicated as antithrombotic agents; however, studies of their antithrombotic activity have been conflicting. For example, in one study, methyl allyl trisulfide was shown to be the agent responsible for the complete blockage of platelet aggregation in response to serotonin 1 hour after oral ingestion of fresh garlic (100–150 mg/kg). It should be noted that no inhibition was seen at 30 minutes or 2 hours after ingestion.

In addition, components of garlic may activate calcium-dependent nitric oxide synthase, producing increased amount of nitric acid by which the therapeutic actions of garlic may be exerted. This activation does not appear to be dependent upon the alliin-derived products or arginine.

Other Cardiovascular Effects
Garlic's other protective heart effects may include decreasing unstable heart pain, increasing elasticity of blood vessels, and increasing peripheral blood flow in healthy people. Garlic may also play a role in slowing down the progression of coronary calcification (hardening of arteries due to calcium buildup) in patients receiving statin therapy (a type of drug to reduce high cholesterol).

Antimicrobial and Antifungal Effects
Garlic has been used as an antimicrobial for hundreds of years in a variety of cultures. Allicin is considered to be the primary antibacterial constituent of garlic. Garlic has been shown to inhibit the growth of (but not to kill) *Staphylococcus aureus*, *Streptococcus* (alpha- and beta-hemolytic), *Escherichia coli*, *Proteus vulgaris*, *Salmonella eneritidis*, *Citrobacter* sp., *Klebsiella pneumoniae*, *Mycobacteria*, *Helicobacter pylori*, *Proteus mirabilis*, and *Pseudomonas aeruginosa*. However, other researchers have been unable to demonstrate any inhibition of *Staphylococcus aureus*.

In addition, garlic has been shown to have a significant antifungal effect, especially against fungal skin infections. Studies have demonstrated its effectiveness against *Microsporum*, *Epidermophyton*, *Trichophyton*, and *Candida albicans*. In Asia, garlic preparations are used, alone or in combination with amphotericin B, to treat systemic fungal infections and cryptococcal meningitis. In vitro evidence supports garlic's fungistatic and fungicidal activity against *Cryptococcus neoforans*.

Cancer Prevention

Garlic has long had a reputation for providing protection from cancer. Much of the evidence that garlic may reduce cancer deaths comes from epidemiological studies. Several good reviews of the evidence — or lack thereof — for this indication for garlic have been published over the past 10 years. The most recent of these reviews nine epidemiological studies of the association between garlic consumption and cancer. Of these studies, four reported that garlic had a protective effect against cancer (thyroid nodular disease, stomach cancer, cancer of the larynx, colon cancer), two found positive but non-significant trends (cancers of the stomach, nasal cavity, and sinuses), and three found no protective effect for garlic (gastric cancer and two studies of stomach cancer). The authors conclude that "the hypothesis that regular consumption of *Allium* vegetables (including garlic, onions and leeks) reduces the risk of cancer is compelling and would seem to deserve testing in intervention trials."

Two specific studies have garnered attention due to their more rigorous designs. The Iowa Women's Health Study followed 41,837 women aged 55 to 69 years for 5 years and found that garlic consumption was inversely associated with risk of colon cancer. The protective association with garlic was stronger than with any other nutrient analyzed in the study. The second notable study followed 58,279 men and 62,573 women aged 55 to 69 for just over 3 years. This study found no protective effect from garlic against cancers of the stomach or breast.

An ongoing randomized, multi-intervention trial involving 3,599 people to investigate the ability of daily long-term use of 500 mg vitamin C, 200 IU vitamin E, 75 mcg selenium, 800 mg garlic, and 4 mg garlic oil to inhibit the progression of precancerous gastric lesions recently reported that the supplements were well tolerated and that high compliance rates were achieved to date. Clinical outcomes from this study will be reported in the future.

> *Garlic has long had a reputation for providing protection from cancer. Much of the evidence that garlic may reduce cancer deaths comes from epidemiological studies.*

A case-control study at a hospital compared 1,369 patients with benign prostatic hyperplasia to 1,451 control patients who were admitted to the same hospital for a wide range of acute, non-tumor-growth-related conditions and not related to long-term changes in their diet. The validated and reproducible food frequency questionnaire was conducted by trained interviewers and found that there was an inverse relationship between how much garlic and onion is eaten and the likelihood of having benign prostatic hyperplasia. However, there is no well-accepted clinical definition for this condition, and there may have been some misclassification of patients (especially older men) who were without symptoms in the control group. Another non-controlled study found that drinking aqueous garlic extract at the daily amount of 1 mL per kg of body weight for 1 month resulted in significant improvement in disease markers in 27 patients with benign prostatic hyperplasia (non-cancerous prostate enlargement) and 9 patients with prostate cancer.

In a 12-month double-blind, randomized controlled trial, high-dose aged garlic extract (2.4 mL per day) was used as an active treatment and low-dose aged garlic extract (0.16 mL per day) was used as a control for patients with colorectal adenomas (precancerous lesions of the large bowel). Fifty-one patients who were diagnosed as having colorectal adenomas were randomly assigned to the two groups after tumors larger than 5 mm in diameter were surgically removed. Although there was a gradual increase in the number of colorectal adenomas in the control group, the high-dose aged garlic extract treatment showed significant suppression of both the size and number of colon adenomas in patients.

Results from another double-blind, randomized controlled trial with 50 patients with inoperable colorectal, liver, or pancreatic cancer suggest that garlic may prevent a decline in immune function but does not improve the quality of life. Participants in the garlic group took 2 capsules after breakfast and 2 capsules after dinner, for a total of 500 mg of aged garlic extract per day. The rest of the capsule was made of crystalline cellulose and sucrose fatty acid ester, which were the ingredients of the placebo capsules.

Animal studies have shown garlic to be effective at inhibiting chemically induced stomach and colon cancer; suppressing the growth of human colon tumor cell xenografts in mice; protecting against the effects of known gene-damaging agents, both alone and in combination with selenium; inhibiting induced mammary carcinogenesis; and inhibiting gamma-radiation-induced chromosomal damage. In addition, diallyl disulfide has been shown to inhibit the proliferation of human tumor cells in vitro. There are excellent reviews of both the in vivo and in vitro studies in this area.

It has been hypothesized that components of garlic may exert their antitumor effects by modulating gluthione S-transferase-dependent detoxification enzymes. Other researchers have suggested that the sulfur components of garlic may inactivate inside the body and form nitrosamines. Garlic's anticancer properties may also be due to its ability to generate reactive oxygen species that activate enzymes, such as stress kinases and cysteine proteases, that lead to cell death

in tumors. In addition, the antibacterial effect of garlic (especially against *Helicobacter pylori*, which is a major risk factor for stomach cancer) may add to its protective effects. For example, it may limit the formation of potentially carcinogenic nitrosamines by bacterial conversion in the stomach. Based on the Ames test, one author identified ajoene as a primary compound that prevents genetic mutations.

Antidiabetic Effects

Animal studies have demonstrated the hypoglycemic (blood sugar lowering) action of garlic. Allicin has been shown to have a significant hypoglycemic effect because it appears to compete with insulin for insulin-inactivating sites in the liver, resulting in an increase in free insulin in the bloodstream.

Miscellaneous Effects

HIV and AIDS

One small German study of 10 patients with advanced AIDS and severely low natural killer (NK) cell activity (all had opportunistic infections) involved the ingestion of 5 g of garlic (Kyolic) daily for 6 weeks, followed by 10 g daily for another 6 weeks. Three patients died before the trial was completed, but all 7 patients who completed the trial were reported to have normal natural killer cell activity by the completion of the trial. Symptoms from their opportunistic infections were also reported to have improved, including chronic diarrhea and genital herpes.

Anti-Aging Properties

Garlic has a reputation for being able to prolong longevity and youthful appearance. However, few studies support these claims. Researchers report that ingestion of garlic was able to increase the survival of age-accelerated-prone mice (genetically bred to have shorter survival times) but did not affect the survival of another strain of mice bred to have longer survival times. Garlic appears to have improved the performance of mice in several models designed to test learning deficits, memory acquisition, and memory deficits. The applicability of these findings to human physiological aging and age-related memory deficits is unknown.

Common Cold

One double-blind, randomized controlled trial evaluated 146 patients using garlic over the course of 12 weeks between November and February. Participants used a five-point scale to describe their health and kept record of common cold infections and symptoms in a daily diary. Patients took 1 capsule daily of either a placebo or an allicin-containing garlic extract supplement (Allimax, dose not reported). It was found that patients in the treatment group had a significantly lower number of colds and recovered faster from them than those in the placebo group.

Earaches

Garlic oil is a popular folk remedy for the relief of earaches. Traditionally, raw garlic is inserted into the ear. Garlic's usefulness for this indication is thought to be related to the antibacterial action of allicin.

Fatigue

Two studies have been published on the effects of garlic supplementation on fatigue. Both were positive, leading one study to conclude that garlic may be effective in reducing tiredness. In the first study, it was found that taking aged garlic extract (2 mL twice daily) for 22 days improved the subjective symptoms of fatigue and enhanced the threshold of knee reflection in athletes given an exercise load by using a subjective or objective fatigue test. The second study looked at the effects of taking a combination product that contained aged garlic extract with pyridoxine hydrochloride, nicotinamide, pantenol, and liver extract for 4 weeks. There was a significant decrease in measured performance of brain function associated with mental fatigue, but the role of garlic cannot be determined from that of the other ingredients.

> *Two studies have been published on the effects of garlic supplementation on fatigue. Both were positive, leading one study to conclude that garlic may be effective in reducing tiredness.*

Ischemia (Restriction in Blood Supply)

Aged garlic extracts have been shown to provide a protective action in a rat model of brain ischemia (a lack of blood supply resulting in a stroke). The mechanism of action is hypothesized to be either an antioxidant action or an inhibitory action on arachidonic acid metabolism.

Antioxidant Effects

Several in vitro studies have demonstrated the antioxidant activity of garlic. This activity is thought to be related to the mechanisms of action of many of its clinical effects, including decreasing blood cholesterol levels and providing protection in ischemic attacks.

Protection from Acetaminophen-Induced Liver Toxicity

Two animal studies report that pretreatment with garlic provides protection from acetaminophen-induced liver toxicity in a time- and dose-dependent manner.

Tick Repellent

A brief report of a crossover study of 100 Swedish military service personnel suggested that daily consumption of garlic (1,200 mg) for 8 weeks may decrease tick bites. This finding has been questioned. Additional studies are required.

Adverse Effects

Heartburn, flatulence, and gastrointestinal upset have been noted, usually at doses equivalent to 5 or more cloves daily. In addition, the odor of garlic is noticeable in the milk of lactating women. Contact dermatitis caused by direct skin contact with raw garlic is also possible, although most case reports occur in individuals, often young children, where crushed garlic pastes are applied to the skin for extended periods of time.

Several cases of allergic reactions to garlic have been reported in the literature. In one case, a cook developed eczematous eruptions on his hands and was found to have a positive type IV patch test for diallyl disulfide, one of the compounds in garlic. In addition, a single case of IgE-mediated urticaria caused by the ingestion of garlic has been reported. In another instance, a 47-year-old man developed ruptured blisters in a crusted, bloody, erosive, and scaling lesion over a large area on his knee. He had applied garlic under occlusion for about 12 hours on his knee, and the lesions started to appear 2 days later. This had been the first time he tried using garlic to relieve joint pain. Finally, one case of exercise-induced anaphylaxis possibly stimulated by garlic has been described.

Several cases of postoperative bleeding associated with the ingestion of garlic have been reported. A 72-year-old man who had been taking garlic for "many years" experienced unusual bleeding following a transurethral resection (TURP), and laboratory tests confirmed a decrease in platelet coagulation in the presence of collagen. Another case involved a 32-year-old women undergoing elective cosmetic surgery who also experienced increased bleeding postoperatively. Her heavy dietary garlic intake prior to surgery is suspected to have caused her increased blood-clotting time.

Several cases of occupational asthma stimulated by garlic have also been reported in the literature.

In animal studies, rats fed high concentrations of garlic for a prolonged period suffered from anemia, weight loss, and failure to grow. Rats administered 500 mg/kg (equivalent to 10 cloves per day in humans) intraperitoneally once daily were reported to have extensive damage to the lungs (thickening of the alveolar walls) and liver, especially near the organ's surface. The same dose administered orally caused less damage, and those fed low doses of garlic orally (50 mg/kg, which is equivalent to 1 clove or 3–4 g in humans) daily had no significant lung or liver damage.

Cautions/Contraindications

Garlic supplements in doses above those found in the diet should be used with caution by pregnant and lactating women. In addition, due to possible postsurgical bleeding, such doses should be avoided before undergoing surgical procedures. One author also recommends caution after organ transplants, because it has been reported that garlic enhances the activity of natural killer cells, which are largely responsible for tissue rejection.

Attacks of pemphigus, a relatively rare autoimmune disorder resulting in lesions of the mucous membranes and skin, may be induced by drugs that contain active thiol groups. This sulfur-containing group is found in garlic; thus, it is suggested that patients with this condition avoid garlic.

Constant use of garlic and garlic supplements may cause stomach and intestinal discomfort, sweating, bleeding disorders, and allergic reactions.

Drug Interactions

A possible interaction with warfarin has been reported. In addition, it has been suggested that garlic may potentiate the antithrombotic effects of ASA. High doses of garlic may also interfere with existing diabetic therapy because it appears to have a hypoglycemic effect.

> *High doses of garlic may also interfere with existing diabetic therapy because it appears to have a hypoglycemic effect.*

There are two case reports of HIV-infected persons taking garlic who developed severe gastrointestinal toxicity after initiating ritonavir-containing antiretroviral therapy. However, a study evaluating the effect of acute dosing of garlic supplements on the single-dose pharmacokinetics of ritonavir did not find any significant changes in the pharmacokinetics of ritonavir in healthy volunteers. The authors caution that their results should not be extrapolated to steady-state conditions, where the possibility of an interaction still needs to be evaluated. Taking garlic at the same time as the HIV drug saquinavir (Invirase, Fortovase) may lower the concentration of the drug in the blood.

On a more positive note, an animal study has found potential in garlic oil to reduce the possible genetic damage that may be associated with taking the anti-HIV drug stavudine (Zerit, d4T).

Garlic did not appear to have any interactions with the cancer drug docetaxel in a prospective study of cancer patients (11 women, aged 40 to 66 years) taking 600 mg garlic tablets (3,600 mcg of allicin per tablet) twice a day by mouth for 13 days while being treated with docetaxel at the same time.

Dosage Regimens

- Fresh garlic: 3–30 g (1–8 cloves) daily.

The German Commission E considers a daily dose equivalent to 4 g of fresh garlic to be therapeutically effective.

The *British Herbal Compendium* recommends:

- Dried cloves: 2–5 g of fresh air-dried daily.
- Dried powder: 400–1,200 mg of fully dried powder daily.
- Garlic oil: 2–5 mg daily.
- Allicin: 2–5 mg daily.

Selected References

Ernst E. Can *Allium* vegatables prevent cancer? Phytomedicine 1997;4(1):79–83.

Rahman K, Lowe GM. Garlic and cardiovascular disease: A critical review. The Journal of Nutrition Mar 2006;163 (Supp 3):736S–40S.

Silagy CA, Neil HA. A meta-analysis of the effect of garlic on blood pressure. Journal of Hypertension 1994;12(4):463–68.

Stevinson C. Garlic for treating hypercholesterolemia: A meta-analysis of randomized clinical trials. Annals of Internal Medicine 2000;133(6):420–29.

Ginger
Zingiber officinale Roscoe

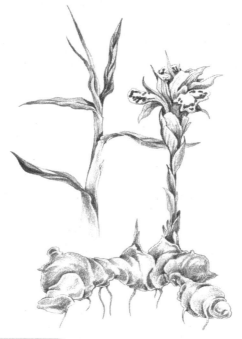

Common Uses
- Digestive aid (dyspepsia and gastrointestinal upset)
- Motion sickness
- Nausea (following anaesthesia)
- Nausea and vomiting due to pregnancy (see Cautions/ Contraindications)
- Inflammatory conditions (such as osteoarthritis, rheumatoid arthritis, and myalgias)

Active Constituents
- Components of the oleoresin portion (notably the gingerols and shogaols)

Adverse Effects
- Heartburn and digestive upset (rare)

Cautions/Contraindications
- Gallstones (use only under medical supervision)
- Pregnancy (doses greater than 1 g daily should be used in pregnancy only when the patient is under medical supervision)

Drug Interactions
- None noted when ginger is taken at the suggested therapeutic doses

Doses
General Use:
- *Dried rhizome:* 0.25–1 g taken orally as a capsule, tablet, powder or decoction three times daily
- *Weak ginger tincture BP (1:5 in 90% ethanol):* 1.5–3 mL three times daily
- *Strong ginger tincture BP (1:2 in 90% ethanol):* 0.25–0.5 mL

General Anti-emetic:
- *Powdered rhizome:* 1–2 g single dose

Motion Sickness:
- *Powdered rhizome:* 2–4 g daily

Introduction

Family
- Zingiberaceae

Synonyms
- Zingiber
- Gan-jiang

Medicinal Forms
- Dried root
- Tincture

Description
While native to southern Asia, ginger is one of the most widely used spices in the world and is now cultivated throughout India, Australia, the Caribbean (notably Jamaica), and parts of West Africa. The plant is an erect perennial, growing up to 1 meter (40 inches) in height, with knife-shaped leaves, white or yellow flowers, and a characteristic gnarled, aromatic rhizome.

Parts Used
The rhizome (underground stem), which is often referred to as the root, is the part used medicinally. Once the rhizomes are harvested, they can be used as fresh ginger (green ginger), candied ginger, dried ginger (as a spice), or an extract (e.g., volatile oil).

Traditional Use
Very few herbs have more of a medicinal history than ginger. Its use originated in the healing models of Asia and quickly spread to the ancient cultures of Europe and the Middle East. It was introduced to North America during the exploration of the "New World" in the 16th century. Historically, it has been used for numerous conditions, ranging from dyspepsia and vomiting to cholera and malaria. Ginger has also been used extensively as a culinary spice.

Current Medicinal Use
A growing amount of evidence, including clinical trials, supports the use of ginger in the treatment of a number of forms of nausea, including motion sickness, nausea from pregnancy, and potentially even after anesthesia. Ginger may also prove useful as a digestive aid in treating dyspepsia and asthma, as well as acting as an anti-inflammatory in the treatment of certain types of arthritis and muscle aches, or myalgias.

Relevant Research

Preventative and Therapeutic Effects

Constituents
- Oleoresin: pungent principles, notably gingerols, shogaols and zingerone. (Proportion of shogaols increases upon drying; these compounds are largely absent in the fresh plant.)
- Volatile oils: complex mixture of various hydrocarbons, including beta-bisabolene, zingiberene, zingiberol, various alcohols, and aldehydes.
- Lipids: free fatty acids, triglycerides, phosphatidic acids, lecithins.
- Carbohydrates: up to 50% starch.

Antinausea Effects
Of all its modern-day applications, ginger is perhaps best known for its suggested use in

the management of nausea. Since nausea can be caused by many different things, the section below reviews the scientific evidence for using ginger to manage motion sickness, nausea associated with anesthesia, nausea associated with chemotherapy, nausea associated with pregnancy, and nausea associated with other drugs.

> *Of all its modern-day applications, ginger is perhaps best known for its suggested use in the management of nausea.*

Motion Sickness

A number of clinical trials have been conducted to investigate the use of ginger in the management of motion sickness. One of the challenges with reviewing these studies is that they used many different doses, dosing schedules, and forms of ginger. A 2007 review and a more comprehensive 2005 meta-analysis agree that there may be benefit in using ginger for motion sickness; however, one suggested that more robust evidence is required before ginger should be routinely recommended.

The 2007 review included six controlled studies, of which five reported positive results when ginger was used to treat motion sickness. Three studies were both double-blinded and randomized and the other two were not randomized. There were between 8 and 662 participants involved in these trials, with most of them having fewer than 70. All of the studies used ginger powder at a daily dosage that ranged from 0.5 to 2 g. The author concluded that people with motion sickness may benefit from using ginger.

Eleven human studies on experimental and clinical motion sickness were identified in the 2005 meta-analysis. Both controlled and uncontrolled clinical studies and preclinical studies were included in this review, with most of these studies being randomized and blinded. The study size ranged from 8 to 662 participants, with 8 of the 11 studies having fewer than 40 participants. Ten of the trials used ginger powder, while one used freshly minced ginger, and the dosage ranged from 0.5 to 3.5 g of ginger per day (most were around 1 g daily). With two exceptions, all the studies in this meta-analysis reported ginger to be superior to a placebo or similarly effective to a comparator anti-emetic treatment. One of the negative studies found scopolamine to be more effective than ginger.

However, only one (positive) study was known to use a validated outcome measure (time to vomit), and this study has been criticized for other aspects of its methodology. The other studies all used non-validated or not-yet-validated outcome measures. Because of this, the authors of the review concluded that "the evidence is insufficient to suggest the effectiveness of ginger beyond reasonable doubt" for this condition.

The Commission E, a German government advisory body, has approved the use of ginger in the management of motion sickness. Their suggested dosage of 2 to 4 g daily is higher than those used in the majority of the studies. In addition, many practitioners suggest that for the prevention of motion sickness, ginger must be ingested for a prolonged period, starting several days before the journey commences.

In conclusion, while ginger is a long-established treatment for motion sickness in complementary health-care circles, its efficacy, especially for severe forms of motion sickness, has yet to be conclusively confirmed by high-quality clinical trials.

> *The Commission E, a German government advisory body, has approved the use of ginger in the management of motion sickness.*

Postoperative Nausea and Vomiting

Many anti-emetics commonly used to control nausea and vomiting following surgery have side effects, which has led to a search for a less toxic agent. Studies of the use of ginger for the prevention of postoperative nausea and vomiting have presented conflicting results. A 2006 comprehensive meta-analysis assessed data from five randomized trials including a total of 363 patients. The authors of this review concluded that when 1 g or more of ginger was taken orally, it could significantly reduce the incidence of 24-hour postoperative nausea and vomiting for patients recovering from gynecologic and lower extremity surgeries. The authors also noted, however, that further research is necessary to clearly define ginger's role in postoperative nausea and vomiting.

> *Overall, ginger appeared to be the best treatment, supporting its role in preventing postoperative nausea and vomiting.*

In contrast, a 2005 meta-analysis report concluded that ginger was not effective at relieving postoperative nausea or vomiting despite the fact that ginger was found to be superior to placebo and/or similar in efficacy of a comparator drug in all six randomized controlled studies included in this review. The authors explain that they reached their negative conclusion because in the studies that compared ginger to another medication, the comparative treatments were either ineffective or only weakly effective (i.e., metoclopramide 10 mg), or their effects were not improved by the addition of ginger (to droperidol and to diazepam), which is thus technically a negative finding for ginger. The comparative meta-analysis of the pooled data from these studies led the authors to conclude that there was "no evidence beyond reasonable doubt that ginger is effective as a postoperative antiemetic." The fact that a larger number of studies was considered in this meta-analysis may contribute to the reasons why this conclusion differs from that of the 2006 review described above.

One additional large double-blind, randomized controlled trial investigating the ability of ginger to prevent postoperative nausea and vomiting compared to four common anti-emetics and a placebo has been published since the reviews described above. In this new trial, patients were given capsules of ginger (containing 250 mg of shavings of fresh ginger), one of four drugs (metoclopramide 10 mg, prochlorperazine 5 mg, promethazine 20 mg, and ondansetron 4 mg), or a placebo 1 hour before the surgical procedure and at 8-hour intervals thereafter for a total of 24 hours. No one in the ginger group experienced nausea, but 15% of patients had vomiting, all of them in first 6 hours postoperatively. The frequency and quantity of vomiting was significantly lower among those in the ginger group than among those in the placebo group. Ginger was significantly more effective than both metaclopramide (40% of patients experienced nausea or vomiting) and prochlorperazine (35% of patients experienced nausea or vomiting) in reducing postoperative nausea and vomiting. The incidence of postoperative nausea and vomiting was slightly less with ginger (15% of patients) than with promethazine (20% of patients) and ondensetron (25% of patients). Overall, ginger appeared to be the best treatment, supporting its role in preventing postoperative nausea and vomiting.

Although additional high-quality trials are needed to determine the optimal dose and dosing regimen, the totality of the evidence suggests that ginger may be helpful in the management of postoperative nausea and vomiting.

Nausea Associated with Pregnancy

Three reviews published in 2005 all agree that there is sufficient evidence to conclude that ginger is effective in the management of nausea associated with pregnancy.

> *There is sufficient evidence for the use of ginger in the management of nausea associated with pregnancy. The only condition for which there is clinical evidence beyond doubt is pregnancy-related nausea and vomiting.*

In a comprehensive review of literature from 1966 to 2004 to evaluate ginger's safety and efficacy during pregnancy, it was concluded that ginger appears to be a fairly low-risk and effective treatment for nausea and vomiting associated with pregnancy. Five double-blind, randomized controlled trials were discussed in the review. Three found ginger treatment to be superior to a placebo, one found ginger to be more effective than vitamin B_6, and one found ginger to reduce symptoms just as well as vitamin B_6. The duration of these studies ranged from 3 days to 3 weeks, with three of the five testing ginger treatment for 3 to 4 days. The number of participants in the studies ranged from 26 to 291, with daily ginger doses in capsule or syrup form ranging between 1,000 mg and 1,500 mg daily. The authors suggest that divided doses ranging between 500 mg and 1,500 mg daily may be appropriate for patients not responding to traditional first-line therapies.

In another 2005 review, two additional studies were found to support ginger's use in the management of nausea associated with pregnancy. The first was a double-blind, randomized controlled trial in which 26 women were treated with either ginger syrup or a placebo. One tablespoon (15 mL) of ginger syrup (250 mg of ginger) in 4 to 8 ounces ($^1/_2$ to 1 cup) of hot or cold water four times daily for 2 weeks appeared to improve vomiting episodes and degree of nausea in the treatment group. However, no statistical analysis of the data was performed due to the small study size. In the other double-blind, randomized crossover trial of 30 women, powdered ginger root (250 mg four times daily for 4 days) was reported to be superior to a placebo treatment for hyperemesis gravidarum.

A third 2005 review concludes that there is sufficient evidence for the use of ginger in the management of nausea associated with pregnancy. The only condition for which there is clinical evidence beyond doubt is pregnancy-related nausea and vomiting. This review contained six of the aforementioned studies.

Chemotherapy-Induced Nausea

There is currently one large randomized controlled study under way that commenced in 2003 and will end in 2009 investigating whether ginger will increase the effectiveness of anti-emetic medications given to treat the effects of chemotherapy for cancer. In addition, an animal study found that an acetone extract of ginger (150 mg/kg) ingested orally by rats was comparable to metoclopramide (25 mg/kg) when administered 60 minutes prior to cyclophosphamide (300 mg/kg, injected). Both provided complete protection from vomiting episodes. The authors suggest that this warrants further investigation.

Mechanism of Action

The exact mechanism responsible for the anti-emetic effects of ginger is unknown. It appears that it is primarily due to a gastrointestinal action, rather than one mediated through the central nervous system. However, several studies have concluded that ingestion of ginger does not affect the gastric (stomach) emptying rate, as has been hypothesized by many investigators. A 2005 comprehensive meta-analysis found five studies that investigated ginger's ability to improve gastrointestinal motility. Three gave positive results, while two reported that ginger had no impact. The authors concluded that that there are not enough data to draw definitive conclusions about ginger's ability to improve gastrointestinal motility.

More recently, it has been suggested that ginger exerts a more generalized action on the entire gastroinestinal tract. In addition, the lack of centrally mediated action is being questioned. For example, ginger has been reported to antagonize 5-HT3 receptors, which are found in both the wall of the gastrointestinal tract and in the brain. Antagonism of these receptors produces antiemetic (antinausea and antivomiting) effects. A recent study suggests that ginger may have a novel antinausea action by decreasing tachygastric activity and preventing the elevation of plasma vasopressin induced by motion sickness caused by circular motion.

Digestive Actions

Ginger has long been praised in the management of digestive conditions. It is classically described as a "stimulating carminative," both aiding digestive function and tonifing the gastrointestinal system. Like many other spices, it has traditionally been used to enhance digestion by those who believed it increased salivary flow and gastric acid secretion.

Gastroprotective Action

Historical wisdom suggests that spices promote or irritate gastric ulcers. However, several animal studies have demonstrated that ginger has potential gastroprotective properties. In these studies, extracts of ginger were administered orally to rats in doses ranging from 500 to 1,000 mg/kg, resulting in significant decreases in the incidence of stress-induced gastric ulcers initiated by various experimental protocols (including HCl/ethanol and NSAIDs). Acetone extracts of ginger compared favorably to cimetidine and misoprostol in one animal study. While an exact mechanism of action has yet to be ascertained, it is suggested that certain components, especially zingiberene and 6-gingerol, may be influencing the activation of a protective action in cells.

In addition, several studies have demonstrated that extracts of ginger increased gastric pH and decreased gastric secretions.

In one study with rabbits, the effect of an aqueous extract of ginger (dose 169 mg/kg) on gastric secretion 3 hours after oral administration was comparable to an oral dose of 50 mg/kg of cimetidine. Another study found that the increase in gastric pH due to the ginger extract was very slight when compared to cimetidine. These actions may play a role in the gastroprotective action noted above.

> *Historical wisdom suggests that spices promote or irritate gastric ulcers. However, several animal studies have demonstrated that ginger has potential gastroprotective properties.*

Digestive Aid

Animal studies have shown that dried ginger added to the diet results in increased digestive enzyme action, especially lipase activity. Other studies have reported that an acetone extract of ginger caused an increase in bile secretion. These studies support the historical use of ginger to aid in the digestion of fatty meals.

Cardiovascular Effects

Ginger has long been praised in many healing models as an effective circulatory stimulant. While clinical evidence confirming ginger's influence on the cardiovascular system is limited, it has been shown that the gingerol portion exerts an inotropic effect on isolated guinea pig atria. One study in rats has found ginger to increase the circulation of cerebral circulation, which may improve the symptoms of cerebrovascular disease. No human studies have yet been conducted, and such results are needed before ginger's usefulness in this condition can be determined.

Inhibition of Platelet Aggregation (Blood Clotting)

Several studies have found that ginger inhibits platelet aggregation induced by various means, including adenosine diphosphate (ADP) and epinephrine. In a 2005 meta-analysis, five human studies that investigated ginger's ability to inhibit platelet aggregation were identified. Two gave positive results, while three found ginger to have no effect. The authors concluded that this was insufficient evidence to recommend ginger for use as a blood thinner.

Cholesterol-Lowering Effects

It has been suggested that ginger may be useful in the management of patients with elevated cholesterol levels. In 1978, a study of cholesterol-fed rats concluded that oral administration of ginger oleoresin (1.5 mg/kg) resulted in significantly lowered serum and hepatic cholesterol levels, as well as increased fecal excretion of cholesterol. These findings have been only partially supported by more recent studies. A 1984 study found that oral ingestion of 1 g of fresh ginger by rats offered no immediate protection against a cholesterol-rich diet. While ginger was shown to have an antihypercholesterolemic effect (it lowers high cholesterol levels in the blood), the study's results suggested that it must be ingested for several days before this action is manifested. A recent report of the isolation and identification of a specific compound, ZT, from ginger, which is assumed to be an HMG-CoA reductase inhibitor, found that ZT exerted an inhibitory effect on cholesterol synthesis in the body.

Musculoskeletal Effects

Ginger has historically been used for its anti-inflammatory properties in many Asian healing models, notably in the Ayurvedic (Indian subcontinent) and Kanpo (Japanese) systems of medicine. Attempts have been made to investigate this action in both animal models and human subjects.

> *Ginger has historically been used for its anti-inflammatory properties in many Asian healing models, notably in the Ayurvedic (Indian subcontinent) and Kanpo (Japanese) systems of medicine.*

Knee Pain

In a 2006 review, three clinical trials were identified that have tested the effects of ginger extract on pain. Two randomized, double-blind, placebo-controlled studies, one lasting for 6 weeks and one for 6 months, found ginger extract to have a statistically significant effect in reducing knee pain, but the size of the effect was only moderate. In contrast, the third randomized, double-blind, placebo-controlled crossover study of 46 patients with knee pain reported that ginger had no effect. The study authors suggested that a carryover effect of the ginger extract may have confounded the results because the statistics before the crossover suggested a positive effect. Although these findings seem promising, there is much more to be done in this area. The relative effectiveness of different extracts is unknown, and there are methodological limitations in measuring this. Given the confounding effects of the total diet, more clinical studies are needed to confirm these results.

Osteoarthritis and Rheumatoid Arthritis

In the same review, five studies, mostly randomized controlled trials, investigating the effect of ginger on symptoms of osteoarthritis and rheumatoid arthritis were assessed. Ginger extracts were tested at dosages ranging from 510 mg to 1 g daily. Arthritis pain was evaluated by various validated measures of pain, such as visual analog scales, the WOMAC (Western Ontario and McMaster universities) Osteoarthritis Index total score, and the SF-12 (12-item short form) Health Survey. The pain level of the participants in the intervention group was significantly lower than that in the placebo group in these trials, indicating moderately strong evidence that ginger may be a useful in treating these conditions. There was also a decreased use of NSAIDs and analgesics observed. However, one trial concluded that the improvement with ginger may not be clinically significant, and one of the other trials reported that ginger treatment was less efficacious than ibuprofen.

An earlier meta-analysis (2005) identified five studies, three of which were included in the aforementioned 2006 review, that assessed ginger's effect in inflammatory pain, including rheumatoid arthritis, knee pain, and swelling. Although the results of all the individual studies were positive, the authors concluded that "further studies are necessary to prove the efficacy of proprietary ginger preparations in the treatment of [inflammatory pain] and to find the optimum daily dosage" because not all of the studies were controlled trials, nor were important details of the preparations disclosed in the trials.

The results from these clinical trials are generally supported by two reviews of case studies, one with 7 and the other with 56 patients suffering from a variety of arthritic conditions and muscle pain. When ginger was ingested, an appreciable decrease in pain and swelling was noted in the majority of cases. The daily doses ingested by these patients ranged from 3 to 7 g of powdered ginger, with one individual ingesting 50 g of raw ginger daily. No adverse reactions were reported in any of these patients, who had taken ginger from periods ranging for 3 months to 2.5 years. Relief was normally noted within 1 to 3 months and remained for as long as the ingestion of ginger continued. Symptoms returned, usually within 2 weeks, when the therapy was discontinued. It should be noted that these reports were not clinical trials but case studies and no attempt was made to standardize the therapeutic protocols.

In one final randomized control trial, ginger was shown to be significantly more effective than a placebo and comparable to ibuprofen in decreasing pain and other symptoms of osteoarthritis. A total of 120 patients with osteoarthritis were assigned to one of three groups receiving ginger extract (1000 mg daily), ibuprofen (1200 mg daily), or the placebo for 1 month.

While no exact mechanism of action is known, the anti-inflammatory action of ginger could be due in part to its influence on eicosonoid production and other inflammatory mediators. Constituents of the oleoresin portion, especially the gingerols, are thought to decrease levels of inflammatory mediators produced from lipid membranes. It has been suggested that by inhibiting cyclo-oxygenase and 5-lipoxygense respectively, the production of both inflammatory prostaglandins and leukotrienes could be prevented. In addition, aromatic components of ginger may inhibit the inflammatory action initiated by pyrogens, such as interleukin 1.

Asthma

Two studies of ginger produced mixed findings about ginger's usefulness for patients who suffer from asthma. One study randomly assigned 92 patients diagnosed with asthma who were receiving therapy for at least 1 year into two groups: one received an alcoholic extract of gingerroot (150 g/mL, or 150 g/drop) of which 20 drops were to be taken every 8 hours and the other received a placebo for 2 months. Significant subjective improvements were observed in the number of patients experiencing dyspnea (difficulty in breathing), wheezing, and chest tightness. The study report did not identify whether the participants or the investigators of this study were blinded.

More high-quality clinical trials are necessary before ginger's benefits (or lack thereof) for asthma can be conclusively determined.

Another randomized, placebo-controlled, double-blind crossover study involved 32 adults with mild to moderate asthma who were given either a combination product containing ginger (as well as ginkgo and katuka, or *Picrorhiza kurroa*) or a placebo in addition to their usual treatment for 12 weeks. No significant improvements in lung function, symptoms, or quality of life were seen, although consistent trends were seen to improvements in patient-centered outcomes such as asthma symptom control, asthma health status, and cough health status. However, since this was a combination product, it is difficult to determine what, if any, role ginger played in determining these results. More high-quality clinical trials are necessary before ginger's benefits (or lack thereof) for asthma can be conclusively determined.

Migraines

Given its proposed anti-emetic action and the fact that the treatment of headaches is one of ginger's traditional uses, some have suggested that it may play a role in the management of migraines. The evidence to support this is limited to a single published paper reviewing one case history. In this case, 500 to 600 mg of powdered ginger was ingested by the patient at the first sign of an aura and then every 4 hours for 3 to 4 days thereafter. The development of the migraine was halted within 30 minutes. Subsequently, the patient began adding ginger to her diet, which resulted in a decreased incidence of migraines over the next 13 months.

Miscellaneous Effects

Cancer Prevention and Treatment

In a 2008 review, ginger is identified as possibly having protective effects against cancer. In addition, several studies using animals, human breast cancer cells, and human blood samples have demonstrated ginger's potential to treat or prevent cancer. However, these effects have not yet been studied in any human clinical trials.

Type 2 Diabetes

The only studies that have looked at ginger's effects on type 2 diabetes have used animal models. Although the results are positive, they cannot be extrapolated to human subjects.

Liver Protection

Ginger may have protective effects for the liver, but this has been demonstrated only in animal studies. In mice, orally injected ginger decreased the injury to the liver produced by excessive alcohol intake, decreased the effects of cadmium toxicity in mice liver cells, and decreased the genetic damage caused by parabens in the liver.

Antimicrobial and Antifungal Action

Certain constituents of ginger, notably the shogaols and zingerone, appear to exert an antimicrobial action against specific pathogens, including *Salmonella typhi*, *Vibrio cholerae*, and *Tricophyton violaceum*, in vitro. However, it does not appear that crude ginger extract is able to inhibit *Bacillus* species, *Escherichia coli*, or *Salmonella* species. The clinical relevance of these finding is unknown. Ginger essential oil has also been shown to have antifungal activity against fluconazole-resistant *Candida albicans*, often responsible for vaginal infections.

Memory Enhancement

Recent studies in animals suggest that ginger may have positive effects on memory. However, further research is warranted, as these data may not be directly extrapolated to the human population.

Weight Loss

A combination herbal product, NT, which contains ginger, rhubarb, astragalus, red sage, and turmeric combined with gallic acid, was assessed for its ability to enhance weight loss. The 24-week randomized controlled study involved 105 volunteers who were given either divided doses of 1.2 g of gallic acid and 300 mg of NT (containing 6% to 7% ginger) daily, 2.4 g of gallic acid and

600 mg of NT (containing 6% to 7% ginger) daily, or a placebo. All were given in capsule form. The results indicated that both high- and low-dose treatments were ineffective in inducing weight loss. It needs to be noted that, being a combination product, the effects cannot be exclusively attributed to ginger. More research using ginger as a single ingredient would be necessary before its effect in reducing weight can be determined.

Mosquito Repellent

A study using the arms of one human volunteer suggests that ginger may be an effective mosquito repellent. Essential oil of ginger was applied at levels of 1, 2, 3, and 4 mg/cm^2 separately in the exposed area of the forearm. Ethanol was used as a control. The volunteer inserted the treated and control arm into the same cage for 1 full minute every 5 minutes. The results showed that essential oil of gingerroot has significant repellent activity. Further testing in larger clinical trials is required before ginger can be recommended for this use.

Adverse Effects

Adverse effects of ginger appear to be so rare that the majority of Western European pharmacopoeias fail to mention any observed cases at all. In practice, unwanted side effects appear to be limited to gastric burning and dyspepsia (stomach upset). This is found more often when ginger preparations, which are not packaged into capsules, are taken and the individual lies down soon after taking the preparation. While some have cautioned against the prolonged use of ginger due to its anticoagulant properties (see Cardiovascular Effects, above), the use of ginger for culinary purposes or at therapeutic doses of less than 1 g daily do not appear to be associated with any significant adverse affects.

Cautions/Contraindications

The use of ginger in pregnancy has been questioned. This concern arises mainly from two sources: the use of ginger is "contraindicated" during pregnancy within the traditional Chinese medical (TCM) model, and several animal studies performed in the 1980s suggested that large doses of the gingerol portion may exert a mutagenic action in vitro. One study in rats found increased early embryo loss but increased growth of surviving fetuses. Finally, ginger has been anecdotally reported to induce labor during childbirth in western Uganda. However, it should be noted that the doses given within TCM therapeutic protocols are normally far higher (approximately 9 g daily) than those suggested for therapeutic purposes in North America (1–2 g daily). In addition, while it has been shown that 6-gingerol possesses mutagenic properties, antimutagenic components were also found to be present in the total ginger extract. Moreover, in the only study in pregnant women (with hyperemesis gravidarum), no teratagenic effects (i.e., birth defects) or increased rates of abortion were observed. Ginger has also been shown in both animal and human studies to be devoid of any negative effect on sperm.

While the Commission E monographs — which identify a higher therapeutic dose than other texts — do caution against the use of ginger in pregnancy, this concern is not shared by the other major pharmacopeias, such as the *British Herbal Compendium*. Consequently, it is reasonable to conclude that ginger can be taken for a limited period during pregnancy in doses within the North American standard therapeutic range.

Due to the reported inhibition of thromboxane synthetase, concerns have been raised over the possibility of increased bleeding time following surgery if the patient is taking ginger preparations. It appears unlikely that this presents a problem when the plant is taken in standard North American therapeutic doses, as described in the management of postsurgical nausea.

While the Commission E monographs – which identify a higher therapeutic dose than other texts – do caution against the use of ginger in pregnancy, this concern is not shared by the other major pharmacopeias, such as the British Herbal Compendium.

Given ginger's cholagogic properties (i.e., it increases the flow of bile), some authors caution against its use without medical supervision in people with gallstones.

Drug Interactions

There is one case report of a 76-year-old white European woman on long-term phenprocoumon (anticoagulant) therapy with an international normalized ration (INR) within the therapeutic range who began regularly using ginger products (pieces of dried ginger, tea from ginger powder). She had a history of heart problems and osteoporosis. Several weeks later, she developed an elevated INR up to 10 and nose bleeding. No other specific interactions could be found between ginger and conventional medications. Given the described pharmacological actions of ginger, it should be used with caution in situations of concurrent conventional cardiac, diabetes, and anticoagulant therapy.

Dosage Regimens
General Use:
- Dried rhizome: 0.25–1 g taken orally as a capsule, tablet, powder, or decoction three times daily.
- Weak ginger tincture BP (1:5 in 90% ethanol): 1.5–3 mL three times daily.
- Strong ginger tincture BP (1:2 in 90% ethanol): 0.25–0.5 mL.

General Anti-Emetic:
- Powdered rhizome: 1–2 g single dose.

Motion Sickness:
- Powdered rhizome: 2–4 g daily.

Selected References

Boone SA, Shields KM. Treating pregnancy-related nausea and vomiting with ginger. Annals of Pharmacotherapy 2005 Oct; 39(10):1710–13.

Chaiyakunapruk N, Kitikannakorn N, Nathisuwan S, Leeprakobboon K, Leelasettagool C. The efficacy of ginger for the prevention of postoperative nausea and vomiting: A meta-analysis. American Journal of Obstetrics and Gynecology 2006 Jan; 194(1):95–99.

Chrubasik S, Pittlerc MH, Roufogalis BD. Zingiberis rhizoma: A comprehensive review on the ginger effect and efficacy profiles. Phytomedicine 2005;12:684–701.

Cohen M. Traveller's "funny tummy" — Reviewing the evidence for complementary medicine. Australian Family Physician 2007 May;36(5):335–36.

Tapsell LC, Hemphill I, Cobiac L, Patch CS, Sullivan DR, Fenech M, et al. Health benefits of herbs and spices: The past, the present, the future. Medical Journal of Australia 2006 Aug 21;185(Supp 4):S4–S24.

Ginkgo

Ginkgo biloba L.

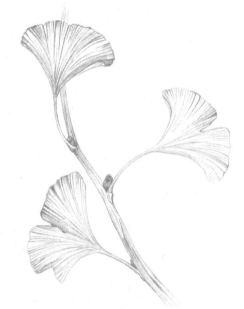

THUMBNAIL SKETCH

Common Uses
- Cerebral insufficiency
- Intermittent claudication
- Raynaud's syndrome
- Memory impairment and dementia
- Tinnitus
- Vertigo

Active Constituents
- Ginkolides
- Bilobides
- Flavone glycosides

Adverse Effects
- Extremely infrequent, but include gastrointestinal disturbances and headache
- Very rarely, spontaneous bleeding

Cautions/Contraindications
- Pregnancy and breastfeeding (safety not established)

Drug Interactions
- May potentiate the effect of anticoagulants (theoretical)

Doses
- Ginkgo biloba *extract (standardized for 24% ginkgo-flavone glycosides and 6% terpenoids):* 40 mg three times daily
- *Dried leaves:* 300 mg daily

Note: Treatment for many conditions must be continued for 1 to 3 months before positive results can be expected.

Introduction

Family
- Ginkgoaceae

Synonyms
- Maidenhair tree

Medicinal Forms
- Standardized extracts
- Dried leaves

Description
It has been estimated that the ginkgo tree has existed for more than 200 million years, making it the oldest known tree species on earth. Charles Darwin is reported to have called the ginkgo tree a living fossil. A given tree may live for 1000 years, growing to a height of 30 meters (100 feet) and up to 120 centimeters (40 inches) in diameter. The fan-shaped leaves attach to short, horizontal branches. The foul-smelling fruit is inedible but contains an edible seed that resembles an almond. Ginkgo trees are now extensively cultivated to meet the growing medicinal demand, and they continue to be favored by city planners because they flourish in adverse conditions in urban environments.

Parts Used
The leaves of the ginkgo tree are the part used medicinally in North America. Products standardized for 24% flavone glycosides and 6% terpenoids have been available for several decades as non-prescription agents. To date, the majority of the research has been conducted using one specific extract of ginkgo, EGb 761. However, several trials using a similar extract, LI 1370, are also reviewed here.

Traditional Use
Although ginkgo has been used in traditional Chinese medicine (TCM) for such indications as "benefiting the brain," as an astringent to the lungs, and for the relief of asthma symptoms and coughs, it is not generally regarded as a particularly important herb in TCM. However, ginkgo is considered a conventional drug in Europe, where annual sales are estimated as being more than US$500 million.

Current Medicinal Uses
Ginkgo biloba is one of the most widely used and best researched herbal medicines. While more evidence is needed, *Ginkgo biloba* products are used for a variety of conditions, many associated with aging, including peripheral vascular disease, tinnitus, dementia, cases of trauma to the brain, and "chronic cerebral insufficiency." The vast majority of research supporting the use of *Ginkgo biloba* refers to standardized extracts (*Ginkgo biloba* extract, or GBE) made from the leaf. While many people take GBE to enhance memory, there is currently little scientific evidence that it will work unless you have significant memory impairment.

Relevant Research

Preventative and Therapeutic Effects

Constituents

- **Terpenes:** diterpene ginkgolides (A, B, C, J, and M), sesquiterpenes (bilobalides).

- **Flavonoids:** ginkgo-flavone glycosides (e.g., bilobetin, gikgetin, isoginkgetin, sciadopitysin), glycosides of quercetin and kaempferol, isorhamnetin derivatives.

- **Organic acids:** 6-hydroxykynurenic acid, kynurenic acid, shikimic acid, protocatechic acid, vanillic acid, p-hydroxybenzoic acid.

- Essential oils.

- Tannins.

Cardiovascular Effects

Blood Flow

Many studies have demonstrated the ability of extracts of ginkgo (EGb 761) to increase blood flow. EGb 761 has been shown to increase skin perfusion, decrease blood viscosity, decrease blood vessel elasticity, increase blood flow in nail-fold capillaries, decrease erythrocyte aggregation, increase coronary blood flow in isolated guinea pig heart, and increase cerebral blood flow. However, plasma viscosity, packed cell volume, haematocrit, and thrombocyte aggregation do not appear to be affected by this ginkgo extract. The specific compounds in the ginkgo extract responsible for these effects have not yet been identified, although much attention has been focused on the flavonoids and the ginkolides.

Ginkgo extracts appear to have the ability to relax blood vessels in spasm and constrict those that are abnormally dilated by increasing their tone. Several authors have noted the ability of these extracts to produce dose-dependent relaxation of the aorta in animal models. This relaxant effect appears to be at least partially mediated by a factor that is released from endothelial cells. Other studies suggest that ginkgo extracts cause the relaxation of contracted blood vessels by prolonging the half-life of endothelium-derived relaxing factor. The flavonoids are thought to be primarily responsible for this action.

Interestingly, ginkgo seems to act preferentially at ischemic (oxygen-deprived) sites. For example, administration of extracts of ginkgo in animals subjected to cerebral ischemia increased glucose consumption, normalized mitochondrial respiration, diminished cerebral edema, preserved neurological function, and decreased the accumulation of free polyunsaturated fatty acids. In another animal study, *Ginkgo biloba* extract was found to be comparable to methylprednisone and more effective than thyroid-releasing hormone at providing a protective effect against ischemic spinal cord injury. This effect was thought to be due to its antioxidant actions.

> *Many studies have demonstrated the ability of extracts of ginkgo (EGb 761) to increase blood flow.*

Hypoxia

In addition, ginkgo has been shown to protect healthy volunteers from the effects of hypoxia. Animal studies have confirmed this finding. One study reported that both *Ginkgo biloba* extract and bilobalide alone were able to inhibit a hypoxia-induced decrease in ATP content and an increase in total lactate production in endothelial cells in test tube studies.

Antioxidant

The flavonoid components of *Ginkgo biloba* are reported to possess the potent antioxidant activity exhibited in its extract. Ginkgo's activity as an antioxidant is thought to play a role in many of its therapeutic actions, especially its postulated neuroprotective effect and its protection from ischemia-reperfusion damage. Several studies have demonstrated that the ginkgo extract EGb 761 has both hydroxyl radical scavenging and superoxide dismutase-like activity.

Cerebral Insufficiency

A variety of studies report the effectiveness of ginkgo in the treatment of chronic cerebral insufficiency. Symptoms typical of cerebral insufficiency include memory loss, difficulty concentrating, confusion, fatigue, decreased physical strength, anxiety, dizziness, tinnitus, headache, and depressive mood. It is hypothesized that these symptoms may be associated with some impairment of the cerebral circulation. One study reviewed 40 controlled trials studying the use of *Ginkgo biloba* in cases of "cerebral insufficiency" and concluded that although only 8 trials were of "good quality," all the trials reviewed except one showed clinically relevant positive effects for ginkgo when compared with a placebo. For example, in an open trial of 112 patients suffering from symptoms of chronic cerebral insufficiency (mean age 71 years) taking 40 mg *Ginkgo biloba* extract three times daily for 1 year, significant improvements in short-term memory, alertness, mood disturbances, vertigo, headaches, and tinnitus were reported. A more recent double-blind, placebo-controlled trial of 90 patients suffering from "cerebral insufficiency" found that those taking ginkgo scored significantly higher on a variety of tests of cognitive function.

> *A variety of studies report the effectiveness of ginkgo in the treatment of chronic cerebral insufficiency. Symptoms typical of cerebral insufficiency include memory loss, difficulty concentrating, confusion, fatigue, decreased physical strength, anxiety, dizziness, tinnitus, headache, and depressive mood.*

Peripheral Arterial Occlusive Disease

One of the most heavily studied peripheral arterial occlusive diseases is intermittent claudication. In 2000, a meta-analysis assessed the efficacy of ginkgo extract for intermittent claudication, based on the results of randomized, double-blind, placebo-controlled trials. Eight trials met their inclusion criteria (which included using pain-free walking distance as a primary outcome measure). The authors concluded that "*Ginkgo biloba* extract is superior to placebo in the symptomatic treatment of intermittent claudication. However, the size of the overall treatment effect is modest and of uncertain clinical relevance."

Another study reviewed 15 placebo-controlled trials that investigated the use of ginkgo extracts in the treatment of intermittant claudication. They report that only two were of "acceptable" quality and that all 15 indicated positive effects for treatment with ginkgo. A double-blind, placebo-controlled study of 79 patients given either ginkgo (40 mg) or a placebo three times daily for 1 year reported reduction in pain that was four times greater in the ginkgo group (p < 0.001). Given the overall poor quality of trials in this area, further research into the use of ginkgo extract for this indication was recommended.

Other clinical trials focus more on peripheral arterial occlusive diseases in general. A randomized, double-blind study designed to compare two different doses of ginkgo (extract EGb 761, 240 mg vs 120 mg daily) in patients with peripheral arterial occlusive disease Fontaine stage IIb reported that both dosage regimens led to clinically relevant improvement in pain-free walking distance after 24 weeks of treatment and that the higher dose (240 mg) produced a statistically significantly superior effect. Another double-blind, placebo-controlled trial investigated the use of ginkgo in 20 patients suffering from stage II claudicating arterial occlusive disease. Each patient ingested 160 mg *Ginkgo biloba* extract (EGb 761) or a placebo twice daily for 4 weeks. The main outcome measure of this trial was measurement of the transcutaneous partial pressure of oxygen both at rest and after a treadmill test. The areas of ischemia decreased by 38% in the ginkgo group but did not change in the placebo group ($p < 0.04$).

Not all the trials for peripheral arterial occlusive diseases were in general positive. For example, a double-blind, placebo-controlled trial randomized 22 subjects with peripheral arterial disease to receive 12 weeks of either 240 mg *Gingko biloba* tablets or a placebo and then 12 weeks of supervised treadmill exercise program combined with their randomized treatment. The authors measured parameters, such as walking capacity, oxygen consumption, and blood viscosity at baseline, several times during exercise. They reported that the only parameter significantly improved was walking duration; however, the benefit was seen in both the treatment and placebo groups. The authors concluded that administration of *Ginkgo biloba* treatment did not improve the effects of supervised exercise training in this test population.

While overall these results are promising and *Ginkgo biloba* extract may be of use in the conditions listed above, more research is needed before a definitive conclusion can be reached.

Ischemic Heart Disease

It is suggested that *Ginkgo biloba* extract may have a beneficial effect in patients who have experienced an ischemic stroke. A 2008 review identified 10 randomized controlled trials with a total of 792 patients who had recently experienced ischemic stroke. The outcome of interest in all the studies was the number of patients with neurological improvement after a selected time span ranging from 14 to 35 days. After assessment of the articles, the authors concluded that only 1 out of 10 trials was of high methodological quality. This high-quality trial randomized 55 patients who had experienced an acute ischemic stroke more than 48 hours previously to receive either 40 mg of *Ginkgo biloba* extract or a placebo during 6-hour intervals, with all patients receiving routine management. The patients were assessed on the Mathews scale at baseline, 2 weeks, and 4 weeks, and improvement was seen in both the placebo and the treatment groups. The authors suggested that a trial using a different dosage of *Gingko biloba* that was started more quickly after the ischemic stroke may be more beneficial. This trial was unique because it used a sliding evaluation scale to assess neurological improvement, whereas the other nine trials in this review used a dichotomous method of

> *It is suggested that* Ginkgo biloba *extract may have a beneficial effect in patients who have experienced an ischemic stroke.*

assessment. A meta-analysis of the nine trials using the same outcome measure indicated a statistically significant improvement among patients treated with *Ginkgo biloba* compared to control patients. However, due to the methodological flaws in the available studies, the authors of the review concluded that more high-quality trials are needed to provide convincing evidence that *Ginkgo biloba* is an effective treatment for neurological recovery following stroke.

Ginkgo extracts have been reported to improve cardiac mechanical recovery, suppress leakage of lactate dehydrogenase, and diminish the decrease of myocardial ascorbate during reperfusion. It is hypothesized that this action of ginkgo may be attributed to its antioxidant properties. In addition, ginkgolide B has been shown to provide dose-related protection comparable to diltiazem and superior to metoprolol against dysrhythmias (disturbances of heart rhythm) induced by ischemia, which the authors hypothesize may be related to an antagonism of an increase in slow calcium influx induced by platelet aggregating factor (PAF) in myocardial cells. This study noted that ginkgolide B did not produce any changes in heart function, even when given in high doses.

Anticoagulant Effects

Ginkgo's ability to competitively inhibit platelet activating factor has been documented in a number of animal and test tube studies. One review completed in 2002 cited three clinical trials evaluating the use of *Ginkgo biloba* for inhibiting platelet aggregation. One trial administered a single oral dose of 600 mg *Ginkgo biloba* extract to 6 healthy male individuals, and another trial administered a lower dose of 240 mg daily for 7 days to 12 healthy individuals. The third study administered 87.5 mg of intravenous solution containing ginkgo extract to patients with atherosclerotic disorders. All of these studies reported an inhibition of induced platelet aggregation, the first study reporting that this effect was most pronounced 2 hours after consuming the extract. The authors of the review concluded that while this herb may show clinical potential, further research is necessary. There are also excellent reviews of this action.

Ginkgo extracts have been shown to decrease microvascular permeability, cause bronchodilation, and inhibit thromboformation in test tube studies and in animal studies to a degree comparable to acetylsalicylic acid (ASA). It is thought that the ginkgolides (especially ginkgolide B) are responsible for this action. However, several researchers have reported that ginkgo extracts do not affect coagulation or skin bleeding time.

Neurological and Psychiatric Effects

Neuron Metabolism

Animal studies have shown that extracts of *Ginkgo biloba* can influence neuron metabolism and have a positive effect on neurotransmitter disturbances. It appears to increase the production of dopamine and noradrenaline, as well as increasing the number of acetylcholine and serotonin receptors. In addition, one study demonstrated that chronic oral treatment with ginkgo prevented decline in muscarinic (cholinergic) receptor density in the hippocampus of rats as they aged. Test tube and animal studies indicate that the *Ginkgo biloba* extract EGb 761 increases synaptosomal uptake of 5-hydroxytryptamine and decreases the synaptosomal uptake of dopamine and serotonin.

It has been suggested that the bilobalides may aid in the regrowth of damaged neurons in the central nervous system; however, an exact mechanism of action has yet to be proven. *Ginkgo biloba* extract EGb 761 was also reported to prevent dopaminergic neurotoxicity in an animal study. It has been suggested that the neuroprotective effects of ginkgo are caused by its effect on glucocorticoid biosynthesis — it appears to decrease glucocorticoid levels and increase ACTH release. This mechanism of action has been described in detail, and other possible mechanisms for the neuroprotective properties associated with ginkgo have been described by many other authors.

The effect of ginkgo on cerebral glucose utilization continues to be controversial, with some studies reporting increases in cerebral glucose utilization, some reporting no change, and others reporting decreases.

Dementia

In recent years, much attention has been focused on the role of *Ginkgo biloba* in the management of various forms of dementia and other forms of moderate to severe memory impairment. A 2008 review of randomized double-blind trials using ginkgo (dose ranging between 120 and 500 mg daily) to treat dementia or cognitive decline identified 29 trials of varying durations (2 to 15 weeks) to be included in a meta-analysis. The outcome measures of these trials included cognitive function, activities of daily living, behavior, quality of life, safety, viability of treatment, and dependency. The meta-analysis reported no consistency in patterns of improvement, with some symptoms showing improvement earlier but not later in treatment and others showing improvement only after a period of 24 weeks. The conclusion of this review was that there are substantial discrepancies in trials concerning

> *In recent years, much attention has been focused on the role of Ginkgo biloba in the management of various forms of dementia and other forms of moderate to severe memory impairment.*

this topic and that further well-designed trials are needed to determine if *Ginkgo biloba* improves symptoms of dementia.

A review article published in 2000 compared placebo-controlled efficacy studies of cholinesterase inhibitors and ginkgo extracts that were at least 6 months in duration. The authors concluded that ginkgo extract Egb 761 and second-generation cholinesterase inhibitors (donepezil, rivastigmine, metrifonate) should be considered equally effective in the treatment of mild to moderate Alzheimer's dementia. This conclusion is supported by the results of a 2006 double-blind 24-week trial in which patients with Alzheimer's-associated dementia were randomized to receive either placebo, 160 mg daily dose of EGb 761, or a 5 mg daily dose of donepezil. Analysis of Clinical Global Impression (CGI) scores indicated that the clinical efficacy of EGb 761 was comparable to that of denepezil.

Memory Enhancement
There is growing interest in whether ginkgo might provide memory enhancement among individuals without memory impairment. Although improvement of short-term memory, simple reaction time, attention, speed of processing abilities, and other neuropsychological tests in healthy volunteers and improved retention of learned behavior in healthy rats have been reported, the evidence supporting these effects remains controversial. This is because other studies have reported negative results — that ginkgo did not have a beneficial effect on neuropsychological tests of learning, memory, attention, concentration, or verbal fluency. Several studies have also reported enhanced cognitive function in healthy volunteers who ingested combination products that included ginkgo and Asian ginseng, although the magnitude of ginkgo's effect in these products is unknown.

Given the wide range of neuropsychological outcomes assessed, it is difficult to compare the results of different studies. Additional research is required to determine if ingesting ginkgo will have any clinically significant effect on the cognitive function and memory of healthy individuals. This is particularly important because memory enhancement is frequently the reason people take ginkgo.

> *Although improvement of short-term memory, simple reaction time, attention, speed of processing abilities, and other neuropsychological tests have been reported, the evidence supporting these effects remains controversial.*

Depression
One randomized, placebo-controlled trial with 40 patients aged 51 to 78 years diagnosed with resistant depression found that *Ginkgo biloba* extract (EGb 761) was significantly more effective than a placebo. Patients in the trial had shown insufficient improvement when taking tri- and/or tetracyclic antidepressants for a minimum of 3 months before being enrolled in the trial. During the trial, patients continued to take antidepressant therapy but were also given either EGb 761 (80 mg) or a placebo three times daily. The main outcome measure was the sum score of the Hamilton Depression Rating Scale (HAMD). After 4 weeks, a significant (50%) decrease in the severity of depression for the EGb 761 group, compared to a 10% decrease in the placebo group, was noted. A further significant decrease in the HAMD scores was noted after 8 weeks for the ginkgo group.

However, another randomized, double-blind, placebo-controlled study of 27 patients with seasonal affective disorder (SAD) did not support this claim. Treatment with ginkgo (1 tablet twice daily of ginkgo extract PN246, Bio-Biloba) for 10 weeks starting in a symptom-free period about 1 month prior to the expected onset of symptoms did not prevent the development of the symptoms of seasonal affective disorder, and no significant differences were found between the ginkgo and the placebo groups. One study found that extracts of ginkgo leaves caused reversible inhibition of rat brain MAO-A and MAO-B, suggesting a mechanism for reported antidepressant effects.

Sudden Hearing Loss

Two studies have investigated the effects of ginkgo in patients with sudden hearing loss. One randomized, double-blind trial compared two doses (120 mg vs 12 mg twice daily over 8 weeks) of ginkgo extract EGb 761 in 106 outpatients with acute idiopathic sudden hearing loss of at least 15 decibels (dB) at one frequency within speech range occurring less than 10 days before inclusion in the study. A majority of both treatment groups recovered completely. The authors conclude that a "higher dose of EGb 761 (oral) appears to speed up and secure the recovery." In this case, while promising, it is important to realize that, without a placebo group, it is difficult to determine whether these results would be greater than those seen with a placebo.

The second randomized, double-blind study compared non-oral admisnitration of ginkgo extract EGb 761 (200 mg IV infusion) to pentoxifylline (300 mg IV infusion) for 10 days in 72 patients with sudden deafness. The authors concluded that ginkgo extract EGb 761 given by IV was as effective a treatment for sudden deafness as pentoxifylline.

Trauma to the Brain

Numerous animal studies have suggested that ginkgolide B has a protective effect against neuronal damage following trauma, probably related to its platelet-activating factor (PAF) antagonist action. A study with rats suggests that treatment with *Ginkgo biloba* extract reduced the extent of brain swelling in response to injury (bilateral frontal cortex lesions) and was associated with less impairment following the injury. In addition, it has been shown in rat experiments that EGb 761 treatment prior to electroconvulsive shock (ECS) treatment reduces the extent and duration of the remodeling of membrane phospholipids that traditionally results from seizures.

Schizophrenia

Two clinical trials have investigated the effects of ginkgo in addition to haloperidol in individuals diagnosed with schizophrenia. One randomized, double-blinded, placebo-controlled study used ginkgo (360 mg EGb 761 extract daily) as an adjunctive treatment to haloperidol (0.25 mg/kg/day) on the symptoms experienced by 82 patients with treatment-resistant chronic schizophrenia according to ICD-10 criteria. Both groups' scores on the Scale for the Assessment of Negative Symptoms (SANS) improved compared to baseline, but only those taking ginkgo had improved scores on the Scale for the Assessment of Positive Symptoms (SAPS). The authors concluded that these results suggest that ginkgo may "enhance the efficacy of the classic antipsychotic haliperidol in patients with schizophrenia, especially on their positive symptoms."

A similar study randomized 109 schizophrenic patients to receive either 360 mg daily EGb 761 or a placebo while receiving 0.25 mg/kg/day haloperidol. The authors stated that there was a significantly lower peripheral immune support cell population in schizophrenic patients than in healthy controls at baseline and that the group treated with ginkgo and haloperidol had a more marked increase in immune cell status compared to the group taking a placebo and haloperidol.

While these preliminary studies are promising, additional research is necessary to confirm the findings.

> *Two clinical trials have investigated the effects of ginkgo in addition to haloperidol in individuals diagnosed with schizophrenia.*

Eye Effects

Ginkgo biloba extract is believed to protect the eye from damage by reducing free-radical damage to the retina. Animal studies suggest that ginkgo may be useful in the prevention of retinal damage in diabetes and in cases of lesions, inflammations, or degenerative insults of the retina. In addition, several small clinical studies provide preliminary evidence that ginkgo may be beneficial in the management of glaucoma.

A double-blind trial involving 10 individuals with senile macular degeneration found ginkgo to be significantly better than a placebo at improving long-distance visual acuity. An additional randomized, double-blind, placebo-controlled crossover study reported that ingestion of ginkgo (40 mg of Ginkoba three times daily) for 2 days resulted in a significant increase in end diastolic velocity in the ophthalmic artery in 11 healthy volunteers. The authors suggested that ginkgo deserves further investigation as a possible treatment of glaucomatous optic neuropathy and other ischemic ocular diseases.

These data are supported by another placebo-controlled study that used either 40 mg ginkgo extract daily with a topical ocular beta blocker or the topical ocular beta blocker alone in 30 participants with primary open angle glaucoma. The authors reported a significant increase in ocular blood flow and end diastolic velocity after 3 months in the group taking both ginkgo and the beta blocker, compared to the group taking only the beta blocker. Finally, a fourth randomized, placebo-controlled, double-blind crossover study assessed the effect of ginkgo (40 mg extract standardized for 24% flavinoid glycosides and 6% terpenes three times daily) for 8 weeks on pre-existing visual field damage in 27 patients with normal tension glaucoma. In this study, ginkgo treatment resulted in significant improvement in visual field indices compared to baseline, while no significant changes were noted in the placebo group.

Ear Effects

The effects on the ear appear to be related to the ability of ginkgo to increase cochlear blood flow (CBF). One study of *Ginkgo biloba* extract (EGb 761) in guinea pigs demonstrated that after 4 to 6 weeks of treatment, EGb 761 partly counteracted sodium salicylate-induced decreases in CBF. In a double-blind trial of ginkgo for the treatment of acute cochlear deafness, ginkgo was found to be more effective than nicergoline (an alpha blocker), but significant improvement was seen with both treatments.

Tinnitus

A 2008 review of the use of *Ginkgo biloba* to treat tinnitus initially identified 172 trials for critique, although many were excluded for methodological reasons and only three were included in the final meta-analysis. The inclusion criteria for the meta-analysis were: participants experiencing tinnitus were 18 years of age or older, tinnitus was a primary complaint, and tinnitus was the result of "cerebral insufficiency." The three randomized, double-blind, placebo-controlled trials included in the review involved a total of 1,137 patients who took ginkgo extracts (from 120 to 150 mg daily) for from 12 weeks to 5 years.

One trial found that ginkgo was no more effective at treating stable tinnitus than the placebo. The second reported that the group receiving treatment with ginkgo showed a statistically significant decrease in loudness compared to the placebo group. The final study reported no significant difference between the placebo group and the treatment group in any improvement parameters measured. Based on these studies, the authors of the review concluded that the evidence does not indicate that *Ginkgo biloba* is effective for treating tinnitus and further research is necessary.

Vertigo

Several animal studies have demonstrated that the administration of ginkgo extracts speeds vestibular compensation. For example, accelerated postural, locomotor balance recovery, spontaneous neck muscle activity, vestibulo-collic reflexes, and spontaneous firing rates of vestibular units on the lesioned side were noted in unilateral vestibular neurectomized cats. One clinical study of patients with recent-onset idiopathic vertigo found that ginkgo significantly decreased the intensity, frequency, and duration of symptoms of vertigo when compared with a placebo.

Urological Effects

Impotence

Ginkgo biloba extract has been suggested in the treatment of impotence. One study of 60 patients with proven arterial erectile dysfunction who had not responded to papaverine injections were given 60 mg per day of ginkgo extract for 12 to 18 months. Improvement in blood flow (as measured by duplex sonography) was noted after 6 to 8 weeks, and 50% of the men gained potency after 6 months. In another 20% of the sample, a new trial with papaverine proved successful. This trial was not blinded, and given the large psychological component of impotence, additional studies are required to confirm these results.

These positive results were not supported by another study of the use of ginkgo in the management of antidepressant-induced sexual dysfunction. In this randomized, double-blind, placebo-controlled study involving 37 individuals, ingestion of ginkgo (120 mg

> *Further research in this area is needed to determine whether ginkgo may provide some benefit to patients with sexual dysfunction.*

daily for 2 weeks, followed by 160 mg for the second 2 weeks, followed by 240 mg daily for the final 4 weeks) was not associated with any significant improvement in sexual dysfunction compared to the placebo, although both patient groups did improve from baseline, confirming the presence of a placebo effect.

One laboratory study reported that fractions of *Ginkgo biloba* extract had a relaxing effect on corpus cavernosum tissue in test tube studies. Further research in this area is needed to determine whether ginkgo may provide some benefit to patients with sexual dysfunction.

Respirological Effects

Asthma

Several preliminary studies suggest that *Ginkgo biloba* extracts may have a beneficial effect in patients with asthma. A study of the smooth muscle relaxant activity of *Ginkgo biloba* on guinea pig trachea noted a concentration-dependent relaxation in test tube studies and antagonism of bronchoconstriction induced by various agonists in animal studies. One single-blind, randomized crossover study with 10 patients found that ingestion of 240 mg of *Ginkgo biloba* extract (BN 52063) 1 hour prior to induction of bronchoconstriction by hyperventilation with dry cold air did not result in any reduction in bronchoconstriction. On the third day of treatment with either BN 52063 or a placebo, asthma was induced by exercise in these patients. There was no effect on the initial bronchoconstriction of those receiving ginkgo; however, the prolonged reduction of peak expiratory flow was attenuated. The rise in plasma concentrations of platelet factor 4 and beta-thromboglobin seen in the placebo group was inhibited in the group treated with ginkgo extract ($p < 0.01$).

Miscellaneous Effects

Ginkgolide B (BN 52021) administered intravenously (120 mg twice daily for 4 days) was found to be useful as an adjunct to standard intensive care support in the treatment of patients with severe gram-negative bacterial sepsis, as determined by a randomized, double-blind, placebo-controlled, multi-center phase III clinical trial. There was a significant reduction in mortality of patients treated with ginkolide B compared with those taking the placebo. The authors suggest that this was due to the extract's ability to prevent a systemic inflammatory response to infection through platelet-activating factor antagonism, inhibition of amplification of sepsis-induced tumor necrosis factor and thromboxane B2 release, plasma trypsin-like activity, and several other steps of the immuno-inflammatory cascade associated with gram-negative bacterial sepsis.

Persons irradiated, either for therapeutic reasons or accidentally, have clastogenic factors in their plasma. Thirty workers accidentally exposed to radiation were given 40 mg of *Ginkgo biloba* extract (EGb 761) three times daily for 2 months, at which time the clastogenic activity of their plasma had returned to the same level as controls. This effect persisted for at least 7 months. This anticlastogenic effect was also demonstrated in test tube studies. Another study demonstrates the ability of ginkgo to protect microsomal fatty acids and proteins from UVC radiation-induced peroxidative degradation.

Ginkgo biloba extract was shown to inhibit cyclosporine A-induced peroxidation in human liver microsomes in a dose-dependent manner. Thus, it may have some use in the prevention of damage to human membranes caused by cyclosporine A.

Several components isolated from *Ginkgo biloba* have been reported to have antitumor activity.

Ginkgo is reported to have beneficial effects in cases of cyclic edema. The flavonoids are thought to normalize excessive capillary permeability, and one clinical study found complete elimination of edema in 3 patients and partial elimination of the edema in 6 patients. Ginkgo has also been reported to be effective against the "congestive" symptoms of PMS, especially breast symptoms.

One open-label, uncontrolled clinical trial involving 48 participants reported that ginkgo (extract GBE 761 ONC) administered intravenously once every 3 weeks in conjunction with 5-fluorouracil may enhance the response to treatment of patients with locally or metastatic advanced pancreatic cancer. Additional studies are needed to confirm these preliminary findings.

Adverse Effects

All three of the 2008 reviews by the Cochrane database discussed in this section have concluded that no major adverse effects have been associated with *Ginkgo biloba* and that minor effects that do arise are not significant compared to those associated with a placebo. Most sources suggest that side effects from ginkgo are extremely infrequent but include gastrointestinal disturbances, headache, and allergic skin reactions. Two systematic reviews report no serious side effects in any trial reviewed. Headaches, although relatively rare, appear to be the most common side effect. Some authors have suggested that these adverse effects may be decreased by slowly increasing to the therapeutic dose level.

> *Most sources suggest that side effects from ginkgo are extremely infrequent but include gastrointestinal disturbances, headache, and allergic skin reactions.*

Skin reactions are thought to be caused only by direct contact with the fruit of the ginkgo tree, which is not the part used medicinally. However, there is one case of a women who ingested 2 doses of a ginkgo preparation (brand and dose not known), as well as a ginkgo-containing product called

One-A-Day Memory and Concentration (Bayer Pharmaceuticals), prior to hospital admission for an exfoliative rash, blistering, and other symptoms consistent with Stevens-Johnson syndrome. The content of the products ingested by the patient was not analyzed, and the role of ginkgo in this case cannot be confirmed.

Several cases of spontaneous bleeding associated with ingestion of ginkgo have been reported; however, the role of ginkgo in these cases remains unclear. In one case report, a healthy 33-year-old woman with a long-term history of use of *Ginkgo biloba* (60 mg twice daily for 2 years) was reported to have an increased bleeding time and suffered bilateral subdural hematomas. Her bleeding times had returned to normal 35 days after discontinuation of ginkgo ingestion. In another case, a 70-year-old man presented with spontaneous bleeding from the iris into the anterior chamber of the eye 1 week after beginning treatment with 40 mg *Ginkgo biloba* extract daily. The patient had also been taking acetylsalicylic acid (ASA) 325 mg daily for 3 years. Given the large number of individuals ingesting *Ginkgo biloba* worldwide, this appears to be a relatively rare phenomenon; however, ginkgo has been shown to be a platelet-activating factor antagonist in in vivo and in vitro studies.

Cautions/Contraindications

Safety in pregnant and nursing mothers has yet to be established. One review suggests that ginkgo products should be used with caution around the time of labor because it may increase bleeding time.

Drug Interactions

Most authors suggest that there are no known drug interactions. Although there is little clinical evidence, theoretically *Ginkgo biloba* may potentiate the action of anticoagulants.

Dosage Regimens

Almost all of the research has been conducted using a standardized extract (SE): ginkgo-flavone glycosides (24%) and terpenoids (6%). A recent pharmacokinetic study found no significant differences between the bioavailability of three different formulations of *Ginkgo biloba* (capsules, drops, and tablets). There is an excellent review of the quality control and standardization of ginkgo preparations.

- **_Ginkgo biloba_ extract (standardized for 24% ginkgo-flavone glycosides and 6% terpenoids): 40 mg three times daily.**
- **Dried leaves: 300 mg daily.**

Note: Treatment for many conditions must be continued for 1 to 3 months before positive results can be expected.

Selected References

Birks J, Grimley, EJ. *Ginkgo biloba* for cognitive impairment and dementia. Cochrane Library 2008;2.

Drew S, Davies E. Effectiveness of *Ginkgo biloba* in treating tinnitus: Double-blind, placebo-controlled trial. British Medical Journal 2001;322(7278):73.

Mahady G. *Ginkgo biloba* for the prevention and treatment of cardiovascular disease: A review of the literature. The Journal of Cardiovascular Nursing 2002;16(4):21–32.

Pittler MH, Ernst E. *Ginkgo biloba* extract for the treatment of intermittent claudication: A meta-analysis of randomized trials. American Journal of Medicine 2000;108(4):276–81.

Zeng X, Liu M, Yang Y, Li Y, Asplund K. *Ginkgo biloba* for acute ischaemic stroke (Review). Cochrane Library 2008;3.

Ginseng
(Asian and American/Canadian)
Panax ginseng C.A. Meyer;
Panax quinquefolius

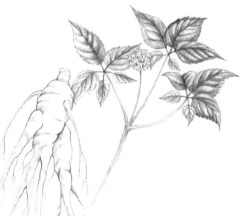

THUMBNAIL SKETCH

Common Uses
- Stress and fatigue (both physical and mental)
- Exercise (increased endurance and performance)
- Immune system (strengthening the immune system in cases of inadequate resistance to infection and in convalescence)
- Hyperglycemia (as an adjunct in the treatment of mild conditions)

Active Constituents
- Ginsenosides
- Panaxans

Adverse Effects
- Insomnia (most common), restlessness, and nervousness
- Euphoria
- Hypertension
- Diarrhea
- Skin eruptions

Cautions/Contraindications
- Hypertension, acute illness, premenopausal women (with unstable hormonal cycles), controlled diabetics, concomitant use of stimulants
- Children, pregnancy, breastfeeding (safety not established)

Drug Interactions
- Possible with many centrally acting drugs (e.g., phenalzine, pentobarbital, and haloperiol) and stimulants, including caffeine

Doses
- *Standardized extract (4% to 8% ginsenosides):* 100–500 mg daily in two or three divided doses
- *Raw root decoction (boiled in water or broth):* 0.6–4 g, usually taken in the morning

Note: In cases of long-term administration, ginseng is usually taken for a period of 2 to 3 weeks, followed by a 2-week resting period.

Introduction

Family
- Araliaceae

Synonyms
- *Panax ginseng*
- Asian ginseng
- Chinese ginseng
- Ginseng
- Korean ginseng
- Panax schinseng
- Nees
- Asiatic ginseng
- Oriental ginseng
- *Panax quinquefolius*
- American ginseng
- Canadian ginseng

Description
Although many different kinds of ginseng may be sold in Canadian and American retail outlets, two species are commonly seen in pharmacy practice: *Panax ginseng* C.A. Meyer (also called Panax ginseng, Chinese ginseng, Korean ginseng, or Oriental ginseng) and *Panax quinquefolius* (also called American or Canadian ginseng). Other closely related species include *Panax pseudoginseng* Wallich var. *japonicus* (C.A. Meyer) G. Hoo & C. J. Tseng (Japanese ginseng), *Panax pseudoginseng* Wallich var. *notoginseng* (Burkill) G. Hoo & C.J. Tseng (Sanchi ginseng), and *Panax trilolius* L. (Canadian dwarf ginseng); however, these three species are rarely seen. Another product widely available is *Eleutherococcus senticosus* (Rupr. & Maxim.) Maxim. (Siberian ginseng or eleuthero), which is in the same family (Araliaceae) but is not a true ginseng (member of the *Panax* genus). *Panax ginseng* (Chinese/Korean ginseng) and *Panax quinquefolius* (Canadian/American ginseng) will be discussed in this chapter, while *Eleutherococcus senticosus* (Siberian ginseng) will be reviewed in the next.

Panax ginseng C.A. Meyer is the most widely used and most extensively studied species of ginseng. Native to and now widely cultivated in both Korea and China, this herbaceous shrub grows to a height of 60 to 70 cm (20 to 25 inches) from a tap root and produces a cluster of small, green-yellow flowers. The fully grown tap roots are approximately 2 centimeters (1 inch) in diameter and 8 to 20 centimeters (3 to 8 inches) long. Many ginseng products available in North America are made from *Panax ginseng* grown in Asia.

Panax quinquefolius is a smaller plant, growing to 30 centimeters (1 foot), with oval leaflets, green flowers, and kidney-shaped red berries. Native to eastern North America, it is now cultivated to be sold primarily for medicinal products in Asia. *Panax quinquefolius* tastes sweeter and is considered to be more "yin" than *Panax ginseng* in the traditional Chinese medicine paradigm.

Parts Used
The roots from 4- to 6-year-old plants are harvested in September or October and used medicinally.

Traditional Use
"Panax" is derived from the Greek roots *pan*, meaning "all," and *akos*, meaning "cure," and refers to the cure-all or panacea quality generally attributed to the herb. The name "ginseng" means "essence of the earth in the form of a man" and refers to the resemblance of the root to a human form.

Ginseng has been an important part of traditional Chinese medicine (TCM) for more than 5,000 years. It is considered a bittersweet herb with a warming character. In traditional Chinese medicine, ginseng was used to restore "yang" quality and to treat general weakness, deficient *qi* (chi) patterns, anemia, lack of appetite, nervous agitation, thirst, and impotence. It is classified as an adaptogen, which is thought to increase non-specific resistance to adverse influences, such as stress and infection. Traditionally, it was used as a tonic to "increase strength, increase blood volume, promote life and appetite, quiet the spirit, and give wisdom." It was generally thought to improve vitality.

Current Medicinal Use

As with its traditional uses, Asian ginseng is primarily used as a tonic in the treatment and prevention of stress and fatigue and in strengthening the immune system. While Asian ginseng has been the subject of many clinical trials, the quality of the trials has often been poor and the results often conflicting. American/Canadian and Asian ginseng may be useful in stabilizing blood sugar levels.

Medicinal Forms

In North America, ginseng is commonly sold in two forms, white and red, which represent different processing procedures. White ginseng is obtained by drying the root, often peeling the external skin in the process. In contrast, red ginseng root is steamed, which produces a color like caramel. According to traditional Chinese medicine philosophy, red ginseng is more "heating," or more "yang," in nature than white ginseng.

Relevant Research

Preventative and Therapeutic Effects

Constituents

Panax ginseng

- Triterpenoid glycosides (saponins): ginsenosides Rb1, Rb2 = panaquilin B, panaxoside E

  ginsenoside Rc = panaquilin C, panaxoside D

  ginsenoside Rd = panaquilin D, panaquilin E2, ganaxoside C, ginsenoside Re2

  ginsenoside Re = panaquilin E3, panaxoside B, ginsenoside Re3

  ginsenoside Rg1 = panaquilin G1, panaxoside A

  ginsenoside Rg2 = panaquilin G2

  ginsenoside Ra = panaxoside F.

- Other ginsensides: Ra1, Ra2, Rb3, Rf, Rh1, Rh4, Ro.

- Peptidoglycans: panaxans.

- Volatile oil: panacene.

- Polysaccharides.

- Vitamins (e.g., thiamin, riboflavin, B_{12}, nicotinic acid, pantothenic acid, and biotin).

Panax quinquefolius

- Triterpenoid glycosides (saponins): ginsenosides (also called panaxosides), including, Rb1, Rb2, Rb3, Rc, Rd, Re, Rg1, Rg2, Ro, which produce 20-S-protopanaxadiol and 20-S-protopanaxatriol in alkaline conditions.

Note: There are both qualitative and quantitative differences in the ginsenoside content of various species and varieties, allowing easy verification of the identity and quality of commercial ginseng products by high-performance liquid chromotography.

Qualifications

Although hundreds of studies since the 1950s have attempted to separate factual from fictitious therapeutic properties of ginseng, there are many inconsistencies among the results, primarily due to different extraction procedures, use of different plants, adulterants, and lack of quality control. To compound this problem, few of the studies involve the use of human subjects.

A systematic review of 16 randomized clinical trials that assessed the efficacy of ginseng for a variety of different medicinal uses, including enhancing physical and psychomotor performance, as well as cognitive function, immunomodulation, diabetes mellitus, and herpes simplex type II infections, concluded that the efficacy of ginseng is "not established beyond reasonable doubt for any of these indications." Because many of the studies completed with ginseng are animal studies that often examine the effects of a single ginsenoside, it is not possible to extrapolate the results to the human ingestion of commercial ginseng products. Unless noted otherwise, all studies discussed here were completed with *Panax ginseng*, which is the most well-researched *Panax* species.

> *Although hundreds of studies since the 1950s have attempted to separate factual from fictitious therapeutic properties of ginseng, there are many inconsistencies among the results.*

Adaptogenic Activity

Historically, ginseng has been used as a general tonic, relying on its adaptogenic action. An adaptogen works in a non-specific manner, drawing the patient toward normal function irrespective of the direction of the pathologic state. For example, ginseng has been found to increase blood pressure in cases of hypotension or shock but restored blood pressure to normal in cases of hypertension. Other researchers have noted that there are at least three components of *Panax ginseng* root that can depress central nervous system (CNS) activity and at least two other constituents that stimulate the CNS. It appears that different constituents of *Panax ginseng* have opposing action, generally stimulating or sedating respectively. Thus, different doses of ginseng can have opposite effects clinically and the same dose of ginseng given to

> *Historically, ginseng has been used as a general tonic, relying on its adaptogenic action. An adaptogen works in a non-specific manner, drawing the patient toward normal function irrespective of the direction of the pathologic state.*

individuals with differing physiological states can have different clinical actions. This is a defining feature of an adaptogenic herb.

Antistress Activity

Ginseng has been reported to enhance a person's ability to cope with various mental and physical stressors (e.g., exposure to heat or cold, environmental toxins, physical trauma, and emotional responses to various stimuli). One of the few double-blind clinical studies to date investigated the effects of taking a multivitamin, compared with taking 40 mg of ginseng in addition to the same multivitamin, on the quality of life of 501 city dwellers. After 4 months, the study found that those ingesting the ginseng and multivitamin had a significant improvement in all 11 quality of life measures, while those ingesting the vitamins alone had no significant improvement.

Ginseng's antistress effects have been linked primarily to its effects on the adrenal glands. It has been suggested that, rather than a direct stimulation, ginseng influences the higher control centers, including the hypothalamus and pituitary gland, which in turn influence the adrenals. Studies suggest that *Panax ginseng* has the ability to increase both ascorbic acid and cholesterol stores in the adrenal gland while decreasing the 17-ketosterol and increasing adrenocorticotropic hormone (ACTH) excreted in the urine. An increase in plasma ACTH and corticosteroids following administration of ginseng is well documented. All of these effects are blocked by the administration of dexamethasone. It is hypothesized that the end-organ effects of the ACTH and related substances, whose release ginseng stimulates, can explain many of its antistress and antifatigue actions. However, another study reported that ingestion of ginseng (2 g daily) by competitive athletes for 6 weeks was not associated with any change in hormonal indices of stress, such as cortisol and testosterone levels.

Physical Performance Enhancement

Two reviews conclude that, due to poor methodological quality of existing studies, conflicting results, and the use of 10 to 100 times the usual human dose in many animal studies, there is currently insufficient scientific evidence to demonstrate enhancement of physical performance by ginseng. Overall, the evidence is conflicting, and larger studies that assess clinically significant outcomes are needed.

Animal studies report that mice taking ginseng were shown to swim longer, run up a seemingly endless rope for a longer time, and run on a treadmill longer. Other animal experiments found no significant antifatigue action for ginseng compared to a placebo. The majority of the animal trials in this area were not blinded or placebo-controlled.

Several clinical experiments with humans have also been published, most of which did not find ginseng to enhance physical performance significantly. Early, often-quoted studies were small and negative. One found, for example, that 12 nurses switching from day to night duty reported improvement in 11 of 16 mood variables and 8 of 14 somatic symptoms while taking 1.2 g of Korean ginseng as opposed to a placebo. Contrary to the description of this study in many lay publications, however, none of these differences was statistically significant. It has been suggested that the lack of significant results in this study was due to the relatively low dose and short study period.

Another study comparing 11 army cadets ingesting 2 g of *Panax ginseng* daily for 4 weeks found no difference in performance during heavy, prolonged exercise when compared to cadets taking a placebo. Another

double-blind, placebo-controlled trial with 43 male triathletes taking either 200 mg of ginseng or a placebo twice daily found no significant differences in the physical fitness of the two groups after 10 weeks; however, at a follow-up 10 weeks later, the group taking the ginseng had significantly better maximal oxygen uptake, which suggested that ginseng may retard the loss of physical fitness.

> *Several clinical experiments with humans have also been published, most of which did not find ginseng to enhance physical performance significantly.*

A more recent randomized, placebo-controlled study of ginseng (200 mg, 7% standardized extract daily) for 3 weeks found that ginseng did not enhance peak aerobic exercise, nor did maximal oxygen uptake change, in 28 healthy young adults with moderate exercise capabilities. To some extent, these findings were supported by a subsequent randomized, double-blind, placebo-controlled trial of ingesting 350 mg ginseng daily for 6 weeks. This study found that while ginseng did not influence maximal oxygen uptake or lactate threshold, it did shorten multiple choice reaction time (a measure of psychomotor performance) in 15 soccer players.

Several small studies have reported more positive effects. For example, a double-blind, placebo-controlled crossover study with 50 male sports teachers found that total workload and maximal oxygen uptake were increased, while plasma lactate levels, carbon dioxide production, and heart rate were all significantly lower when the individuals were ingesting a product containing ginseng, vitamins, and trace elements than when they were taking the placebo. A smaller open-label, uncontrolled trial enrolled 7 healthy male participants to perform an exhaustive treadmill exercise before and after taking 6 g of *Panax ginseng* extract daily for 8 weeks.

The authors reported a 1.5-minute increase in exercise endurance, a decrease in MDA (a marker for oxidative stress), and an increase in scavenger enzymes after ginseng treatment. A positive randomized, double-blind, placebo-controlled trial involving 70 elderly participants demonstrated that taking 1,200 mg of red ginseng daily for 12 weeks promoted reduced heart rate, lower body fat, and a self-reported increase in muscle strength when combined with a weekly 60-minute strength training session. Over 80% of the participants in the ginseng treatment group also reported stronger vitality after the trial. Larger studies are needed to confirm any of the effects documented in these small studies.

Several mechanisms of action have been postulated for ginseng's antifatigue effects including stimulation of nerve impulses, an ability to affect the hypothalamus/pituitary/adrenal axis, an ability to spare glycogen utilization in exercising muscle, and improved oxygen utilization. Biochemical studies have noted increased blood glucose levels and decreased levels of both lactic acid and pyruvic acid in ginseng-treated animals after exercise when compared with saline controls (no differences were noted at rest). However, much of this work has been criticized for lack of proper control animals and for making little attempt to guarantee the purity and quality of the ginseng products tested.

Cognitive Enhancement

The trials investigating ginseng's ability to enhance cognitive activity, including learning and memory, have reported mixed results. Most have been very small and have tested such a wide array of outcome measures that it is difficult to draw any conclusions. More research is definitely needed in this area.

Several much-quoted studies have reported that ginseng enhances mental activity and decreases mental fatigue. For example, radio operators who ingested ginseng extract were reported to transmit text faster and make fewer errors than those on a placebo, and university students in Italy were reported

to perform better on a series of mental tests (including attention, mental arithmetic, logical deduction, integrated sensory-motor function, and auditory reaction time) while taking ginseng in comparison to those on a placebo. However, a closer look at the second study reveals that although positive trends were noted in some of the other tests, the only test in which the ginseng-treated group performed significantly (statistically) better than the control group was the mental arithmetic test and no difference at all was found between the placebo and the ginseng group on three other tests: pure motor function, recognition, and visual reaction time.

> *The trials investigating ginseng's ability to enhance cognitive activity, including learning and memory, have reported mixed results.*

Another randomized, placebo-controlled study involving 27 healthy participants allocated them to receive one of four combinations of 200 mg *Panax ginseng* G115 extract and 25 g glucose drink. The glucose drink was administered 30 minutes after the ginseng extract or placebo was taken. A cognitive demand test was taken at baseline and 30 minutes after the drink was administered. Both the glucose drink and the *Panax ginseng* were reported to enhance mental arithmetic performance and decrease feelings of mental fatigue caused by sustained demanding cognitive tests in these participants.

Animal studies have demonstrated the ability of ginseng to modify brain wave tracings, to improve metabolic activity in the brain, to affect the hypothalamus/pituitary/adrenal axis, and to have favorable effects on learning and memory.

Anti-Aging Effects

Ginseng's "anti-aging" effects have yet to be proven; however, it does seem to exert an action on cellular function. It appears to stimulate protein synthesis and decrease cellular destruction. As well, it has been shown to promote Kupffer cell activity, which increases liver detoxification and thus may decrease cellular damage caused by external pollutants.

Hepatic (Liver) Effects

Many of the adaptogenic effects of ginseng appear to be related to its effects on the liver. Ginseng has been reported to enhance the activity of the Kupffer cells, which are primarily responsible for detoxification of the blood; provide protection against carbon tetrachloride-induced hepatotoxicity in rats; induce tyrosine aminotransferase gene expression in vitro; and decrease AST and ALT levels in dexamethasone-treated rats. Ginseng has also been reported to increase protein synthesis in the liver of animal models. This has yet to be confirmed in clinical trials. In addition, ginseng is thought to have a significant antihepatotoxic action.

Cardiovascular Effects

Blood Pressure

It appears that ginseng has a dose-related action on blood pressure. In low doses it slightly increases blood pressure and in high doses it appears to decrease blood pressure in animal models. One study of dogs given 10 to 20 mg per kg of ginseng intravenously reported an initial increase in blood pressure, which was followed by slight decrease in blood pressure. Another study of 40 mg/kg ginseng extracts administered intravenously to dogs reported significant decreases in mean arterial pressure, cardiac output, stroke volume, and central venous pressure. Clinically, increased blood pressure has been reported as a side effect.

However, several clinical trials have reported that ginseng may decrease blood pressure. One clinical trial of 26 participants with essential hypertension found that ingestion of 4.5 g of red ginseng daily in three divided doses for 8 weeks resulted in a significant reduction in mean systolic blood pressure but only a trend toward a decline in diastolic blood pressure. However, in 8 participants with "white coat hypertension" (high blood pressure induced by anxiety experienced in a clinical setting), no significant blood pressure change was observed. Another clinical study suggests that Korean red ginseng can improve vascular endothelial dysfunction in patients with hypertension, possibly through increasing synthesis of nitric oxide. Additional research studies are needed to confirm these results.

Platelet Aggregation

Several in vitro and in vivo studies have noted ginseng's ability to decrease platelet aggregation. Ginsenosides Rg2 and Ro were found to significantly inhibit the conversion of fibrinogen to fibrin induced by thrombin in experimental models. Other studies suggest that components of ginseng inhibit thromboxane A2. However, the clinical effects of oral ingestion of commercial ginseng products by humans is unknown. Prolonged thrombin time (TT) and activated partial thromboplastin time (APTT) have been reported in animal studies. Decreases in blood-clotting time in humans do not appear to have been reported in the literature.

Other Cardiovascular Effects

Children with congenital heart disease receiving cardiopulmonary bypass surgery were randomized to receive either ginseng (1.35 mg/kg ginsenosides intravenously before and during the operation) or a placebo. The ginseng treatment was found to prevent changes in gastric intramucosal pH and plasma diamine oxidase. Patients in the treatment group were reported to need less inotropic medications and to have shorter hospital stays than those in the placebo group. The authors concluded that this effect may have been caused by an inhibition of the inflammatory process that usually occurs following cardiopulmonary bypass.

Ginseng has also been reported to cause vasodilation of the coronary vessels and to have a cardioprotective action against catecholamine tachycardia. Under experimental conditions, *Panax ginseng* was found to delay induced heart mitochondrial impairment and muscle contraction deterioration. When administered to patients with hyperlipidemia, ginseng has been shown to increase serum HDL cholesterol levels while at the same time decreasing total serum cholesterol, triglyceride, and fatty acid levels. Other studies have found that *Panax ginseng* may protect against myocardial ischemia-reperfusion damage and cerebral damage caused by ischemia. It has been suggested that the cardioprotective effects of ginseng may be mediated by the release of nitric oxide, a potent antioxidant.

Immunostimulating Effects

Ginseng appears to enhance antibody response, increase natural killer cell activity, stimulate macrophage activity, stimulate lymphocytes in vitro, stimulate the reticuloendothelial system (RES), increase proliferation of T and B cells, and increase the production of interferon.

Prevention of Colds

In laboratory animals, ginseng has been shown to reduce the incidence of viral infections. This finding has been confirmed by a multi-center, double-blind, randomized, placebo-controlled trial in 227 individuals. Each participant was given 100 mg of Ginsana daily for 12 weeks, while receiving an anti-influenza polyvalent vaccination at week 4. In the placebo group, 42 cases of colds or

The ginseng treatment group had a significantly lower occurrence of two or more cold episodes during the study period, their colds were shorter in duration, and their symptoms were less severe than for those in the placebo group.

flus were reported in the final 8 weeks of the trial, in comparison with 15 reports in the ginseng group, which represents a statistically significant difference. In addition, the group receiving ginseng had significantly higher antibody titers and natural killer cell activity levels. In another double-blind, placebo-controlled trial, 323 subjects were randomized to receive either 400 mg of North American ginseng extract daily or a placebo for 4 months during influenza season. The ginseng treatment group had a significantly lower occurrence of two or more cold episodes during the study period, their colds were shorter in duration, and their symptoms were less severe than for those in the placebo group.

Neurological Effects

Emotional Disorders

Although *Panax ginseng* has reportedly been used in the treatment of a variety of emotional conditions, this clinical application is supported by very little research. Ginsenoside Rb1 has been shown to decrease aggressive behavior (between resident and intruder mice) when given to the resident mouse at doses of 25 to 100 mg of ginsenoside per kg intraperitoneally (IP). However, when ginsenoside Rb1 was given to the intruder mouse, no change in activity was noted. In addition, ginsenoside Rg1 produced no change in behavior when given to either mouse. Another study reported that a crude extract of ginseng (50 and 100 mg/kg) and ginsenoside Rb1 (2.5 and 5 mg/kg) given IP significantly decreased maternal aggression in female mice without causing motor dysfunction; however, ginsenoside Rg1 appeared to increase maternal aggression. None of these studies were blinded and there have been no studies reporting similar effects in humans.

A study of *Panax ginseng* 50 mg/kg showed that it was as effective as diazepam 1 mg/kg in decreasing experimentally induced anxiety in mice. However, another study using 50 to 100 mg per kg given orally to mice found no effect on the pentobarbital sleep of

> *Although* Panax ginseng *has reportedly been used in the treatment of a variety of emotional conditions, this clinical application is supported by very little research.*

psychologically stressed mice. This is supported by an additional study that also found no effect on pentobarbital sleep induction.

Miscellaneous Neurological Effects

Several animal studies have investigated the effects of ginseng on the development of tolerance to and dependence on a variety of narcotics, including morphine, cocaine, and methamphetamine. Other in vitro studies have reported the ability of ginsenoside Rb1 to potentiate nerve growth and of ginsenosides Rg1, Rb2, Rd, Re, and Rf to protect cerebellum growth in vivo. Another in vivo study suggests that ginsenosides directly affect the activity-dependent synaptic plasticity in the brain.

Effect on Diabetes

Ginseng has had a long history of folk use in the treatment of diabetes. Most of the recent studies have focused on *Panax quinquefolius* (Canadian or American ginseng). Overall, the findings from clinical trials are not consistent, but a number of studies have documented the hypoglycemic effects of American ginseng in both healthy participants and individuals diagnosed with type 2 diabetes mellitus. However, not all studies have been positive. One study could not reproduce these findings, and the authors suggest that this may have been because the extract they tested varied in its total ginsenoside content, as well as in key ratios of different ginsenosides, when compared to another extract that was shown to have hypoglycemic effects.

One randomized, double-blind, placebo-controlled crossover trial assigned 19 participants with well-controlled type 2 diabetes to receive either 6 g Korean red ginseng (*Panax ginseng*) daily or a placebo for 12 weeks. Participants were instructed to take the study medication with meals and to continue their usual diet or medication therapy for the duration of the study. The authors reported that no change was seen in their primary outcome measure, HbA1C, measured to indicate recent blood sugar levels. Results did, however, show a maintenance in glycemic control and improvements in both insulin and glucose control. The authors concluded that this dose of Korean ginseng, taken in conjunction with conventional diet or medications, did not show a long-term improvement in HGA1C, although improvements were seen in these other clinically relevant parameters. Two studies conducted by the same authors using different balances of G115 (*Panax ginseng*) and glucose in healthy individuals both reported that G115 significantly lowers fasting blood glucose.

> *A number of studies have documented the hypoglycemic effects of American ginseng in both healthy participants and individuals diagnosed with type 2 diabetes mellitus.*

Other studies suggest that the hypoglycemic effects of ginseng may depend on when the ginseng is taken in relation to food. One study reported that a single 3 g dose of American ginseng (*Panax quinquefolius*) attenuated postprandial glycemia (blood sugar after eating) in 10 non-diabetic participants and in 9 participants diagnosed with type 2 diabetes mellitus when the ginseng dose was ingested 40 minutes prior to the glucose challenge. When the ginseng dose was ingested at the same time as the glucose challenge, the hypoglycemic effect was found only in those with type 2 diabetes mellitus. In another study, American ginseng reduced postprandial glycemia in 10 type 2 diabetes individuals irrespective of the dose (3 g, 6 g, or 9 g) or the time of administration (120, 80, 40, or 0 minutes before the glucose challenge).

One study found that a fraction isolated from ginseng (DPG-3-2) stimulated insulin secretion, but only in diabetic mice and non-diabetic controls who had been loaded with glucose. There was no effect on insulin secretion in non-diabetic mice on a standard diet. These findings reinforce the adaptogenic character — an ability to restore balance — of ginseng. Research suggests that the ginseng components responsible for these effects include panaxans A, B, C, D, and E, adenosine, and a fraction designated DPG-3-2.

Miscellaneous Effects

Reproductive Effects

Although ginseng has a reputation as an aphrodisiac, no human studies support this belief. However, *Panax* species have been shown to increase the formation of sperm and the growth of the testes in rabbits, enhance ovulation and the growth of the ovaries in frogs, stimulate egg laying in hens, and increase the mating activity in male rats. Ginseng has been shown to increase sperm count and motility in men, as well as increasing plasma total and free testosterone, DHT, FSH, and LH levels. An in vitro study suggests that extracts from *Panax ginseng* may relax the corpus cavernosum by releasing nitric oxide.

In addition, the estrogenic action of ginseng has been demonstrated in postmenopausal women who experienced reduced atrophy and dryness of the vaginal epithelium. It should be noted that breast tenderness has been reported in women taking ginseng.

Anticancer Properties

Ginseng has been reported to decrease the incidence of some human cancers and to have a protective effect against the adverse effects of radiation, but studies in humans were not found. Other studies have reported that components of *Panax ginseng* caused inhibition of lung metastasis of B16-BL6 melanoma and colon 26-M3.1 carcinoma in mice, inhibition of the growth of human ovarian cancer cells in mice, and induction of differentiation in teratocarcinoma cells in vitro. Two case-control epidemiological studies and one prospective study in populations with high rates of ginseng use (70% users) suggested that oral ingestion of ginseng may decrease the incidence of some human cancers. It has been hypothesized that the possible anticancer effects of ginseng may be due to its stimulating effects on the immune system.

Effects on Symptoms of Menopause

A randomized, double-blind, placebo-controlled study that assessed the effects of ginseng (Ginsana, containing 100 mg G115 standardized extract) in 384 healthy postmenopausal women found a trend toward overall symptom improvement that was not statistically significant. Those ingesting ginseng scored significantly better on the depression, well-being, and health subscales. However, no significant differences were seen between the ginseng and the placebo group on the Women's Health Questionnaire (WHQ) and visual analog scales used to assess specific symptoms (i.e., hot flashes). The study also reported that physiological parameters, such as follicle stimulating hormone (FSH), estradiol levels, endometrial thickness, maturity index, and vaginal pH, were also not affected by ginseng treatment.

Effects on Quality of Life and Mood

A randomized, double-blind, placebo-controlled study of ginseng (200 mg or 400 mg G115 extract daily) ingested for 60 days by 83 healthy volunteers reported that ginseng supplementation has no effect on positive affect, negative affect, or total mood disturbance. The authors concluded that their findings "do not support claims that chronic ginseng supplementation — at either its clinically recommended level or at twice that level — enhances affect or mood in healthy young adults." In contrast, another randomized, double-blind, placebo-controlled study involving 30 participants reported that ingestion of ginseng (200 mg Ginsana) for 4 weeks was associated with an increase in mental health and social functioning, as measured by a health-related quality of life questionnaire. However, these effects were attenuated after another 4 weeks of ginseng use, so no differences between the ginseng and placebo group were noted at the end of the 8-week study.

This review was limited to the scientific and clinical evidence available within the biomedical model. However, it would be a disservice to this herb to discount its historical use within the traditional Chinese medical paradigm. In using this herb, it is important to remember that extensive empirical evidence exists. This is reviewed thoroughly in several texts.

> *This review was limited to the scientific and clinical evidence available within the biomedical model. However, it would be a disservice to this herb to discount its historical use within the traditional Chinese medical paradigm.*

Adverse Effects

The most common adverse effect noted is insomnia. Other reported effects included diarrhea, skin eruptions, vaginal bleeding, and breast tenderness. One case each of Stevens-Johnson syndrome, mania, fugax amaurosis, and cerebral arteritis possibly associated with ingestion of ginseng have been reported. However, the ginseng products were not tested for purity; thus, these reactions may have been caused by adulterated products. In addition, given the widespread use of ginseng products worldwide, such reactions are very rare indeed.

The term "ginseng abuse syndrome" has been used to describe symptoms of overstimulation, including hypertension, diarrhea, restlessness, nervousness, euphoria, insomnia, and skin eruptions, which may occur in the overuse of the product. However, this description has been criticized because the majority of the individuals in the study that coined the term were also ingesting high levels of caffeine.

Cautions/Contraindications

Ginseng should be used with caution in patients diagnosed with hypertension or acute illness, premenopausal women with unstable hormonal cycles, controlled diabetics, and patients also using stimulants. As well, given that ginseng is considered a tonic, its use may not be appropriate in young, robust individuals. Ginseng should not be ingested in the evening due to its ability to induce insomnia.

A 2008 review on the safety of ginseng consumption during pregnancy identified a total of 10 clinical and animal studies discussing safety parameters. One human trial involving pregnant women experiencing intrauterine growth retardation reported no adverse effects using Chang Bai Shan ginseng saponin tablets, although several animal studies reported a risk of mutation and toxicity when embryos were exposed to isolated components of ginseng. These animal studies have been criticized because they use higher doses of ginseng constituents than would be attainable from routine supplementation. Authors of another review report that active components in ginseng can cross the placenta during gestation. It was concluded that although there is not enough evidence to identify any specific negative effects of ginseng consumption during pregnancy, it should be recommended with caution, especially during the first trimester, until more research is available.

This review also investigated the safety of *Panax ginseng* during breastfeeding. No clinical trials could be found, although three animal studies suggest minimal risk during lactation.

> *Ginseng is generally considered to have an additive effect when used concomitantly with monoamine oxidese inhibitors (MAOIs).*

Drug Interactions

Ginseng is generally considered to have an additive effect when used concomitantly with monoamine oxidese inhibitors (MAOIs). This caution is derived from a case study describing symptoms of headache and tremulousness in a 64-year-old woman who was taking phenelzine and added ginseng to her regimen. Three years later, a rechallenge with ginseng in the same woman resulted in the same symptoms. A second possible case of an interaction between ginseng, contained as an ingredient in an herbal tea, and phenelzine has also been reported.

One study found that ginseng augmented the hypnotic effect of pentobarbital, while others have found no effect. However, potentiation of an amphetamine-induced increase in motility and stereotypy, as well as potentiation of haloperidol catalepsy, have been reported in animal studies. Caution with concomitant use of centrally acting medications is recommended.

A recent randomized, controlled, open-label trial to evaluate the potential interaction between *Panax ginseng* and warfarin has been conducted. Twenty-five participants who had recently been diagnosed with ischemic stroke were randomized to receive either warfarin treatment alone (2 mg daily for 1 week and then 5 mg daily for 1 week) or the same warfarin treatment plus *Panax ginseng* (1.5 g daily in 3 doses) for 2 weeks. Results showed no significant difference between the prothrombin time and international normalized ratio of these two groups, and the authors concluded that no pharmacological interaction was found between this dosage of warfarin and *Panax ginseng* in ischemic stroke patients.

However, another case report suggested a different reaction. The authors describe a clinically significant decrease in the international normalized ratio (from 3.3 to 1.5) of a 47-year-old man with a history of cardiac problems who had been taking warfarin (5 mg daily) along with several other medications for 7 years. This reaction occurred 2 weeks after he started taking 300 mg of ginseng (Ginsana standardized capsules) daily in an attempt to boost his energy. Two weeks after discontinuing ginseng use, his international normalized ratio returned to 3.3.

Quality of Dosage Forms

Premium ginseng root is extremely expensive, often costing thousands of dollars per kilogram, which leads one to question the quality of cheaper brands of the product. Commercially, ginseng is available in a wide range of forms, including teas, capsules, extracts, tablets, roots, chewing gum, cigarettes, and candies. It is extremely difficult to determine the quality and quantity of ginseng present in some of these dosage forms. A study done in the late 1970s — and currently being repeated by the American Botanical Council — reported that 60% of the 54 North American ginseng products tested did not contain enough ginsenosides to be considered pharmacologically active and that 25% contained no ginsenosides at all. Another study of 17 commercial ginseng products available in Sweden found that only one out of the five brands that listed their ginsenoside content on the label met the label claim.

> *Premium ginseng root is extremely expensive, often costing thousands of dollars per kilogram, which leads one to question the quality of cheaper brands of the product.*

In a follow-up study of 50 ginseng products from 11 countries, the same team of researchers reported a range of 1.9% to 9.0% ginsenoside content, with six products (gathered from Sweden, the US, and the UK) that did not contain any ginsenosides. Several cases of athletes consuming adulterated ginseng products (e.g., with ephedrine, psuedophedrine) that have resulted in doping charges have been reported.

Dosage Regimens

- Standardized extract (4% to 8% ginsenosides): 100–500 mg daily in two or three divided doses.
- Raw root decoction (boiled in water or broth): 0.6–4 g, usually taken in the morning.

Note: In cases of long-term administration, ginseng is usually taken for a period of 2 to 3 weeks, followed by a 2-week resting period.

Selected References

Predy GN, Goel V, Lovlin R, Donner A, Stitt L, Basu TK. Efficacy of an extract of North American ginseng containing poly-furanosyl-pyranosyl-saccharides for preventing upper respiratory tract infections: A randomized controlled trial. Canadian Medical Association Journal 2005;173(9):1043–49.

Seely D, Dugoua JJ, Perri D, Mills E, Koren G. Safety and efficacy of *Panax ginseng* during pregnancy and lactation. Canadian Journal of Clinical Pharmacology 2008;15(1):e87–e94.

Vogler BK, Pittler MH, Ernst E. The efficacy of ginseng: A systematic review of randomised clinical trials. European Journal of Clinical Pharmacology 1999;55(8):567–75.

Ginseng
(Siberian)
Eleutherococcus senticosus (Rupr. & Maxim.) Maxim

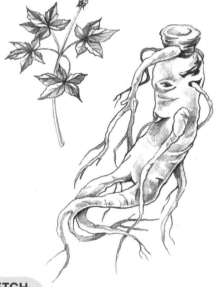

Introduction

Family
- Araliaceae

Synonyms
- Eleuthero
- *Acanthopanax senticosus*
- Touch-me-not
- Devil's shrub
- Eleuthero ginseng
- Wild pepper

Medicinal Forms
- Dried root
- Tincture
- Fluid extract
- Solid extract

Description
Eleutherococcus senticosus is native to the Russian far east, as well as the parts of Korea, China, and Japan north of the 38th latitude. This shrub grows to approximately 2 to 3 meters (7 to 10 feet) in height, with several leaflets on each stem.

Parts Used
The root, which is the part used medicinally, is normally harvested in the fall, when the medicinally active constituents are the most concentrated. The leaves can also be used medicinally.

Traditional Use
Although historical documentation of the medicinal use of plants in the Araliaceae family (which also includes *Panax ginseng* C.A. Meyer and *Panax quinquefolium* L.) can be confusing, it appears that *Eleutherococcus senticosus* has been used in traditional Chinese medicine (TCM) for more than 4,000 years to increase longevity, improve general health, improve appetite, and aid memory. Traditional Chinese medicine indications for Siberian ginseng also include benefiting *qi* (chi), or the vital energy, and treating "yang" deficiency, especially of the spleen and kidney, as well as normalizing body functions.

Although documentation of *Eleutherococcus senticosus* in Russia dates back to 1855, when two Russian scientists began studying the plant, interest in its medicinal use began only in the 1960s, when researchers in that country became aware of its potential as a substitute for the more expensive and difficult to obtain *Panax* species (e.g., *Panax ginseng* and *Panax quinquefolium*). Although some of the adaptogenic properties of Siberian ginseng are thought to be similar to those of *Panax ginseng*, it is not the same botanical species, nor are the main active constituents the same. Marketing in North America under the common name "Siberian ginseng" only compounds the confusion surrounding these species. Today, this species is becoming more commonly known by its abbreviated scientific name, eleuthero, in an attempt to reduce this confusion.

Current Medicinal Use
Siberian ginseng is primarily used as a tonic in cases of stress and fatigue. Although Siberian ginseng may be used in attempts to increase endurance and enhance athletic performance, current scientific evidence suggests that it is not effective for this indication. Preliminary research with rats indicates that Siberian ginseng may decrease the adverse effects of radiation used in cancer therapy.

Relevant Research

Preventative and Therapeutic Effects

Constituents

The main active chemical constituents are a group of chemically dissimilar compounds that have been called eleutherosides. Tyler argues that this was done to make Siberian ginseng appear more similar to the true ginsengs from the *Panax* species, whose active constituents are the ginsenosides — a group of triterpenoid saponins. Siberian ginseng does not contain any of the ginsenosides found in *Panax* species.

Roots

- **Coumarins**: eleutheroside B1 (isofraxidin-7-0-alpha-L-glucoside, also known as beta-caly canthoside), isofraxidin, coumarin X.

- **Lignans**: eleutheroside B4 ((-)-sesamin), eleutheroside D ((-)-syringarsinol di-0-beta-D-glucoside), eleutheroside E (different crystal form of D, also known as acanthoside D).

- **Phenylpropanoid**: eleutheroside B (syringin), caffeic acid, caffeic acid ethyl ester.

- **Polysaccharides**: eleutheroside C (methyl-alpha-D-galactoside), eleutherans A-G.

- **Sterols**: eleutheroside A (daucosterol).

- **Triterpene**: oleanolic acid.

- **Miscellaneous eleutherosides**: eleutheroside B2, eleutheroside B3, eleutheroside F, eleutheroside G.

Leaves

- **Triterpenes**: eleutheroside I (also known as mussenin B), eleutheroside K, eleutheroside L, eleutheroside M (also known as hederasaponin B), senticosides A to D (may be identical to eleutherosides I, K, L, and M).

Research Note

Numerous in vivo, in vitro, and human clinical trials have been conducted on this species in Russia. Unfortunately, few have been translated into English. This monograph includes information from review articles (the review by Farnsworth is the most extensive encountered), as well as any original articles available in English.

Adaptogenic Activity

Historically, Siberian ginseng has been used as a general tonic, relying on its adaptogenic action. An adaptogen is thought to work in a non-specific manner, drawing the patient toward normal function irrespective of the direction of the pathologic state. One study reports that Siberian ginseng is widely used in Russia by such diverse populations as deep-sea divers, mine and mountain rescue workers, soldiers, factory workers, cosmonauts, and athletes, largely for its perceived ability to increase endurance and promote the body's ability to tolerate stressful conditions.

Antistress Activity

An early study suggested that Siberian ginseng increases non-specific development of resistance to stress, as well as inhibiting the alarm reaction to stress, including decreasing the activation of the adrenal cortex.

Antifatigue (Physical)

Perhaps the most common use of Siberian ginseng in North America is to increase physical endurance and stamina. Most of the Russian studies of this indication, however, were neither double-blinded nor controlled adequately, making it difficult to assess its true clinical effect. Several animal studies found no significant difference between the length of time that mice ingesting Siberian ginseng could swim in comparison with placebo. One animal study also found no difference in plasma lactic acid, glucagon, insulin, or liver glycogen levels in exercised rats who had ingested Siberian ginseng. Yet in one single-blind, placebo-controlled clinical trial in 6 healthy males, all four parameters of physical capacity (oxygen uptake, oxygen pulse, maximal work capacity, and exhaustion time) were significantly increased in the group taking the Siberian ginseng as compared to those a taking placebo.

In a more recent double-blind, placebo-controlled study of 20 highly trained long-distance runners, no significant differences were noted between the group who took the Siberian ginseng extract daily for 6 weeks and the placebo group. The authors caution that while Siberian ginseng may not enhance the physical ability of highly trained athletes, it may still provide some benefit to the average individual.

Immunostimulating Effects

A placebo-controlled, double-blind study of healthy volunteers who were given 30 to 40 mL of an Siberian ginseng extract (0.2% w/v eleutheroside B) reported that those ingesting Siberian ginseng experienced a significant increase in total lymphocyte count, with the most pronounced effect noticed with the T lymphocytes. Granulocyte and monocyte levels were unchanged in these individuals.

Neurological Effects

Siberian ginseng has been reported to have both a sedative action and a stimulant effect in animal experiments. One study found that mice given Siberian ginseng exhibited significantly more aggressive behavior than those given distilled water.

Miscellaneous Effects

Social Functioning

One clinical study suggests that Siberian ginseng may enhance social functioning in the elderly. In the study, 20 elderly hypertensive participants were randomized to receive either 300 mg of Siberian ginseng or a placebo daily for 8 weeks. The authors reported that a significant improvement was seen in social functioning at 4 weeks in the group taking Siberian ginseng, but these results were not present at 8 weeks. No effect was seen on blood pressure.

Bipolar Disorder

One randomized, double-blind clinical trial compared the addition of either Siberian ginseng (750 mg three times daily) or fluoxetine (20 mg daily) to lithium (500 mg daily) for 6 weeks in 76 Chinese adolescents diagnosed with biopolar disorder. The authors reported no significant differences on scales of depression and mood changes between the two groups, although both treatments were well tolerated. Unfortunately, since there was no control group that was administered lithium alone, it is not clear if either additional therapy (Siberian ginseng or fluoxetine) had a clinical effect beyond that of lithium alone.

Chronic Fatigue Syndrome

Investigators in one trial randomized 96 participants who had experienced chronic fatigue for over 6 months to receive either 2,000 mg of standardized Siberian ginseng daily or a placebo. At 2 months, a statistically significant improvement in self-reported symptoms was seen in a subset of participants taking Siberian ginseng who had experienced mild to moderate fatigue, compared to a placebo. Overall, an improvement was seen in the Siberian ginseng group within the first month compared to the placebo, but these results were not present at the second month. The authors conclude that although clinical efficacy was not demonstrated, further studies should be conducted concentrating on the treatment of moderate, short-term chronic fatigue.

Diabetes

Hypoglycemic activity has been reported in animal studies with some forms of induced hyperglycemia; however, another study found no effect of Siberian ginseng on alloxan-induced hyperglycemia in rats. Positive effects appear to be due to the polysaccharide components, also known as eleutherans A-G.

Platelet Aggregation

An anti-aggregatory compound, 3,4-dihydroxybenzoic acid (DBA), has been identified in Siberian ginseng, which is reported to be as potent as ASA in inhibiting collagen- and adenosine-induced platelet aggregation but less potent at inhibiting arachidonic acid-induced platelet aggregation.

Anticancer Properties

Several Russian in vitro and in vivo studies suggest that Siberian ginseng may have direct cytostatic activity and metastasis-preventing effects. In a review of these studies, it was reported that aqueous extracts of Siberian ginseng, in combination with cytarabine, provided additive antiproliferative effects against L1210 murine leukemia. No human clinical trials could be found for this indication.

Protection from Radiation

Siberian ginseng is noted for its ability to provide protection in animals subjected to both single-exposure and long-term X-ray radiation. In one study, rats given Siberian ginseng survived twice as long as control rats when exposed to long-term radiation (total dose 1,620 to 7,000 rads). When the rats were given both Siberian ginseng and antibiotics and exposed to radiation (total dose 3,000 rads over 60 days), they survived three times as long. An in vitro study noted only slight radioprotective effects of Siberian ginseng on the survival of cultured mammalian cells, while *Panax ginseng* was found to have significant effects in the same test system. Although no human trials were available for review, Siberian ginseng is thought to be useful as an adjunctive treatment for those undergoing radiation treatment for a variety of cancerous conditions.

> *Siberian ginseng is thought to be useful as an adjunctive treatment for those undergoing radiation treatment for a variety of cancerous conditions.*

Adverse Effects

Two reviews of clinical trials in which over 6,000 individuals ingested Siberian ginseng for up to 60 days reported no incidences of serious toxicity. In addition, no long-term toxicity was reported in mice at a dose of 5.0 mL/kg of fluid extract. Another comprehensive review of the literature concluded that unlike *Panax ginseng*, Siberian ginseng never produces excitation or a stress-like syndrome in patients.

However, another review cites one study in which an unspecified proportion of 64 atherosclerotic patients (taking 4.5 to 6.0 mL of an ethanolic root extract daily for 25 to 30 days, repeated 6 to 8 times with 3- to 4-month intervals) experienced hypertension, cardiac problems (e.g., extrasystole, shifts in cardiac rhythm, tachycardia), and insomnia. This review cites a second study in which 2 of 55 patients with rheumatic heart lesions reported headaches, hypertension, pericardial pain and palpitations. In contrast, no effect was seen on blood pressure in a recent randomized controlled trial of 20 elderly hypertensive patients given Siberian ginseng.

Siberian ginseng products have been commonly misidentified or adulterated in the past, most commonly with a plant known as *Periploca sepium* Bunge, Asclepiadaceae (the bark of silk vine). The Chinese name for Siberian ginseng is ci-wu-jia, while the Chinese name for *Periploca sepium* is wu-jia, which may explain the original source of confusion. *Periplocia sepium* is known to contain cardiac glycosides and chemicals with steroidal bases, which may explain many of the side effects that have previously been attributed to Siberian ginseng products.

The most famous Canadian case is one of maternal-neonatal androgenization attributed to "Siberian ginseng." The "Siberian ginseng" product was later determined to contain no *Eleuthercoccus senticocus* but almost certainly *Periploca sepium* instead. However, oral administration of the original adulterated material to rats in a bioassay for androgenization failed to produce positive results. Thus, either the androgenizing effects noted in mother and infant were not due to the implicated herbal product, or the effects were specific to humans or idiosyncratic to the individuals involved. Another study reports a further Canadian incident in which a Siberian ginseng product, adulterated with 0.5% caffeine, provided a stimulant effect to the user.

Clinically, ingestion of true Siberian ginseng products is associated with very few adverse effects.

Cautions/Contraindications

Some authors suggest that Siberian ginseng should not be given to individuals with hypertension (greater than 180/90 mmHg), asthma or emphysema, diabetes, cardiac disorders, or those receiving anxiolytic or sedative treatment. Another study also suggests caution when treating individuals with acute illness or fever, individuals suffering from mania or schizophrenia, or premenopausal women. Safety has not been established for use in children and in pregnant or lactating women.

Clinically, Siberian ginseng appears significantly less likely to cause problems in most individuals than *Panax* species (e.g., *Panax ginseng* and *Panax quinquefolium*).

Drug Interactions

Some authors suggest caution with concomitant use of Siberian ginseng and a variety of other therapies, including cardiac, anticoagulant, hypoglycemic, and hypo- or hypertensive agents. Siberian ginseng has been reported to both increase and decrease barbiturate sleeping time in in vitro and in vivo experiments.

In addition, a recent Canadian case study reported that Siberian ginseng may be responsible for elevated serum digoxin levels in a 74-year-old man who presented with elevated levels with no signs of toxic effects at a routine checkup. The authors suggested that there were three possible explanations for

> *Siberian ginseng products have been commonly misidentified or adulterated in the past, most commonly with a plant known as* Periploca sepium *Bunge, Asclepiadaceae (the bark of silk vine).*

this finding: (1) some chemical constituent of Siberian ginseng was converted to digoxin in vivo; (2) some component of Siberian ginseng interfered with digoxin elimination; or (3) the Siberian ginseng caused a false serum assay result.

A Canadian expert on herbal products argues that the eleutherosides are in no way chemically similar to cardiac glycosides, such as digoxin, and have not been observed to have any cardiotonic effects. He argues that this case is most likely another one in which *Periploca sepium* had been substituted for *Eleutherococcus senticosus*, because the former contains several cardiac glycosides, which provides a more rational explanation for the rise in serum digoxin noted in the patient. It should be noted that the "Siberian ginseng" product in this case was never tested for eleutheroside content.

Dosage Regimens

- Dried root: 2–4 grams in one to three divided doses daily.
- Tincture (1:5): 10–20 mL in one to three divided doses daily.
- Fluid extract (1:1): 2–4 mL in one to three divided doses daily.
- Solid extract (20:1): 100–200 mg in one to three divided doses daily.

Note: Most human studies involving long-term administration of Siberian ginseng have involved ginseng-free periods of 2 to 3 weeks every 30 to 60 days.

Selected References

Baldwin CA, Anderson LA, Phillipson JD. What pharmacists should know about ginseng. The Pharmaceutical Journal 1986;November 8:583–86.

Hartz AJ, Bentler S, Noyes R, Hoehns J, Logemann C, Sinift S, Butani Y, Wang W, Brake K, Ernst M, Kautzman, H. Randomized controlled trial of Siberian ginseng for chronic fatigue. Psychological Medicine 2004;34:51–61.

Goldenseal

Hydrastis canadensis L.

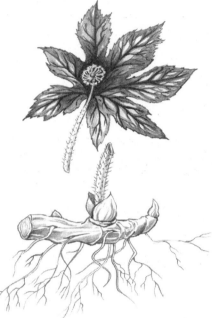

THUMBNAIL SKETCH

Common Uses
- Infections and inflammation (mucous membranes of the digestive tract, upper respiratory tract, and genitourinary tract)

Active Constituents
- Isoquinoline alkaloids (including hydrastine and berberine)

Adverse Effects
- Few at therapeutic doses, but there is a potential of poisoning

Cautions/Contraindications
- Pregnancy
- Hypertension

Drug Interactions
- None noted in clinical practice

Doses
- *Dried root and rhizome:* 0.5–1 g dry, or as decoction, three times daily
- *Hydroalcoholic tincture (1:10 in 60% ethanol):* 2–4 mL three times daily
- *Liquid extract (1:1 in 60% ethanol):* 0.3–1 mL three times daily
- *Solid extract (4:1):* 250 mg three times daily
- *Standardized extract (5% hydrastine):* 250–500 mg three times daily

Introduction

Family
- Ranunculaceae

Synonyms
- Hydrastis
- Yellow root
- Orange root
- Indian turmeric
- Eye root
- Jaundice root
- Indian dye
- Yellow puccoon
- Ground raspberry
- Turmeric root

Medicinal Forms
- Dried root and rhizome
- Tincture
- Liquid, solid, and standardized extracts

Description
Goldenseal is a perennial and a member of the buttercup family that stands up to 30 centimeters (1 foot) in height and produces a single white or green flower. While it was once commonly found throughout the woodlands of the central and eastern United States and southern Ontario, overcollection has now seriously diminished its numbers. Goldenseal is now considered an endangered species.

The berberine alkaloid found in goldenseal is common to several related plants that are used medicinally, including bayberry (*Berberis vulgaris* L., Berberidaceae) and Oregon grape, also known as trailing mahonia (*Mahonia aquifolium* (Pursh) Nutt., Berberidaceae).

Parts Used
The knotty, distinctively yellow rhizome is used medicinally.

Traditional Use
Goldenseal has enjoyed a long medicinal history, having originally been used by First Nations peoples for a variety of conditions, including skin diseases, ulcers, liver conditions, digestive conditions, and infections. While herbalists use goldenseal for many conditions, it is considered especially useful in the management of infections and conditions of mucous membranes. Goldenseal is often referred to by herbalists as the king of the tonics of the mucous membranes. Given its bright yellow color, it was also used commonly as a dye. The early Eclectic physicians continued to use goldenseal into the beginning of the 20th century, and goldenseal is now mentioned in most of the world's herbal pharmacopoeias.

Current Medicinal Use
Goldenseal has astringent action that may be of use in managing a variety of inflammatory and infectious conditions of the gastrointestinal tract (gastritis, digestive problems, infectious diarrhea), upper respiratory tract, eyes, and genitourinary system. Based primarily on traditional evidence, goldenseal is often used to treat the common cold, either alone or in combination with other herbal medicines, notably echinacea. The berberine alkaloid found in goldenseal is antimicrobial and is possibly effective against a large number of common bacteria, though it is unlikely that it is absorbed into the body's general circulation.

Relevant Research

Preventative and Therapeutic Effects
Constituents
* **Alkaloids:** isoquinoline alkaloids (berberine, hydrastine, canadine), canadaline, hydrastidine, isohydrastidine, berberastine.
* **Miscellaneous:** meconin, saturated and unsaturated fatty acids, chlorogenic acid, carbohydrates (D-fructose, D-galactose, sucrose).

> *Goldenseal is often used to treat the common cold, either alone or in combination with echinacea, though its effectiveness in the management of this condition has been questioned.*

Common Uses
Astringent Action
Goldenseal has been used for a variety of indications, including inflammatory and infectious conditions of the gastrointestinal tract (gastritis, digestive problems, infectious diarrhea), upper respiratory tract, eyes, and genitourinary system. As a bitter and a chola-gogue, it is used to aid digestion and treat dyspepsia.

Given its astringent action, goldenseal is also used to treat menorrhagia (abnormally heavy menstrual bleeding) and postpartum hemorrhage (see Cautions/Contraindications). External uses include the treatment of various skin conditions, such as eczema, ringworm, athlete's foot, impetigo (a bacterial skin infection), and pruritus (itching).

Common Cold
Goldenseal is often used to treat the common cold, either alone or in combination with echinacea, though its effectiveness in the management of this condition has been questioned. The active antimicrobial agent (berberine) is poorly absorbed following oral administration, and there is a lack of historical data to support this indication. Its popularity in this situation is more likely due to an inappropriate transposition of modern antibiotic protocols. It has been suggested that goldenseal acts, in these cases, not as an "antibiotic-like" agent but rather as an alterative, aiding the body's inherent defensive processes.

Excretion
Goldenseal has often been used to mask detection of illegal substances, such as marijuana and heroin, by urinalysis. However, there are no data to support this use. It has been shown that even large doses of goldenseal have no influence on the excretion of narcotics. In a review article, it was concluded that this myth originated from a fictional novel written by a prominent 19th-century Eclectic physician.

Antimicrobial Effect
Most of the evidence used to support the antimicrobial action of goldenseal is actually taken from information relating to the use of berberine salts, especially sulfate. In vitro studies have shown berberine to be effective against a large number of bacteria, including members of the *Bacillus* species, *Streptococcus* species, *Staphylococcus* species, *Klebsiella* species, *Proteus* species, *Corynebacterium diptheria*, *Enterobacter aerogenes*, *Salmonella typhi*, *Vibrio cholerae*, *Shigella boydii*, *Pseudomonas aeruginosa*, *Mycobacterium tuberculosis*, *Escherichia coli*, and *Xanthomonas citri*. In addition, it is active against a wide variety of fungi (including *Candida albicans*, *Cryptococcus neoformans*, *Saccharomyces cerevisiae*, *Trichophyton mentagrophytes*, *Sporothrix schenkii*) and parasites (including *Giardia lamblia*, *Entamoeba histolytica*, *Leishmania donovani*). Using chick embryos, berberine at a dose of 0.5 mg per egg offered protection from *Chlamydia trachomatis*. This action was comparable to that

afforded by a dose of 1 mg of sulphadiazine per egg.

Berberine sulfate has been shown to prevent the adherence of streptococci to host cells, and this could in part explain its "antibiotic" properties. In vitro experiments have shown that the pH of the medium influences the antimicrobial action of berberine salts, with the action increasing with the basic nature of the medium used (e.g., when pH is 8, antimicrobial activity is two to four times greater than when the medium has a pH of 7.5) Both berberine sulfate and berberine hydrochloride appear to have similar antimicrobial properties.

In determining the use of goldenseal for its reputed antimicrobial properties, it must be remembered that the above information comes from the use and applications of berberine salts. Some authors have suggested that the claims made for this botanical medicine are exaggerated.

Gastrointestinal Effects

Several clinical studies suggest that berberine may be useful in managing the symptoms of diarrhea. However, it is not clear whether these effects will also be seen by patients who ingest goldenseal supplements. In a randomized controlled trial, a single dose of berberine sulfate (400 mg) was shown to decrease the mean stool volume and duration of diarrhea when given to 165 adult individuals suffering from acute diarrhea due to *E. coli*. In patients with diarrhea caused by *Vibrio cholerae*, the decrease in stool volume was slight and was not additive to the effects of tetracycline.

In another randomized, double-blind placebo-controlled clinical trial of 400 adults presenting with acute watery diarrhea, the effects of berberine hydrochloride (HCl) (100 mg four times daily), berberine HCl (100 mg four times daily) plus tetracycline (500 mg four times daily), and tetracycline (500 mg four times daily) alone were studied. In the subgroup of 186 participants suffering from cholera, a significant reduction in duration, frequency, and need for rehydration fluid was noted in the tetracycline and tetracycline/berberine group. Berberine HCl by itself was not shown to have antisecretory action (a reduction of stool volume by 1 L/ 1 quart), which was not clinically significant, but did decrease the number of excreted bacteria in the stool. The authors suggest that an antisecretory action may not have been demonstrated because the dose given was too low. Both berberine HCl and tetracycline were shown to be ineffective in 215 patients suffering from non-cholera diarrhea.

An uncontrolled study showed that berberine administered orally in 137 children aged 5 months to 14 years was comparable to other medications in the management of giardiasis (a type of diarrhea often contracted by travelers). The author suggested that it could be of use in this situation, especially due to the ease of administration and lack of unpleasant adverse effects. There was also an increased rate of relapse after 1 month when compared to conventional treatments, such as metronidazole.

> *Several clinical studies suggest that berberine may be useful in managing the symptoms of diarrhea. However, it is not clear whether these effects will also be seen by patients who ingest goldenseal supplements.*

Cardiac Action

Two studies — one positive, well-designed, randomized controlled study and one positive open-label study — showed that berberine might be of benefit to patients with congestive heart failure if used in conjunction with conventional therapy. It is clear from these studies that lower doses were not beneficial and that high doses (oral: 1.2–2.0 g daily; intravenous: 0.2 mg/kg/min) may be required for berberine to be effective. Larger studies are still required to prove the efficacy of berberine as an adjunct therapy for congestive heart failure.

In vitro studies have produced contradictory results. While hydrastine has been shown to have a vasoconstrictive action and thus raises blood pressure, it has also been noted that berberine and hydrastine lower blood pressure. In addition, berberine has been shown to have anticoagulant properties in human blood, to have dose-dependant action on cardiac function, to increase coronary blood flow, and to exert a protective effect in dogs following ventricular failure.

Anticancer Activity

Berberine sulfate has been shown to inhibit the tumor-promoting action of 12-0-tetradecanoylphorbol-13-acetate and telecodin in vitro. In addition, berberine was shown to have antineoplastic activity in vivo against malignant human and rat brain tumors' cell lines.

Hepatic Activity

Stimulation of bile production is a key historical use of berberine. Berberine has been shown to decrease elevated tyramine levels commonly associated with liver cirrhosis by inhibiting tyrosine decarboxylase produced by gut flora. More research is needed to determine whether these findings will translate to any positive effects in humans.

Miscellaneous Effects

While not exhibiting a hypoglycemic effect, goldenseal has been shown to decrease excessive thirst in streptozotocin-induced diabetic mice.

Animal studies have suggested that berberine is effective in decreasing cholesterol levels by up-regulating liver receptors for low-density lipoproteins (LDL). One of these studies has shown a goldenseal root extract to have a stronger cholesterol-lowering effect than refined berberine alone. Clinical trials are needed to investigate this use.

Adverse Effects

Possible adverse effects are due to the isoquinoline alkaloids, notably hydrastine and berberine. In high doses (details not given), goldenseal has been noted to cause oral and pharyngeal irritation, nausea, vomiting, diarrhea, parasthesia, convulsions, weak pulse, hypotension, and death from respiratory or cardiac paralysis. Given the lack of cases of adverse reactions, some authors suggest that the dangers posed by the use of this herb medicinally have been exaggerated. Some authors argue that the trials mentioned above support this position; however, most were conducted using berberine alone, not whole goldenseal products, which are those normally seen in clinical practice.

Contact ulceration has been noted when goldenseal root is applied externally to mucous membranes, such as in the form of vaginal douches. In addition, drying of the mucous membranes has been noted after the oral administration of goldenseal, even at doses within the therapeutic range.

There has been one reported case of goldenseal potentially enhancing the symptoms of diabetic ketoacidosis in an 11-year-old child with type 1 diabetes. The patient had taken a 500 mg supplement of goldenseal two to three times daily for 2 weeks in an attempt to treat frequent urination before her admission to the hospital with severe ketoacidosis symptoms. It is unclear what role the goldenseal supplement played with respect to these symptoms because the girl was readmitted with diabetic ketoacidosis 11 months after discharge, with no consumption of goldenseal since her first episode.

High doses of plants rich in berberine may cause functional vitamin B problems due to altered metabolism. The administration of a plant rich in berberine (*Coptis chinensis* Franch., Ranunculaceae) to neonates suffering from glucose-6-phosphate dehydrogense deficiency has resulted in jaundice and hemolytic anemia. While the exact mode of action is not yet known, berberine appears to exert a bilirubin-displacing action. These reported adverse effects have, in part, led to a restriction of sale of berberine-rich herbs in general, though the applicability of these cautions to the use of goldenseal has been questioned.

The risk of complications due to the destruction of gut flora commonly seen with conventional antibiotics has yet to be completely determined. Many authors suggest this to be unlikely, a possible explanation being that berberine salts are also active against opportunistic fungi, such as *Candida albicans*.

In theory, goldenseal may cause light-sensitive reactions because light-exposed tissues treated with goldenseal have revealed phototoxic properties of this herb. However, cell studies indicate that this is likely only relevant for eyewashes and lotions and not applicable to orally ingested goldenseal.

Cautions/Contraindications

Due to the fact that the isoquinoline alkaloids are reputed to have a stimulant action on the uterus, goldenseal is contraindicated in pregnancy. Animal studies show mixed results regarding this theory. Goldenseal should also be used with caution in cases of hypertension. One study cautions that the myth that goldenseal is a "natural antibiotic" has led to the herb being used inappropriately in a large number of cases. In addition, liquid products containing goldenseal are bright yellow in color and will stain clothing if spilled accidentally.

Drug Interactions

While no specific drug interactions could be found for goldenseal, theoretically it may impact the liver's metabolism of drugs by altering enzyme activity. Berberine has been noted to increase the sleeping time induced by barbiturates in rats, and a 2006 review found that the goldenseal may also increase antiretroviral drug concentrations, but to clinically insignificant amounts. One open-label study of 20 healthy volunteers randomized for supplementation or medication sequence found goldenseal (3,210 mg daily) intake did not interfere with digoxin levels in the body.

Dosage Regimens

- Dried root and rhizome: 0.5–1 g dry, or as decoction, three times daily.
- Hydroalcoholic tincture (1:10 in 60% ethanol): 2–4 mL three times daily.
- Liquid extract (1:1 in 60% ethanol): 0.3–1 mL three times daily.
- Solid extract (4:1): 250 mg three times daily.
- Standardized extract (5% hydrastine): 250–500 mg three times daily.

Selected References

Khin-Maung U, Myo-Kin, Nyunt-Nyaunt-Wai, Aye-Kyaw, Tin-U. Clinical trial of berberine in acute watery diarrhoea. British Medical Journal 1985;291:1601–5.

Marin-Neto JA, Maciel BC, Secches AL, Gallo JL. Cardiovascular effects of berberine in patients with severe congestive heart failure. Clinical Cardiology 1988;11(4):253–60.

Rabbani G, et al. Randomised controlled trial of berberine sulphate therapy for diarrhoea due to enterotoxigenic *Escherichia coli* and *Vibrio cholerae*. Journal of Infectious Disease 1987;155:979–84.

Zeng XH, Zeng XJ, Li YY. Efficacy and safety of berberine for congestive heart failure secondary to ischemic or idiopathic dilated cardiomyopathy. American Journal of Cardiology 2003;92(2):173–76.

Hawthorn

Crataegus laevigata (Pois) DC.,
Crataegus monogyna (Jacq.)

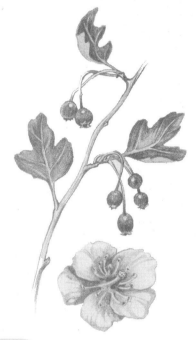

THUMBNAIL SKETCH

Common Uses
- Congestive heart failure (mild)

Active Constituents
- Triterpene glycosides
- Oligomeric procyanidins

Adverse Effects
- Nausea, dizziness, headache (rare)

Cautions/Contraindications
- Pregnancy and breastfeeding

Drug Interactions
- Heart condition medications

Doses
- *Standardized extract (2.2% flavonoids or 18.75% oligomeric procyanides):* 900 mg daily
- *Dried fruit:* 0.3–1 g taken as an infusion
- *Liquid extract (1:1 in 25% alcohol):* 0.5–1 mL three times daily
- *Solid extract:* 1–2 mL daily
- *Tincture (1:5 in 45% alcohol):* 1–2 mL three times daily
- *Syrup:* 5 mL two to three times daily

Introduction

Family
- Rosaceae

Synonyms
- Whitethorn
- Haw
- Mayherb
- Hagadorn

Medicinal Forms
- Dried fruit
- Liquid and solid extracts
- Water ethanol extract
- Tincture
- Syrup

Description
Hawthorn is a thorny deciduous tree native to Europe, where it was often grown as a hedge, reaching a height of 8 meters (25 feet). Clusters of white flowers bloom in the spring, and the berries turn bright red in autumn.

Parts Used
Flowers, leaves, and even bark have been used medicinally, but the bright red berries are the part most commonly used.

Traditional Use
Various species of hawthorn have been used traditionally for their healing powers by many different cultures. In ancient Britain, the hard wood and berries of hawthorn were thought to have magical powers. Many Christians believe that the crown of thorns worn by Christ was made of hawthorn. In Europe, hawthorn is considered one of the most important medicinal herbs and is used to treat heart, blood, kidney, and memory disorders. Its universal appeal is evident when you consider that it is also consumed as a food in the form of jams, preserves, and syrups.

Current Medicinal Use
Under the supervision of a trained health-care provider, hawthorn products are used for cardiovascular conditions, notably mild congestive heart failure and hypertension.

Relevant Research

Preventative and Therapeutic Effects

Constituents
- Triterpene acids: flavonoglycosides, vitexin, isovitexin, crataegolic acid.
- Oligomeric procyanidins: B-2, epicatechin, catechin.
- Miscellaneous: fatty esters, amines.

Traditional Uses
Traditionally, hawthorn is considered to be one of the most important cardiac tonics and is used to treat conditions resulting from heart or circulation problems. It has also been used as to treat such conditions as asthma, diabetes, nervous tension, anxiety, and kidney stones. While many different forms of hawthorn have traditionally been used, in Western herbalism *C. laevigata* and *C. monogyna* are the most common species.

Cardiovascular Effects
Hawthorn contains a number of medicinally active constituents, but most attention has been focused on the triterpene acids and oligomeric procyanidins and their cardiovascular properties. While specific actions differ depending on the constituent investigated, in general it is safe to say that hawthorn products appear to increase the force of heart

> *It appears likely that the way hawthorn products exert their action is similar to several conventional heart medications.*

contractions (inotropic) and have little or a slightly negative effect on heart rate (chronotropic). Specific extracts of hawthorn and its constituents have been shown to increase the force of contraction and blood flow to the heart muscles, protect the heart muscle from decreased blood flow, increase the refractory time between heart beats, and decrease the potential for arrhythmia (irregularities in heart beat).

It appears likely that the way hawthorn products exert their action is similar to several conventional heart medications. By decreasing the action of a group of enzymes called phosphodiesterases, the amount of a cell messenger called cyclic AMP is increased. This increases the ease with which calcium can enter the cells, which in turn causes increased action of the myocardium (heart muscles) and vasodilation (relaxation) of the coronary blood vessels, as well as vasodilation in peripheral blood vessels. In addition to this, the antioxidant properties of the oligomeric procyanidins and triterpene glycosides, such as vitexin, protect the cells from oxidative damage.

Congestive Heart Failure
There is a growing body of evidence from studies of various designs, including systematic reviews, randomized clinical trials, observational studies, and case series, that show hawthorn products are effective in treating mild cases of congestive heart failure (New York Heart Association levels I and II). Improvements are reported in a number of different outcome measures, including exercise performance, quality of life measures, symptom severity, and electrocardiogram (ECG or EKG) readings. Individuals ingesting hawthorn have experienced these benefits when compared with others ingesting placebos or using conventional care, including drug therapy, such as digitalis, nitrates, and angiotensin converting enzyme (ACE) inhibitors, such as captopril.

One of the most detailed systematic reviews published by the Cochrane Collaboration included 14 double-blind, placebo-controlled, randomized trials using hawthorn leaf and flower extract monopreparations as an adjunct to conventional treatment in patients with chronic heart failure (NYHA levels I to III). Compared with the placebo, patients treated with hawthorn extracts showed a significant improvement in symptoms, such as shortness of breath and fatigue. This result is supported by several other systematic reviews. In addition, long-term, multi-center, randomized controlled trials are currently under way, including one with 2,300 patients suffering from class II and class III congestive heart failure, comparing standardized extracts of hawthorn to conventional care.

While this evidence appears compelling, especially for mild cases, there is still a need for longer-term studies and research investigating the role of hawthorn products in more severe cases of congestive heart failure, as well as more information on precise mechanisms of action.

> *There is a growing body of evidence from studies of various designs, including systematic reviews, randomized clinical trials, observational studies, and case series, that show hawthorn products are effective in treating mild cases of congestive heart failure.*

Hyperlipidemia
Evidence from animal studies suggests that hawthorn berry products may reduce blood cholesterol. Additional research in humans is necessary to confirm these findings.

Antioxidant Activity

While hawthorn's antioxidant activities have been demonstrated in animal models, there is currently no evidence to support the use of hawthorn products as a long-term antioxidant supplement in humans.

Hypertension

Extracts of hawthorn have been shown to reduce blood pressure in animal and test tube studies. Evidence in humans is positive but still preliminary. For example, results from one small pilot study of 36 mildly hypertensive patients found some beneficial results associated with ingesting hawthorn. After taking baseline anthropometric, dietary assessment and blood pressure measurements at rest, as well as after exercise and a computer "stress" test, volunteers were randomly assigned to receive 600 mg of magnesium, a 500 mg extract of hawthorn, a combination of both magnesium and hawthorn, or a placebo. While no statistically significant differences were seen between the four groups, a trend toward lowered systolic and diastolic blood pressure, as well as toward decreased anxiety, was noted in the groups taking hawthorn. In addition, a 16-week randomized, placebo-controlled study demonstrated that 1,200 mg hawthorn daily in patients with type 2 diabetes who were taking prescribed medication can result in significant reduction in diastolic blood pressure. The herb was well tolerated, with no contraindications or reports of adverse effects.

Miscellaneous Effects

Psychological Problems

The fact that many of the oligomeric procyanidins found in hawthorn are also found in other herbal medicines with central nervous system (CNS) properties has led many to think that hawthorn may be useful in mental illness. Results from one small placebo-controlled, double-blind trial of 182 patients comparing a proprietary herbal combination product (Euphytose) containing hawthorn to a placebo during a 28-day period showed a significant improvement in the Hamilton Anxiety Scale (HAS or HAMA). Since Euphytose contained more than one herb, it is not possible to determine how much of the effect noted in the trial can be attributed to hawthorn. More research is definitely needed in this area.

Adverse Effects

A series of reviews of the acute toxicity of commercial hawthorn products in animals found the LD50 to fall between 18 and 24 mL per kg following intravenous administration and 1.5 to 33.8 mL per kg when taken orally. The LD50 for various hawthorn constituents following oral and intravenous administration was found to fall between 6 g per kg and 50 to 2,600 mg per kg respectively.

Hawthorn appears to be quite well tolerated, with adverse effects rare. Results from one postmarketing surveillance of 3,664 patients with congestive heart failure (NYHA I and II) taking a commercial hawthorn extract showed that only 22 patients suffered side effects that could be attributed with certainty to the herbal products. When adverse effects do occur, they are largely limited to nausea, palpitations, fatigue, sweating, and skin irritation of the extremities.

The most recent systematic review assessed the safety data of all available human studies on hawthorn monopreparations up to January 2005 and identified 24 clinical trials (5,577 patients) with 166 adverse events. The daily dose and duration of treatment ranged from 160 to 1,800 mg and from 3 to 24 weeks. Most adverse events were mild, except for 8 severe cases (heart palpitations, gastrointestinal complaints, vertigo, chest pain, and migraine). Similar to the results of a previous meta-analysis, nausea, dizziness, and digestive disorders were the most common adverse effects reported. The authors concluded that hawthorn is well tolerated despite some reports of severe adverse events. Further studies are needed to better assess the safety of hawthorn-containing preparations.

Cautions/Contraindications

Since constituents found in hawthorn have been shown to affect uterine muscle in animal models, hawthorn berry products should be avoided in pregnancy and breast-feeding. Hawthorn should only be taken on the advice of a health-care provider if it is being taken for heart conditions. Given the fact that hawthorn products are not appropriate for self-medication, hawthorn should not be used without the supervision of a health-care provider.

Drug Interactions

The potential exists for hawthorn berry products to potentiate the effects of cardiac glycosides, nitrates, and other drugs used to treat cardiovascular conditions. Although the evidence from clinical trials suggests a potential beneficial role for hawthorn in patients taking cardiovascular drugs, they should only be taken together on the advice of an appropriately trained health-care provider. Procyanidins in general may augment the coronary-dilating action of a number of common drugs, including caffeine and theophylline.

> *Although the evidence from clinical trials suggests a potential beneficial role for hawthorn in patients taking cardiovascular drugs, they should only be taken together on the advice of an appropriately trained health-care provider.*

Dosage Regimens

- Dried fruit: 0.3–1 g taken as an infusion three times daily.
- Liquid extract (1:1 in 25% alcohol): 0.5–1 mL three times daily.
- Solid extract: 1–2 mL daily.
- Tincture (1:5 in 45% alcohol): 1–2 mL three times daily.
- Syrup: 5 mL two to three times daily.
- Water ethanol extract of flowers and leaves (equivalent to 3.5–19.8 mg of flavonoids): 160–900 mg two to three times daily.
- Standardized extract (2.2% flavonoid or 18.75% oligomeric procyanides): 900 mg daily in divided doses.

Selected References

Chang Q, Zuo Z, Harrison F, Chow M. Hawthorn. Journal of Clinical Pharmacology 2002;42(6):605–12.

Pittler MH, Guo R, Ernst E. Hawthorn extract for treating chronic heart failure. Cochrane Collaboration 2008;2.

Tauchert M. Efficacy and safety of *Crataegus* extract WS 1442 in comparison with placebo in patients with chronic stable New York Heart Association class-III heart failure. American Heart Journal 2002;143:910–15.

Hoodia

Hoodia gordonii

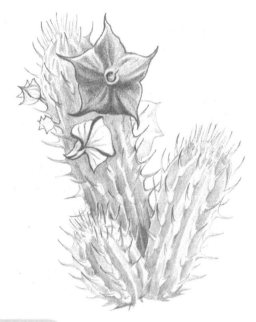

THUMBNAIL SKETCH

Common Uses
- Appetite suppressant

Active Constituents
- Hoodiogosides A-U
- Gordonosides A-L
- Oxypregnane steroidal glycoside P57
- Minerals (including calcium, magnesium, potassium)

Adverse Effects
- Liver problems (possible)

Cautions/Contraindications
- Diabetes
- Liver conditions
- Individuals who are underweight

Drug Interactions
- None known

Doses
- *Adult daily dose:* 300 mg twice daily. Individuals should not exceed 600 mg daily.
- *Child's daily dose:* There is insufficient evidence available to recommend use in children. Hoodia is not intended for use in children under 18 years of age.

Introduction

Family
- Apocynaceae

Synonyms
- Bushman's hat
- *Cactus dillenii*
- Kalahari cactus
- *Opuntia anahuacensis*
- *Opuntia melanosperma*
- *Opuntia nitens*
- *Opuntia stricta dillenii*
- *Opuntia zebrine*
- Queen of the Namib
- *Stapelia gordonii*
- Xhoba

Medicinal Forms
- Capsules
- Liquid extract
- Advertised as an ingredient in gum, patches, and tea

Description
Hoodia is a protected plant found in the Namib Desert. The flowers of this succulent plant exude a very strong smell.

Parts Used
The aerial parts of the plant are dried and powdered to be used medicinally.

Traditional Use
Hoodia has traditionally been used as a thirst quencher, as a cure for abdominal cramps, hemorrhoids, tuberculosis, indigestion, and hypertension, and to help prevent diabetes. The herb has become popular because of stories of the Kalahari bushmen of sub-Saharan Africa using this plant to ward off hunger and thirst when they were traveling in the desert.

Current Medicinal Use
Currently, the most common use for hoodia is as an appetite suppressant. However, there is no scientific evidence from published human clinical trials to support this use.

Relevant Research

Preventative and Therapeutic Effects

Constituents
- Minerals: Ca, K, Mg, P, Na, Cr, Fe, Zn, Co, Mo, Ni, Bo, Mn, Cu.

Stem
- Hoodiogosides A to U.
- Gordonosides A to L.
- Oxypregnane steroidal glycoside P57.

Note: Little precise information is currently known about the chemical constituents of *Hoodia gordonii*.

Appetite suppressant
There is limited information on hoodia's mechanism of action. Specific steroidal glycosides in hoodia extract, commonly called P57, have been hypothesized to be responsible for its appetite suppressant properties because P57 appears to affect certain neuropeptides

exerting appetite suppressant effects. Reduction of food intake may also be seen as a result of increases in ATP, which acts as a signal of energy-sensing satiety, in the hypothalamus.

One human study reported that *Hoodia gordonii* was able to suppress appetite and reduce body fat content, but this study was not published in the peer-reviewed literature. This result is supported by three animal studies, one of which reported that fractionations of the dried stems of *Hoodia gordonii* resulted in a reduction in food intake and a decrease in body weight. Another study found that injection of steroidal glycosides in hoodia into the brains of mice can lower food intake by 40% to 60%. It is not clear whether any of these findings will be relevant to humans.

A press release from Phytopharm described a multi-stage clinical study of the effectiveness of the steroidal glycoside and collective analogs of *Hoodia gordonii* for weight loss in humans. In the double-blind, placebo-controlled study involving 18 individuals, preliminary data indicated that there was a statistically significant reduction in the average daily calorie intake of the treatment group compared with the placebo group. There was also a statistically significant reduction (exact amount not specified) in the body fat content of the treatment group compared with the placebo group at the end of the study. The lack of published clinical trials make the true effects of hoodia difficult to assess, and conclusions cannot be made without further investigations.

Adverse Effects

Some individuals have reported unwanted effects on the liver after the ingestion of *Hoodia gordonii*. The exact nature and severity of the liver problems have not been detailed. This side effect is most likely caused by chemicals other than P57, but these unwanted constituents cannot be easily removed from the formulation.

Cautions/Contraindications

Individuals with diabetes should use hoodia with caution because it can possibly affect blood sugar levels via disruption of neuropeptides in the brain. Theoretically, blood sugar may drop while taking hoodia. If the regular hunger mechanism is turned off, the brain may not be able to sense changes in blood sugar. Therefore, hoodia should be avoided in people with diabetes.

Because hoodia belongs to the Apocynaceae family, people with known allergy or hypersensitivity to the Apocynaceae family should avoid using it. Due to reports of adverse effects on liver function associated with the use of *Hoodia gordonii*, it should also be avoided in individuals with liver abnormalities.

Because hoodia is commonly used as an appetite suppressant, there is a potential danger if it is used to promote weight loss among individuals with eating disorders. It is not intended for use by those who are underweight or within a normal weight range.

Drug Interactions

No known drug interactions could be found.

Dosage Regimens
- **Adult daily dose:** 300 mg twice daily. Individuals should not exceed 600 mg daily.
- **Child daily dose:** There is insufficient available evidence to recommend use in children. Hoodia is not intended for use in children under 18 years of age.

Selected References

Holt S, Taylor TV. *Hoodia gordonii*: An overview of biological and botanical characteristics: Part I. Townsend Letter for Doctors and Patients. Nov 2006.

Van Heerden FR, Horak RM, Maharaj VJ, Vleggaar R, Senabe JV, Gunning PJ. An appetite suppressant from *Hoodia* species. Phytochemistry 2007 Oct;68(20):2545–53.

Hops

Humulus lupulus L.

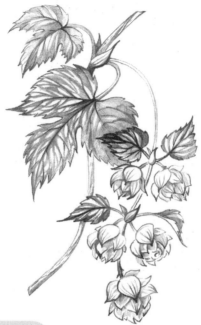

Common Uses
- Insomnia
- Agitation
- Nervous tension ailments (such as irritable bowel syndrome, poor digestion)

Active Constituents
- Volatile oil
- Resinous components
- Flavonoid glycosides

Adverse Effects
- Contact dermatitis and respiratory difficulties (following exposure to the herb itself)
- Menstrual cycle (disruption)

Cautions/Contraindications
- Depression
- Pregnancy

Drug Interactions
- May potentiate the action of hypnotics and alcohol

Doses
- *Dried strobiles:* 0.5–1 g three times daily and before bed
- *Liquid extract (1:1 in 45% ethanol):* 0.5–1 mL three times daily and before bed
- *Tincture (1:5 in 60% ethanol):* 1–2 mL three times daily and before bed

Introduction

Family
- Cannabaceae

Synonyms
- Humulus
- Lupulus
- Common hops
- European hops

Medicinal Forms
- Dried strobiles
- Liquid extract
- Tincture

Description
Hops is a climbing perennial herb standing up to 6 meters (20 feet) in height and is found in marshy areas throughout North America, Europe, and Asia. It produces a yellowish green male flower and a catkin-like, cone-shaped female flower, or strobile. These strobiles have glandular hairs that are rich in volatile oils, producing a characteristic heavy aroma.

Parts Used
The strobiles are the parts used medicinally.

Traditional Use
Hops is an essential plant in the brewing of beer, making it arguably one of the most commonly used herbs. Hops has a long medicinal history and is used primarily as a mild sedative. In addition to being taken orally, "hops pillows" are also often used to aid sleep, with the aroma allegedly having a calming action. Hops is also said to influence both male and female sexual function. It was noted that menarche often occurred early in female hop pickers, and in men a decrease in "sexual excess" was seen.

Current Medicinal Use
Hops is used primarily for its hypnotic and anti-anxiety properties in the treatment of insomnia, nervous tension, and conditions with a psychological component, such as irritable bowel syndrome. These uses are primarily supported by traditional evidence and a few clinical trials of combination herbal products that contain hops along with other active ingredients.

Relevant Research

Preventative and Therapeutic Effects
Constituents
- Volatile oils: include humulene, myrcene, beta-caryophyllene.
- Chalcones: include xanthohumol, xanthohumol.
- Resinous component: alpha-bitter acids, including humulone, cohumulone, adhumulone; beta-bitter acids, including lupulone, colupulone, adlupulone; 2-methyl-3-buten-2-ol.
- Flavonoid glycosides: include astargalin, quercetin, rutin.
- Miscellaneous: condensed tannins, "estrogenic substances."

Note: While 2-methyl-3-buten-2-ol exists in small amounts in the plant, the amount is thought to increase on storage from the auto-oxidation of other resinous components. This component is thought to be one of the active sedative constituents.

Common Uses

Hops is considered to be a mild sedative and is indicated in the management of insomnia and agitation or restlessness. It has also been used in the treatment of conditions related to nervous tension, such as irritable bowel syndrome, palpitations, and nervous coughs. Given the bitter nature of the resinous material, it is used as a digestive aid and to help stimulate appetite.

Antimicrobial and Antifungal Activity

Components of hops have been shown to exert antibacterial action, primarily against gram-positive bacteria. Humulone and lupulone appear to be particularly responsible for this action. The activity against gram-negative bacteria is low due to the presence of a phospholipids-rich membrane, leading to an increased inactivation of the active principles.

Clinically, aqueous extracts of hops have been used to treat various infections, including acute bacterial dysentery and pulmonary tuberculosis. However, no clinical trial investigating these uses could be found.

Activity against a number of fungi and yeasts, including *Trichophyton*, *Candida*, *Fusarium*, and *Mucor* species, has been demonstrated. The action of one component, 3-isopentenylphlorisovalerophenone, was compared favorably to griseofulvin in potency against *Trichophyton* species. A more recent evaluation noted no action against the yeast *Candida albicans*.

> Components of hops have been shown to exert antibacterial action, primarily against gram-positive bacteria.

Sedative Action

A sedative and hypnotic action has been attributed to 2-methyl-3-butene-2-ol in vivo. The sedative action of commercial products containing hops could be due to the in vivo formation of 2-methyl-3-butene-2-ol. This volatile product can induce an hypnotic effect when inhaled and exists in relatively high concentrations in bath products, giving possible credence to the use of items such as "hops pillows." However, it has been questioned whether there is enough 2-methy-3-buten-2-ol in most commercial products to support the use of hops as a sedative.

Oral administration of a commercial product (Seda-Kneipp), which contains valerian in addition to hops, has been shown to decrease the impact of noise on sleep patterns, both slow-wave and REM. Combination products containing both valerian and hops have been shown not to cause morning "hangover" effects but may impair performance a few hours after ingestion. In both the above scenarios, it should be noted that valerian (*Valeriana officinalis* L., Valerianaceae) has been shown to possess hypnotic characteristics of its own.

Miscellaneous Effects

Metabolism

Both colupulone and 2-methyl-3-buten-2-ol have been shown to induce cytochrome P4503A in mice and rats and cytochrome P4502B in rats.

Anti-Inflammatory

Humulone has been shown to possess anti-inflammatory properties, reducing 12-O-tetradecanoylphorbol-13-acetate-induced inflammatory ear edema in mice. The mechanism of action suggested is an inhibition of arachidonic acid metabolism.

Cancer

Hops has been used historically in the treatment of cancer. Humulone has been shown to inhibit the tumor-promoting effect of 12-O-tetradecanoylphorbol-13-acetate on skin tumor formation in mice.

Menopause Symptoms

One randomized, double-blind, placebo-controlled study with 67 menopausal women concluded that daily intake over 12 weeks of a hop extract enriched with 8-prenylnaringenin (the phytoestrogen component of hops) showed beneficial effects on hot flashes and other menopausal discomforts. It should be noted that this study was funded by a pharmaceutical company, whose aim was to evaluate their supplement product, MenoHop. The authors noted, however, that the study design and analysis were completed without input from the company.

Animal studies of the hormonal effects of hops are conflicting. Using the uterine weight assay of immature female mice as a determinant, no estrogenic properties could be shown for various components of hops, including the essential oil fraction and bitter acids. This finding contradicts others that have stated that hops has "appreciable estrogenic activity" and could aid in the treatment of hot flashes resulting from hormonal imbalance. A disruption of menstrual cycle in female hop pickers and decrease in male libido has also been documented.

> *A disruption of menstrual cycle in female hop pickers and decrease in male libido has also been documented.*

Adverse Effects

Components of hops are known to have allergenic potential, resulting in instances of contact dermatitis, as well as respiratory allergy and distress, following frequent contact with hops.

Cautions/Contraindications

Products containing hops should not be taken by individuals diagnosed with depression. Given its possible "estrogenic" action, hops may disrupt menstrual cycles, and the documentation of in vitro uterine antispasmodic activity suggests that hops should be avoided during pregnancy.

Drug Interactions

While no clinical instances were found, caution is prudent when herbal products containing hops are used with hypnotic medications and alcohol. The implication of induction of components of the cytochrome P450 system on concurrent drug therapy has yet to be evaluated.

Dosage Regimens

- Dried strobiles: 0.5–1 g three times daily and before bed.
- Liquid extract (1:1 in 45% ethanol): 0.5–1 mL three times daily and before bed.
- Tincture (1:5 in 60% ethanol): 1–2 mL three times daily and before bed.

Selected References

Heyerick A, Vervarcke S, Depypere H, Bracke M, Keukeleire DD. A first prospective, randomized, double-blind, placebo-controlled study on the use of a standardized hop extract to alleviate menopausal discomforts. Maturitas 2006;54:164–75.

Muller-Limmroth W, Ehrenstein W. Experimental studies of the effects of Seda-Kneipp on the sleep of sleep disturbed subjects: Implications for the treatment of different sleep disturbances. Medizinische Klinik 1977;72(25):1119–25.

Horsechestnut

Aesculus hippocastanum L.

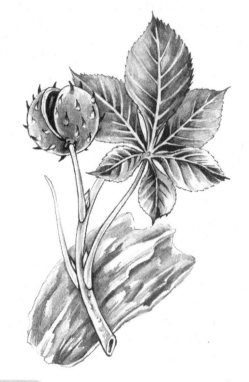

THUMBNAIL SKETCH

Common Uses
- Chronic venous insufficiency

Active Constituents
- Escin (or asecin)

Adverse Effects
- *Horsechestnut seed extract (HCSE):* gastrointestinal upset, calf spasm, headache, nausea, itchy skin
- *Cream or gel:* none reported

Cautions/Contraindications
- Pregnancy and breastfeeding
- Kidney and liver disease

Drug Interactions
- Diabetic drugs and anticoagulants (potential)

Doses
Orally
- *Extract (5:1, 40 mg escin):* 200 mg two to three times daily
- *Escin:* 50–75 mg every 12 hours
- *Dried seed:* 1–2 g daily
- *Fresh seed:* 0.2–1 g three times daily

Cream or gel
- *HCSE gel (2% escin):* three to four times daily

Introduction

Family
- Hippocastanaceae

Synonyms
- Aesculus
- Aesucule
- Eschilo
- Buckeye

Medicinal Forms
- Standardized (for escin) extract
- Fresh and dried seed
- Gel or cream

Description
Native to the Balkans, the horsechestnut tree grows commonly throughout Europe and North America. Standing up to 25 meters (80 feet) in height, with a characteristic domed shape, it is often found on the grounds of English stately homes and in ornamental gardens. The tree has five to seven oval leaflets comprising the leaf, with clusters of white to pink flowers later bearing a spiny-hulled fruit encasing several shiny brown seeds. In the United Kingdom, the hard fruits are referred to by many small boys as conkers and are used in a traditional game. Unlike the fruit of the chestnut tree, this fruit is not edible, though it can be used as fodder for animals.

Parts Used
Medicinally, the seeds and bark, rather than the fruit, are used.

Traditional Use
While horsechestnut products are not widely sold in the North American market, they are very popular in Europe, and especially in Germany, where in 1996 horsechestnut was the third-bestselling herbal product, with estimated sales of US$51 million. Most of these sales are made up of horsechestnut seed extract (HCSE), typically standardized for escin content. In Europe, horsechestnut seed products have been used orally for liver, prostate, kidney, and bladder conditions. It has also been applied in creams to treat bruising and arthritis pain.

Current Medicinal Use
Horsechestnut is now primarily used to treat conditions of cardiovascular insufficiency, notably varicose veins (veins that are enlarged and twisted) and, potentially, hemorrhoids (swelling and inflammation of veins in the anus and rectum).

Relevant Research

Preventative and Therapeutic Effects

Constituents
- Triterpene saponins: aescin (or escin).
- Coumarins: aesculetin, fraxin.
- Flavonoids: kaempferol, quercetin.
- Miscellaneous: tannins, allantoin, amino acids.

Traditional Use
Horsechestnut seed products have historically been used medicinally for a number of conditions, including liver conditions, benign prostatic hypertrophy (enlargement of the prostate), bladder conditions, and applied as a cream for bruising, osteoarthritis, tinnitus (ringing in the ears), ulcers, and upper respiratory conditions.

Chronic Venous Insufficiency

Even though horsechestnut has been used traditionally for a number of conditions, almost all of the modern research has investigated the use of HCSE in chronic venous insufficiency, a common condition resulting from decreased blood flow in the veins, most notably those in the leg. This decrease can cause a number of problems, such as leg pain, itchiness, swelling of the leg, and even generalized fatigue.

The most recent Cochrane review included 17 randomized controlled trials using HCSE as capsules over 2 to 16 weeks. While these studies were typically small and had some methodological challenges, six placebo-controlled studies involving 543 participants concluded that oral administration of HCSE decreases a number of signs and symptoms of chronic venous insufficiency, including ankle swelling, lower leg edema, pain, itchiness, fatigue, and leg tenseness. Other studies comparing the HCSE with rutosides, pycnogenol, or compression stockings indicated that HCSE is as effective as these conventional treatments. Most of these clinical trials used HCSE at a daily dose equivalent to 50 to 100 mg of escin daily.

In contrast to these positive findings, one prospective triple-blind, randomized, placebo-controlled 12-week trial involving 54 patients reported that HSCE may facilitate venous ulcer healing but that the effect was not statistically significant. A review of five clinical studies examining the use of one particular brand of HCSE, Aesculaforce (fresh HCSE available as oral tincture 20 mg or 50 mg tablets and topical gel), suggested that all available preparations provided effective treatment for those with mild to moderate forms of chronic venous insufficiency.

While HCSE creams and gels are often reputed to be of use in chronic venous insufficiency, the evidence supporting these claims is limited. Based largely on horsechestnut's pharmacological properties and the results from small studies, HCSE creams and gels (usually standardized for 2% escin) are also claimed to useful in bruising, sports injuries, varicose veins, and hemorrhoids. At this moment, the evidence supporting the use of oral dosage forms of HCSE (e.g., tablets or capsules) is significantly stronger than that for topical applications, such as gels and creams.

HCSE and escin have been shown to inhibit the inflammation associated with the onset of chronic venous insufficiency. By inhibiting the production of inflammatory mediators produced by the body, leakage from the blood capillaries is decreased. This reduction leads to a decrease in the localized swelling and edema seen with chronic venous insufficiency. While escin is thought to be the primary constituent responsible for this action, the effects appear to be enhanced by the antioxidants found in HCSE. In addition to this anti-inflammatory effect, HCSE appears to increase the muscle tone of the veins found in the leg and to increase blood flow and pressure in the femoral vein.

HCSE has also been shown to reduce the breakdown of proteoglycans, substances that are found in the walls of blood vessels and that affect vessel stability and permeability. Elevated levels of the enzymes known to cause the breakdown of proteoglycans have been found in patients with varicose veins.

HCSE as a whole and some of the individual constituents of the plant have been also shown to influence blood sugar. One constituent, esculin, found in horsechestnut but generally not in available extracts of the plant, has been shown to have antithrombin activity. Escin has also been shown to bind with blood proteins.

> *Even though horsechestnut has been used traditionally for a number of conditions, almost all of the modern research has investigated the use of HCSE in chronic venous insufficiency, a common condition resulting from decreased blood flow in the veins, most notably those in the leg.*

Adverse Effects

Consumption of horsechestnut leaves, twigs, and raw seeds can be potentially harmful and in some cases fatal. Symptoms of horsechestnut poisoning include headache, vomiting, diarrhea, coma, and paralysis.

In contrast, side effects of HCSE are quite rare and are thought to occur in approximately 0.6% of people taking the products. When adverse effects associated with HCSE do occur, they typically include gastrointestinal upset, calf spasm, headache, nausea, and itchiness when HCSE is applied to the skin. More serious adverse effects have been noted following the use of injectable HCSE or escin. Most notable among these are cases of hepatitis and damage to the tubular system in the kidneys. One case of anaphylactic allergic reaction has been reported following intravenous administration of a horsechestnut product.

Cautions/Contraindications

Until more is known, horsechestnut products should not be used during pregnancy or while breastfeeding. Given the potential for serious adverse effects, horsechestnut products should not be used in patients with liver or kidney conditions.

Drug Interactions

While no cases could be found, theoretically horsechestnut products may interact with anticoagulants, drugs which are highly protein bound, and antidiabetes drugs.

For more information, an excellent clinical review of horsechestnut can be found in the *Journal of Herbal Pharmacotherapy*. We would like to thank the authors of this paper for their help with this chapter.

Dosage Regimens

Orally
- Extract (5:1, 40 mg escin): 200 mg two to three times daily.
- Escin: 50–75 mg every 12 hours.
- Dried seed: 1–2 g daily.
- Fresh seed: 0.2–1 g three times daily.

Cream or gel
- HCSE gel (2% escin): three to four times daily.

Selected References

Pittler M, Ernst E. Horse chestnut seed extract for chronic venous insufficiency. Cochrane Database of Systematic Reviews 2005(4).

Suter A, Bommer S, Rechner J. Treatment of patients with venous insufficiency with fresh plant horse chestnut seed extract: A review of 5 clinical studies. Advances in Therapy 2006;23(1):179–90.

Juniper
Juniperus communis L.

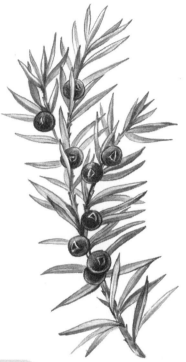

Common Uses
- Reproductive and urinary tract infections (minor, including cystitis)
- Chronic arthritic conditions
- Digestive upset

Active Constituents
- Volatile oils (monoterpenes and sesquiterpenes)

Adverse Effects
- *Internal:* "kidney pain," urination, hematuria, albuminuria, tachycardia (rapid heart beat), hypertension
- *External:* burning, blistering, erythema (redness of the skin), inflammation

Cautions/Contraindications
- Pregnancy
- Chronic or acute kidney disease (disputed)

Drug Interactions
- Avoid with conventional hypoglycemic and diuretic therapy

Doses
- *Dried fruit:* 1–2 g three times daily
- *Liquid extract (1:1 in 25% alcohol):* 2–4 mL three times daily
- *Tincture (1:5 in 45% alcohol):* 1–2 mL three times daily
- *Essential oil (1:5 in 45% alcohol):* 0.03–0.2 mL three times daily

Introduction

Family
- Cupressaceae

Synonyms
- *Buccae juniperi*
- Genievre
- Wacholderbeeren
- Juniper bush

Medicinal Forms
- Dried fruit (berries)
- Tincture
- Essential oil

Description
Juniperus communis is an evergreen shrub native to Northern and Central Europe. The tree itself can stand up to 6 meters (20 feet), with whorls of needles, and produces a distinctive round, deep purple fruit. While the fruits are often referred to as berries, they are in fact fleshy cone scales. For best effect, the berries should be harvested in the second year, when they are dark blue to purple in color. Many adults will be familiar with juniper's distinctive odor and taste because juniper berries are the principal flavoring agent in gin. However, gin contains insufficient amounts of the essential oil to afford it any medicinal properties.

Parts Used
The dried or expressed "berries" are rich in essential oils.

Traditional Use
Juniper berries have been used for centuries, not only for culinary but also for medicinal purposes as a urinary tract antiseptic for treating cystitis (inflammation of the urinary bladder) and as a digestive aid for colic, flatulence, and loss of appetite. In the Middle Ages, it was thought that burning juniper branches in a fire would ward off evil spirits and the plague.

Current Medicinal Use
Based on traditional evidence, juniper is primarily used to treat minor uncomplicated (no kidney involvement) reproductive and urinary tract infections such as cystitis (inflammation of the urinary bladder). Applied as a lotion, it is also used to treat certain arthritic conditions.

Relevant Research

Preventative and Therapeutic Effects

Constituents
- Volatile oil: monoterpenes (including 1,4-cineole, terpin-4-ol, sabinene, limonene, myrcene), sesquiterpenes (including caryophyllene, cadinene and elemene).
- Tannins: proanthocyanins, gallotannins.
- Flavonoid glycosides: include rutin, isoquercitin, quercetin.
- Miscellaneous: sugars, junionone, resin, vitamin C, diterpene acids, glucuronic acid.

Common Effects
While juniper has many medicinal uses, it is primarily considered to be useful in the treatment of conditions of the reproductive and urinary tract and musculoskeletal system. It is also considered a "urinary antiseptic" and diuretic (promotes urination) and is used in such conditions as cystitis (inflammation of the urinary bladder). It may be useful both internally and externally in chronic arthritis, chronic gout, neuralgia (nerve pain), and other rheumatic conditions.

Given its aromatic quality, it is also classified as a bitter and carminative and is used for digestive upset and colic, as well as to stimulate appetite.

Miscellaneous Effects

Most of the evidence supporting the therapeutic usefulness of juniper is empirical, and what little research exits is often not available in English. The diuretic action of juniper is attributed to the terpinen-4-ol portion, which is claimed to stimulate glomerular filtration. Juniper has also been demonstrated to lower blood sugar in both rats and mice. This action appears to be primarily extrapancreatic in origin. In a variety of in vitro and in vivo models, juniper has been shown to have antifungal, antiviral (against herpes simplex virus 1), and anti-inflammatory properties. Finally, oral administration of an extract of juniper berries was seen to decrease experimentally induced foot edema in rats.

Adverse Effects

Adverse effects have been reported following consumption or topical application of the oil. External application has been seen to result in burning, erythema (redness of the skin), inflammation, blistering, and edema. Internally, lower back pain in the kidney area, painful urination, discolored urine, hematuria or albuminuria (blood and proteins in urine), tachycardia (rapid heart beat), and hypertension have been reported. Positive patch test reactions following the topical application of an extract of juniper resulting in dermatitis have also been noted.

Cautions/Contraindications

Juniper berries are generally considered to be contraindicated in cases of chronic and acute kidney disease because of the high concentration of the irritant terpene hydrocarbons, such as alpha and beta pinenes, relative to the diuretic terpenin-4-ol. One review article has challenged this opinion, suggesting that this warning arises from the administration of high doses of juniper and terpentine oil in veterinary medicine. In addition, the author argues that the clouding of urine seen following administration of high doses of the oil probably results from the excretion of juniper oil metabolites and is not an indication of kidney irritation. Oil distilled from the needles, branches, and unripe fruit may be particularly high in the irritant components and should still be of concern to the practitioner. Given the present situation, the oil should be administered only under medical supervision.

Juniper has been shown to have uterostimulant, anti-implantation, and possible antifertility properties and should not be used in pregnancy.

Drug Interactions

Juniper should be used with caution in cases of concomitant conventional hypoglycemic and diuretic therapy.

Dosage Regimens

- Dried fruit (berries): 1–2 g three times daily.
- Liquid extract (1:1 in 25% alcohol): 2–4 mL three times daily.
- Tincture (1:5 in 45% alcohol): 1–2 mL three times daily.
- Essential oil (1:5 in 45% alcohol): 0.03–0.2 mL three times daily.

Selected Reference

Sanchez de Medina F, Gamez M, Jimenez I, Jimenez J, Osuna J, Zarzuelo A. Hypoglycemic activity of juniper "berries." Planta Medica 1994;60(3):197–200.

Kava

Piper methysticum G. Forst

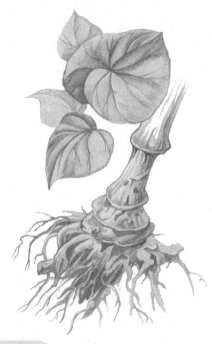

Common Uses
- Anxiety, tension, restlessness
- Muscle tension or spasm and pain

Active Constituents
- Kavalactones (kavapyrones)

Adverse Effects
- Liver toxicity (including cirrhosis, hepatitis, and liver failure)
- Vision disturbances (including photophobia and double vision)
- Skin conditions (including yellowing, itchiness, and allergy)
- Equilibrium (including dizziness and stupor)
- Gastrointestinal discomfort

Cautions/Contraindications
- Liver conditions (pre-existing)
- Pregnancy and breastfeeding
- Not recommended for prolonged use (more than 3 months)

Drug Interactions
- May potentiate the action of other centrally acting drugs

Doses
- *Standardized extract (70% kavalactones):* 100 mg two to three times daily
- *Dried rhizome:* 1.5–3 g daily in divided doses
- *Alcoholic extract (1:2):* 3–6 mL daily in divided doses

Note: Generally, the duration of use should not exceed 3 months.

Introduction

Family
- Piperaceae

Synonyms
- Kawa
- Kava-kava

Medicinal Forms
- Standardized extract
- Dried rhizome (rootstock)
- Alcoholic extract

Description
Kava is a perennial shrub found throughout Polynesia and the Pacific islands. The plant grows to 3 meters (10 feet) in height, with fleshy stems and few leaves, from a knotty, pithy rootstock that has lateral roots extending to 3 meters (10 feet).

Parts Used
The substantial, juicy rootstock (rhizome) is the part used medicinally.

Traditional Use
Kava was first described in the West by British explorer Captain James Cook in the 18th century during his exploration of the South Pacific. Kava has been used as an aphrodisiac, narcotic, and antiseptic, as well as a tonic for pain relief from arthritis, toothache, and other chronic pain conditions.

In addition to its importance as a medicinal agent, kava plays an important role in many social and religious customs of the Polynesian indigenous peoples. A beverage made from kava is consumed during funeral and marriage ceremonies, as well as to honor visiting guests and dignitaries. The preparation of the beverage is a deeply orchestrated procedure that often includes chewing the root to aid extraction. Kava beverage (kava-kava) is considered a social beverage and causes numbness of the mouth, followed by a pleasant mellow and relaxed state. "Hangovers" do not seem to be common.

Current Medicinal Use
Although a significant amount of both traditional and scientific evidence supports the use of kava in the treatment of anxiety, concerns about liver toxicity need to be addressed before it can be widely recommended. Kava may also be useful in treating muscle spasms and pain.

Relevant Research

Preventative and Therapeutic Effects
Constituents
- Kavalactones, including the pyrones: kavain (kawain), dihydrokavain, methysticin, dihydromethysticin, yangonin.
- Alkaloids: cepharadione A (an isoquinoline), pipmethystine (a pyridone, in the leaf only).
- Miscellaneous: flavonoids, benzyl-ketones.

Common Uses
Kava is considered by many to be one of the most effective herbal medicines for the treatment of anxiety. As a muscle relaxant, it is used in conditions associated with muscle tension, such as headaches. It is also reputed

to be effective in the management of mild insomnia and pain and stress and restlessness, as well as in the treatment of urinary tract infections and arthritic conditions. Application of the raw herb has been reported to ease dental pain and canker sores.

Neurological Effects

Most interest and investigation has been focused on the resinous (α-pyrones or kava-lactones. Their affinity for various GABA- and benzodiazepine-binding sites is debatable, with conflicting evidence being found on investigation. Kavalactones are very poorly soluble in water, so for medicinal use they must be placed in colloidal solution or at least converted to a finely divided form to promote absorption of the suspension from the gastrointestinal tract.

Kava, or its constituents, have been reported to exhibit neuroprotective effects against ischemia, produce EEG changes similar to those exhibited by diazepam, block the voltage-dependent sodium ion channel, exert an anticonvulsive action, possess antifibrillatory properties, exert an analgesic effect, relax skeletal smooth muscle, inhibit conditioned reflexes in a number of animal models, have local anaesthetic properties, and possess antispasmodic and tranquilizing characteristics.

Effect on Anxiety and Tension

A number of clinical trials, published primarily in German, have shown that kava extracts may prove beneficial in the management of anxiety and tension of non-psychotic origin. Three systematic reviews have assessed kava as a symptomatic treatment for anxiety.

One review, completed in 2003, has assessed the use of kava to treat generalized anxiety disorder, compared to a placebo. This review conducted a meta-analysis of seven double-blind, randomized controlled trials involving a total of 380 participants. These studies compared a placebo with a kava formula that was administered orally and contained no other active ingredients, and

all except one study used a product called WS1490 (kava extract standardized for 70% kavalactone content). One study chose to use a dose of 140 mg kavalactones daily for 1 week and then 280 mg kavalactones daily for an additional 3 weeks. The trials in this meta-analysis ranged in length from 4 weeks to 24 weeks. The meta-analysis indicated that there was a significant difference in the reduction of the total score on the Hamilton Anxiety Scale (HAS or HAMA) in favor of kava extract compared to a placebo. A previous review by the same authors came to the same conclusion.

> *A number of clinical trials, published primarily in German, have shown that kava extracts may prove beneficial in the management of anxiety and tension of non-psychotic origin.*

Another 2006 review assessed the results of three randomized, double-blind, placebo-controlled trials of varying lengths (4 to 8 weeks) involving a total of 64 participants. The authors note that two of these three studies were not published because the trials were stopped early based on concerns of potential kava-induced liver damage stemming from a case report of two patients. The trial that was published randomized 35 patients to receive either 280 mg kavalactones daily or a placebo for 4 weeks. Of the unpublished trials, one of them also gave 280 mg of kavalactones daily or a placebo to 13 participants for 4 weeks. The other randomized 16 participants to receive either 280 mg kavalactones daily, a placebo, or venlafaxine (225 mg daily). The authors reported no significant difference between any of the test groups and concluded that no clinical efficacy was demonstrated by these trials.

Unlike benzodiazepines, experience with the therapeutic use of kava preparations has shown no evidence of a potential for physical or psychological dependency. In addition, nine double-blind studies have been done with the isolated compound DL-kawain, comparing it to reference drugs and a placebo, with results similar to kava extract.

Effect on Mood and Cognition

One double-blind, placebo-controlled study has evaluated the use of kava to boost general mood and cognitive performance. Twenty healthy participants were randomized to receive one dose of 300 mg standardized kava extract (a total of 90 mg kavapyrones) or a placebo. Tests for cheerfulness and cognition were conducted before and approximately 60 minutes after capsule ingestion. The authors of this trial reported a significant increase in cheerfulness and cognitive performance after ingestion of kava compared to a placebo.

Miscellaneous Effects

Antifungal activity and antimycobacterial activities have been noted in vitro. A number of excellent reviews in English of this plant's medicinal action and historical and cultural importance exist.

Adverse Effects

Kava has been removed from the food supplement market in a number of countries, including Canada, due to concerns about kava-related liver toxicity and the limited regulatory options available at the time to mitigate risk. Health Canada has determined that kava is currently not sufficiently safe to be sold as a food supplement in Canada. This decision may be revisited in the future if any new evidence becomes available that can be reviewed under the Natural Health Products Regulations implemented after this restriction was enacted.

One review of the toxicity of kava completed in 2008 identified more than 30 cases of reported liver toxicity that may be associated with kava in Europe, eight of which had resulted in liver transplantation by 2002. The authors also identified two cases of liver toxicity possibly associated with kava intake in the United States. One case describes a 45-year-old woman who ingested a dietary supplement containing kava for 8 weeks, and the other describes a 14-year-old girl who took two different products containing kava, one of them regularly over a period of 7 weeks. Both cases resulted in hepatitis, leading to liver transplantation.

The reports to date have all been case histories of varying degrees of quality that describe liver toxicity, including cirrhosis, hepatitis, and liver failure, in patients ingesting kava. It is not clear if these effects are dose-related, related to long-term use, or involve specific extracts of kava only. In addition, there has been much criticism of the thoroughness of some of the actual case reports, as well as the fact that many of the patients were taking drugs with potential hepatotoxic (liver damaging) properties at the same time as the kava.

One review has cited three possible mechanisms for the liver damage potentially caused by kava: inhibition of cytochrome P450 and reduction in cyclooxygenase enzyme activity and liver glutathione content. There is also a single case report of a woman who experienced a delayed hypersensitivity reaction to kava that presented as a generalized rash and severe itching. A patch test with kava was strongly positive, suggesting an allergic reaction to kava.

Excessive consumption can result in disturbances of vision (excessive sensitivity to light, double vision, and eye movement disorders), yellowing of the skin, problems with balance, dizziness, and stupor. These effects are seen with consumption of the beverage, and it is unlikely that they are of any

> *Kava has been removed from the food supplement market in a number of countries, including Canada, due to concerns about kava-related liver toxicity and the limited regulatory options available at the time to mitigate risk.*

particular concern in practice. Compared to oxazepam, kava does not adversely affect cognitive function, mental acuity, or coordination as measured by event-related potentials during cognitive testing. One survey of 39 frequent kava beverage users in Australia related intake to malnutrition, weight loss, rashes, and changes to red blood cells. Chronic administration has also been reported to result in a characteristic scaling of the skin on the extremities, associated with intense itching. It was originally hypothesized that this was due to a deficiency in vitamin B$_3$, but symptoms do not appear to be improved following administration of nicotinamide (100 mg daily for 3 weeks). It is now considered most likely to be an allergic skin reaction.

Cautions/Contraindications

Due to its dopaminergic properties, kava should be used with caution in cases of Parkinson's disease. Use is contraindicated in pregnancy, breastfeeding, and depression, as well as in patients with liver conditions or other risk factors for liver disease.

Drug Interactions

Concomitant administration of kava with barbiturates and centrally acting conventional medication may result in a potentiation of their action. Administration of dihydromethysticin is known to potentiate the action of hexobarbital in animal models. While large doses of alcohol are known to potentiate the action of kava in mice, there does not seem to be such a problem in humans. Excessive alcohol consumption is still best avoided among people taking kava.

A possible interaction between kava and a benzodiazepine (alprazolam) has been noted in a 54-year-old man. The individual was admitted to hospital in a "lethargic and disorientated" state soon after introducing kava to his supplement regimen. The patient was also taking cimetidine, which is known to influence the cytochrome P450 system, and terazosin.

In contrast to this reaction, a review paper described a double-blind, randomized controlled study published in German in which 18 healthy volunteers were administered either 9 mg bromazepam (a benzodiapene) daily alone or this dosage of bromazepam as well as 240 mg kavalactones daily. The authors reported no synergistic effects, and participants seemed to maintain motor control, stress tolerance, and alertness. The review paper notes that the small number of participants in this study means that its results should be interpreted with caution. The authors of this review also discuss the potential for kava to alter the body's interaction with many drugs and herbs by affecting cytochrome P450 enzymes, which are essential to the body's drug metabolism.

Dosage Regimens

- Standardized extract (70% kavalactones): 100 mg two or three times daily.
- Dried rhizome: 1.5–3 g daily in divided doses.
- Alcoholic extract (1:2): 3–6 mL daily in divided doses.

Note: Generally, the duration of use should not exceed 3 months.

Selected References

Connor KM, Payne V, Davidson JRT. Kava in generalized anxiety disorder: Three placebo-controlled trials. Psychopharmacology 2006;21:249–53.

Pittler MH, Ernst E. Efficacy of kava extract for treating anxiety: Systematic review and meta-analysis. Journal of Clinical Psychopharmacology 2000;20(1):84–89.

Lemon Balm

Melissa officinalis L.

THUMBNAIL SKETCH

Common Uses

Internal

- Insomnia, anxiety, nervous tension (including digestive and cardiac conditions and pediatric conditions)

Topical

- Cold sores

Active Constituents

- Volatile oils
- Tannins
- Flavonoids (rosmarinic acid)

Adverse Effects

- None reported

Cautions/Contraindications

- Thyroid conditions (existing)

Drug Interactions

- Potential exists for interactions with concomitant thyroid medications

Doses

Oral

- *Dried leaves:* 1–4 g taken three times daily as an infusion or in a comparable dosage for a tincture or fluid extract

Topical

- *Concentrated extract (70:1):* applied two to four times daily in the management of cold sores

Introduction

Description

Native to Mediterranean Europe, North Africa, and Western Asia but now widely distributed, lemon balm is a perennial herb standing up to 1 meter (40 inches) in height, with light green leaves and flowers ranging in color from light yellow to rose and blue-white. Like most members of the mint family, it is aromatic, producing a characteristic lemony scent when bruised or crushed. The name "Melissa" derives from the Greek for "bee," referring to the attraction the plant holds for bees.

Parts Used

The aerial parts, fresh and dried, have many reputed actions.

Traditional Use

Lemon balm has enjoyed a long medicinal and culinary history, with references to it found in Roman, Arabic, and British herbal lore. Brewed as a tea, lemon balm has been enjoyed for its flavor and as a relaxing tonic. It has been used as a mild sedative for anxiety and nervous conditions and as an aid to longevity. Lemon balm is also a key component of perfumes and cosmetics.

Current Medicinal Use

Lemon balm is traditionally used for conditions related to nervous tension. Given its traditional reputation as a gentle herbal product, it is considered particularly well suited to pediatric conditions. Results from clinical trials suggest that creams made from lemon balm may also be of use in treating cold sores. Lemon balm is rarely used as a single agent but is commonly used in herbal formulae.

Relevant Research

Preventative and Therapeutic Effects

Constituents

- Volatile oils (0.1–0.2%): citral a and b, caryophyllene oxide, citronellal, geraniol, linalool, nerol.
- Flavonoids: include isoquercetrin, apigenin-7-O-glucoside, rhamnocitrin, luteolin-7-O-glucoside.
- Henylpropanoids: include triterpenoids, rosmarinic acid.
- Miscellaneous: tannins, ursolic acid, caffeic acid, polyphenolic agents.

Common Effects

Lemon balm is reputed to have sedative, antispasmodic, anti-emetic, antimicrobial, carminative, antihormonal, and diaphoretic properties. Oral consumption is traditionally considered useful in the treatment of anxiety, insomnia, colds, fevers, and digestive upset (bloating). It is considered by many to be especially useful as a children's remedy. Inhalation of the essential oil is reputed to have a direct influence on the nervous system, instilling calmness and improving mood. It is historically thought to be particularly well suited to the management of conditions, often cardiac or digestive, where the etiology has a psychological component.

Nervous System Action

Clinical studies are beginning to provide scientific support for use of lemon balm in the management of stress-related conditions, as a sedative, and perhaps to enhance cognition.

One randomized, double-blind clinical trial has been conducted in which 18 healthy participants were subjected to a 20-minute stress-stimulating cognitive test after ingesting a single dose of either a placebo or 300 mg or 600 mg of standardized lemon balm extract (details not reported). The results showed that both doses of lemon balm were associated with a significant increase in participant-rated calmness. The participants taking the 600 mg dose of lemon balm (but not those on the lower dose) reported a decrease in alertness. Those in the 300 mg lemon balm group appeared to have an increase in cognitive functioning. A randomized, double-blind, placebo-controlled trial involving 42 participants with Alzheimer's disease showed an increase in cognitive function and a decrease in anxiety after treatment with 60 drops of lemon balm extract daily for 16 weeks.

> *Clinical studies are beginning to provide scientific support for use of lemon balm in the management of stress-related conditions, as a sedative, and perhaps to enhance cognition.*

A German trial demonstrated that a combination herbal product containing valerian (160 mg/tablet) and lemon balm (80 mg/tablet), 1 tablet at bedtime, promoted sleep as effectively as triazolam 0.125 mg (Halcion) at a similar regimen. It should be noted that valerian has a long-established hypnotic action of its own. This combination product did not influence concentration or induce daytime sedation and did not potentiate the effects of alcohol. A lyophilized hydroalcoholic extract of lemon balm has also been shown to exert hypnotic and peripheral analgesic activity in mice.

Antimicrobial Effects

The essential oil fraction of lemon balm exerts an antimicrobial action in vitro against a variety of bacteria and fungi. In addition, antiviral properties of lemon balm have been demonstrated on many occasions. The active constituents appear to be primarily the polyphenols and tannins.

> *The essential oil fraction of lemon balm exerts an antimicrobial action in vitro against a variety of bacteria and fungi.*

Most interest has been focused on the action of lemon balm in the management of herpes simplex infections. In a recent placebo-controlled, double-blind study involving 116 participants, the topical application of 1% dried extract of lemon balm appeared effective in the management of herpes simplex. Improvement of symptoms was noted by day 2 of the treatment, and the test agent was considered superior to the placebo by both physicians and patients. For optimum results, the authors suggest that treatment be started at the onset of the infection. Another randomized, double-blind, placebo-controlled trial involving 66 participants reported that lemon balm cream may prolong the intervals between periods of herpes in patients diagnosed with herpes simplex labialis.

Endocrine Effects

Extracts of lemon balm have long been documented to possess antithyrotropic activities, preventing or decreasing stimulation of the thyroid gland. Aqueous extracts contain components, notably certain phenolic agents, that inhibit the extrathyroidal metabolism of both T3 and T4 in a dose-related manner. Test tube studies have demonstrated that a freeze-dried extract of lemon balm inhibits the binding, in a dose-dependent manner, of thyroid stimulating hormone (TSH) to thyroid membrane. It is hypothesized that components present in the freeze-dried extract interact with TSH, preventing its binding to the membrane-bound TSH receptor. In addition, components of the freeze-dried extract of lemon balm inhibit the binding immunoglobulin G found in Grave's disease to TSH receptors. This result may in part support the historical use of lemon balm in the management of certain thyroid conditions.

Miscellaneous Effects

Antioxidant

Hydroalcoholic extracts of lemon balm have been shown to possess antioxidant properties, thought to be due in part to the presence of rosmarinic acid.

Anti-Inflammatory

Rosmarinic acid isolated from lemon balm has been shown to influence complement activity. This action may be explained in part by the component's ability to inhibit the action of C3 and C5 convertase. Studies in animal models suggest that rosmarinic acid also exerts an anti-inflammatory action in complement-dependent inflammatory processes.

Adverse Effects

No examples of unpleasant side effects associated with lemon balm could be found in the literature.

Cautions/Contraindications

While no specific examples could be found, lemon balm should be used cautiously in patients with thyroid conditions. Safety in pregnancy has not been established. Lemon balm appears to have no mutagenic properties.

Drug Interactions

While no clinical examples could be found, products containing lemon balm may interact with conventional thyroid medications. A lyophilized hydroalcoholic extract of lemon balm has been reported to promote the hypnotic action of pentobarbital in mice.

Dosage Regimens

Oral
- Dried leaves: 1–4 g taken three times daily as an infusion or in a comparable dosage for a tincture or fluid extract.

Topical
- Concentrated extract (70:1): applied two to four times daily in the management of cold sores.

Note: Since lemon balm is rich in volatile oils, infusions should be made in a closed container.

Selected References

Akhondzadeh S, Noroozian M, Mohammadi M, Ohadinia S, Jamshidi AH, Khani M. *Melissa officinalis* extract in the treatment of patients with mild to moderate Alzheimer's disease: A double-blind, randomised, placebo-controlled trial. Journal of Neurology, Neurosurgery and Psychiatry 2003;74:863–66.

Kennedy DO, Little W, Scholey AB. Attenuation of laboratory-induced stress in humans after acute administration of *Melissa officinalis* (lemon balm). Psychosomatic Medicine 2004; 66:607–13.

Koytchev R, Alken RG, Dundarov S. Balm mint extract (Lo-701) for topical treatment of recurring herpes labialis. Phytomedicine 1999;6(4):225–30.

Wobling R, Leonhardt K. Local therapy of herpes simplex with dried extract from *Melissa officinalis*. Phytomedicine 1994;1(1):25–31.

Licorice

Glycyrrhiza glabra L.

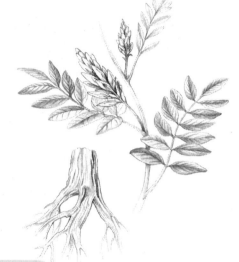

Common Uses
- Gastrointestinal tract inflammation (e.g., peptic and duodenal ulcers, gastritis)
- Skin inflammation (e.g., oral herpes lesions, canker sores)
- Coughs (productive) and bronchitis
- Adrenocorticoid insufficiency (e.g., due to stress and overwork)
- Sweetening and flavoring agent

Active Constituents
- Glycyrrhizin
- Glycyrrhetinic acid

Adverse Effects
- Pseudoaldosteronism (which presents as hypernatremia, hypokalemia, hypertension, headache, edema, and/or lethargy and can lead to congestive heart failure)

Cautions/Contraindications
- Cardiovascular disease (pre-existing)
- Liver or kidney dysfunction
- Pregnancy (safety not established)

Drug Interactions
- Increases the half-life of hydrocortisone and prednisolone
- Possible interactions with medications whose action is closely linked to potassium levels, including cardiac glycosides and both loop and potassium-sparing diuretics

Doses
- *Powdered root:* 1–4 g daily in three divided doses
- *Solid (dry powdered) extract (4:1):* 250–500 mg daily in three divided doses
- *Deglycyrrhizinated licorice tablets:* 380–1,140 mg (1 to 3 chewable tablets) three times daily
- *Licorice extract:* 0.6–2 g daily
- *Decoction:* 2–4 g (5 mL) herb to 120 mL boiling water three times daily after meals
- *Lozenges and candies:* as an expectorant and cough suppressant (make sure they actually contain real licorice)

Introduction

Description

Licorice is a small perennial shrub native to temperate regions, growing to 1 to 2 meters (3 to 6 feet) in height, with dark green leaves, mauve flowers, and a long, round taproot and root branches and runners. Licorice is extensively cultivated as a medicinal herb and as a distinctively flavored sugar for use in making candy and in flavoring botanical formulations because of its distinctive taste and its sweetening action: glycyrrhizin is 50 to 100 times sweeter than sucrose. The amount of licorice in products varies dramatically. Most of the licorice candy available in North America is flavored not with licorice but with anise oil. One study found that authentic licorice candy contained between 0.26 mg per g and 7.9 mg per g of glycyrrhizin, while medicinal products ranged from 0.30 mg per g to 47.1 mg per g of glycyrrhizin. In addition, licorice-flavored chewing tobacco contained between 1.5 mg per g to 4.1 mg per g of glycyrrhizin.

Parts Used

The roots and underground horizontal stems, called rhizomes or stolons, are the parts used medicinally.

Traditional Uses

Licorice has been used medicinally for over 4,000 years as an expectorant, an antitussive, and a mild laxative. It is also a very important herb in traditional Chinese medicine (TCM), where its uses include treating peptic ulcers, asthma, and malaria. In traditional Chinese medicine, licorice (*Glycyrrhiza uralensis* Fisch. & DC.) is considered a sweet, neutral herb that clears phlegm and tonifies the spleen.

Current Medicinal Use

Licorice is arguably the most common herbal medicine because it is frequently added to natural health products as a sweetening and flavoring agent. Based primarily on traditional evidence, licorice is used as an adrenal tonic in cases of stress and fatigue, and as an expectorant in coughs and bronchitis. As an anti-inflammatory, licorice is applied topically to treat various conditions, such as cankers, cold sores, and minor skin abrasions. A growing amount of scientific evidence supports the traditional use of licorice in the treatment of peptic and duodenal ulcers.

Relevant Research

Preventative and Therapeutic Effects

Constituents

- **Terpenoids**: glycyrrhizin (also called glycyrrhizic or glycyrrhizinic acid), which yields glycyrrhetinic acid (also called glycyrrhetic or glycyrretic acid) and glucuronic acid after hydrolysis, glycyrrhetol, glabrolide, licoric acid, liquiritic acid.

- **Flavonoids and isoflavonoids**: include isoflavonol, kumatakenin, licoricone, glabrol, formononetin, chalcone and chalcone derivatives, including isoliquiritigenin, licochalcone A and B.

- **Coumarins**: umbelliferone, herniarin, glycyrin, liqcoumarin.

- **Volatile oils**, including: anethole, benzaldehyde, cumic alcohol, eugenol, fenchone.

- **Miscellaneous**: acetylsalicylic acid, salicylic acid, methylsalicylate.

Metabolic Effects

The pharmacology of licorice has been extensively studied, and several good reviews discuss this in detail. In summary, glycyrrhizin inhibits three enzymes: two (15-hydroxyprostaglandin dehydrogenase and delta13-prostaglandin reductase) are involved in the metabolism of two prostaglandins (E and F2a), and the third (11 beta-hydroxysteroid dehydrogenase), which is found primarily in the kidneys and liver, catalyzes the production of cortisone (inactive) from cortisol (active). Thus, corticosteroid receptors become increasingly activated by cortisol, which may result in hypertension. In addition, glycyrrhizin and glycyrrhetinic acid bind weakly to mineralocorticoid and glucocorticoid receptors, influence aldosterone secretion and elimination, suppress plasma renin activity, and decrease angiotensin levels. Licorice has also been shown to increase atrial natriuretic peptide (ANP) and decrease vasopressin levels.

Licorice is considered a "phytoestrogen"; that is, the steroid-like configuration of several of the components of licorice, including the isoflavones and glycyrrhetinic acid, have the ability to influence estrogen metabolism. Generally, if estrogen levels are high, these constituents inhibit estrogen action by binding to the estrogen receptors and blocking the binding of endogenous estrogen. If estrogen levels are low, however, they appear to potentiate the action of estrogen. For this reason, it is often referred to as being amphoteric (partial agonist) in nature. Phytoestrogens have between $1/20$ and $1/100$ the action of estrogen.

Pharmacokinetics

Peak serum concentration of glycyrrhizin occurs approximately 4 hours after ingestion but varies widely among individuals ingesting the same amount of glycyrrhizin. In contrast, glycyrrhetinic acid levels peak at approximately 24 hours. Glycyrrhizin serum concentration decreases quickly and is no longer detectable by 96 hours. Glycyrrhetinic acid levels decrease more slowly. Consumption of 100 to 200 g licorice daily will result in plasma concentrations of glycyrrhetinic acid of 80 to 480 mg per mL. It appears that the bioavailability (i.e., intestinal absorption) of glycyrrhizin is higher when it is consumed alone than when it is consumed as a constituent of licorice root or licorice root extract, but it does not appear to be influenced by the presence of food. Glycyrrhizin is excreted mainly (80%) by the liver into the bile by a process that can become saturated.

Gastrointestinal Effects

Perhaps one of the best-known uses for licorice is for gastrointestinal conditions. Licorice has been used to treat dyspepsia for centuries. In fact, two pharmaceutical products, deglycyrrhizinated licorice and carbenoxolone, both of which enhance the body's ability to protect the gastrointestinal lining in a variety of ways, including "increasing the number of mucus-secreting cells (thereby increasing the amount of protective mucosubstances secreted); improving the protective nature mucus produced; increasing the life span of the surface intestinal cells; and enhancing the microcirculation of the gastrointestinal tract lining," have been available since the mid-1960s. The mechanism of action is described in detail elsewhere.

> *Perhaps one of the best-known uses for licorice is for gastrointestinal conditions. Licorice has been used to treat dyspepsia for centuries.*

Carbenoxolone

This derivative of glycyrrhetinic acid has been marketed for the treatment of both duodenal and gastric ulcers. Although its exact mechanism of action has not yet been elucidated, it appears to increase the synthesis and secretion of mucus. Although efficacy studies have reported conflicting results, one study showed that maintenance therapy of carbenoxolone decreased the recurrence rate of gastric ulcers significantly more than either antacids or a placebo. Several randomized, double-blind controlled trials have demonstrated that carbenoxolone is also more effective than a placebo in the treatment of duodenal ulcers.

No information could be found comparing the effects of carbenoxolone with standard combination antibiotic therapy in the management of peptic ulcer disease. Carbenoxolone is rarely used today because its adverse effects include water retention, as well as increased blood pressure. These reactions are discussed in detail in the Adverse Effects section (page 299).

Deglycyrrhizinated Licorice (DGL)

Deglycyrrhicinated licorice, or DGL, was developed in an attempt to reduce the adverse effects, which are largely caused by the glycyrrhizin content of licorice products. DGL has a glycyrrhizin content of less than 3% and no known adverse effects. Although the active constituent of DGL has not been identified, it is believed to be a spasmolytic agent (it suppresses cramps and muscle spasms). The majority of randomized, placebo-controlled trials of DGL tested a specific product currently called Caved-S, which is a chewable tablet and is only available in Europe. Another European brand, Ulcedal, which was available in capsule form (it has since been removed from the market) appeared to be ineffective, leading some researchers to hypothesize that DGL must mix with saliva to be effective.

One study involving 100 participants reported that DGL (760 mg three times daily between meals) had comparable efficacy to cimetidine (200 mg three times daily and 400 mg at bedtime) in its ability to increase the healing rate of gastric ulcers. This study also found no significant difference in ulcer recurrence after 1 year when they compared maintenance therapy of DGL (760 mg twice daily) and cimetidine (400 mg at bedtime). In addition, DGL has been shown to be equivalent to ranitidine in treatment of gastric ulcers.

Several studies also report the effectiveness of DGL in the treatment of duodenal ulcers. One trial involving 40 participants showed that both 3 g DGL daily for 8 weeks and 4.5 g daily for 16 weeks provided substantial improvement in most patients within 5 to 7 days; however, the higher dose was reported to be significantly more effective. A

> *Deglycyrrhicinated licorice, or DGL, was developed in an attempt to reduce the adverse effects, which are largely caused by the glycyrrhizin content of licorice products.*

second study involving 874 participants reported no significant difference in the rate of healing at 12 weeks between patients treated with DGL (380 mg three times daily), antacids (15 mL suspension of aluminum-magnesium hydroxide equivalent to 3 g a day) or cimetidine (200 mg three times daily and 400 mg at bedtime).

Anti-Infective Activity
Antiviral
Several studies have found evidence of licorice's antiviral activity. Test tube studies document the ability of glycyrrhizin to directly inhibit the growth of several different viruses, including herpes simplex, herpes genitalis, and herpes zoster, influenza virus A, hepatitis A virus (HAV), and HIV. In addition, both glycyrrhizin and glycyrrhetinic acid have been reported to induce the production of interferon.

A few clinical studies have been conducted indicating that the topical application of glycyrrhetinic acid or its derivatives decreases the pain and increases the rate of healing of oral and genital herpes lesions.

Antibacterial and Antifungal
Extracts of licorice have been shown in test tube studies to inhibit the growth of a variety of bacteria and fungi, including *Candida albicans*, *Staphylococcus aureus*, *Streptococcus mutans*, and *Mycobacterium smegmatis*. The isoflavonoid components appear to be responsible for this action. One in vitro study found that they had activity comparable to streptomycin against *Staphylococcus aureus*, *Mycobacterium smegmatis*, and *Candida albicans*.

Antiparasitic
Licochalcone A, a component of licorice, has been shown to inhibit both chloroquine-susceptible and chloroquine-resistant strains of *Plasmodium falciparum* and *Leishmania* major and *Leishmanian donovani* promastigotes and amastigotes in in vitro studies.

Anti-Inflammatory and Anti-Allergic Activity
The cortisol-like action of licorice confers an ability to inhibit the formation and secretion of inflammatory compounds. A recent study suggests that glycyrrhetinic acid may also have a direct anti-inflammatory action by selectively inhibiting the classical complement cascade, though it has no affect on the alternative pathway. In addition, a recent study reported that glycyrrhizin is a selective inhibitor of thrombin — though it did not effect the clotting activity of thrombin — which may be another mechanism of action for its anti-inflammatory activity. Glycyrrhizin has been shown to inhibit allergenic reactions produced under controlled experimental conditions.

> *The cortisol-like action of licorice confers an ability to inhibit the formation and secretion of inflammatory compounds.*

Hepatoprotective Activity
The role of licorice in liver disease has been reviewed in detail. Intravenous administration of glycyrrhizin is used in the treatment of hepatitis in Japan. This indication is supported by several double-blind, controlled studies that have reported that glycyrrhizin is an effective treatment in the management of viral hepatitis. It has been hypothesized that glycyrrhizin may bind to hepatocytes, modifying the expression of hepatitis B virus (HBV) antigens on their surface, thus suppressing their sialylation. Two long-term studies, one of 15 years' and one of 10 years' duration, have been conducted observing a total of 799 participants diagnosed with chronic hepatitis C (HCV), 328 of whom were treated with glycerrhizin injection and the remaining with other treatments. Both studies observed a significantly reduced incidence (by at least half) of hepatocellular carcinogenesis in the group treated with glycerrhizin.

In addition, several in vitro studies indicate that glycyrrhizin may protect the liver from damage caused by chemical toxins, such as CCl4 (carbon tetrachloride). The mechanism of action for this is hypothesized to be an inhibition of the cytochrome P450 system conversion of CCl4 to CCl3.

Miscellaneous Effects

Premenstrual Syndrome

PMS symptoms have been associated with an increased estrogen:progesterone ratio. Phytoestrogens, such as licorice, are thought to be useful in decreasing the symptoms associated with PMS.

Canker Sores

Licorice has been reported to decrease the pain and speed the healing rate of canker sores in the mouth. One double-blind crossover trial involving 24 participants reported that a mouthwash containing glycyrrhetinic acid reduced the pain associated with mouth ulcers, as well as significantly decreasing the number of new ulcers that developed. Another double-blind trial randomized 46 participants to receive either dissolvable mouth patches with active glycyrrhiza root extract to place over their canker sores or placebo patches and recruited a third group of 23 participants to receive no treatment. By day 8 of the study, ulcer size and pain sensation was significantly decreased in the glycyrrhiza treatment group compared to the two other groups.

> *Licorice has been reported to decrease the pain and speed the healing rate of canker sores in the mouth.*

Expectorant and Antitussive

Although the mechanism of action has not yet been elucidated, licorice has a long historical use as an expectorant and antitussive. Its use for these indications continues to be widespread in North America today.

Erythema

One study has tested the use of a topical preparation containing a compound found in licorice called licochalcone A (0.05% extract) in suppressing erythema. In one study, 45 participants were enrolled in an arm of the study that induced redness through repetitive dry shaving of the skin with a razor, and another 12 patients were enrolled in a different arm in which erythema was induced by UV irritation. The authors reported a significant suppression of erythema in both groups when skin was treated with licochalcone A compared to placebo and suggested that this application may be useful in patients with rosacea.

Diabetes Complications

Many complications of diabetes improve with the addition of inhibitors of aldose reductase (the first enzyme in the polyol pathway) to the therapeutic regimen. Isoliquiritigenin, a component of licorice, has been shown in vitro and in vivo to inhibit aldose reductase, thus decreasing the conversion of glucose to sorbitol and inhibiting sorbitol accumulation.

Burns

Glycyrrhizin has been shown to decrease the generation of burn-associated suppressor T cells (BTs cells) in thermally injured mice. Other reports have found an increasing incidence of septic infections with an increased number of BTs cells. The authors hypothesize that glycyrrhizin may play a role in the future treatment of burns.

Anticancer Properties

A variety of compounds in licorice have been shown to have antimutagenic activity and to decrease the growth of some cancer cell lines in vitro. The clinical significance of these findings is unknown.

Antifatigue Effects

Licorice is considered by some medical herbalists to be an adrenocorticotrophic agent (tonic to the adrenal glands). Consequently, it is used in the management of stress and fatigue.

Hormonal Effects

One clinical trial involving 9 healthy women has shown that regular consumption of licorice (266 mg glycyrrhizic acid daily) for 2 months can increase parathyroid hormone concentrations and urinary calcium secretion. A similar study by the same group of authors found that 0.25 g of glycyrrhizic acid daily for 2 months caused a significant reduction in serum testosterone.

Weight Loss

One trial has investigated the oral ingestion of licorice flavonoid oil to reduce body weight in overweight individuals. In this double-blind, placebo-controlled study, 103 overweight participants received either 300 mg licorice flavonoid oil daily or a placebo for 12 weeks. The authors reported that there was a significant difference in body weight between the two groups at the end of the 12 weeks; however, this was only because the placebo group increased in weight and the group receiving licorice flavonoid oil maintained their pre-treatment weight.

Adverse Effects

Licorice is considered safe in low doses; however, adverse effects are common at doses of more than 20 g of licorice root daily. Adverse symptoms have also been seen in doses significantly lower than this. Because the adverse effects appear at widely differing doses in different individuals, it is important to monitor patients.

The adverse effects most commonly experienced are mineralocorticoid-related, including headache, lethargy, sodium and water retention, excessive excretion of potassium, hypokalemic myopathy, and high blood pressure. Because of the low serum potassium, cardiac arrhythmias and ECG abnormalities may also occur. A few cases of these symptoms have arisen after patients have started taking licorice root long-term after they quit smoking. Together, these effects constitute what has been called pseudohyperaldosteronism. Spironolactone will reverse these adverse effects. Amenorrhea and hyperprolactinemia, possibly resulting in infertility, have also been reported.

> *Licorice is considered safe in low doses; however, adverse effects are common at doses of more than 20 g of licorice root daily.*

Several deaths have resulted from the ingestion of licorice products. Most often adverse effects are caused by the consumption of large amounts of licorice candy and in those with pre-existing cardiovascular or renal impairment. One much-quoted case of severe congestive heart failure and pulmonary edema occurred when a 53-year-old man ate 700 g of licorice candy over 8 days. Another study reports on the successful treatment with licorice of a 63-year-old patient suffering from severe postural hypotension.

It has been suggested that a maximum of 10 mg of glycyrrhizin (approximately 5 g of authentic licorice candy) can be safely consumed daily over long periods. The Dutch Nutrition Information Bureau suggests that no more than 200 mg of glycyrrhizin should be consumed daily.

Deglycyrrhizinated licorice (DGL) does not appear to cause the adverse effects described above.

Cautions/Contraindications

Caution should be used in patients with high blood pressure or any other existing cardiovascular disorders, renal failure, and liver disease. Safety in pregnancy has also been questioned.

Drug Interactions

Licorice may interfere with hormonal therapy or hypoglycemic therapy. It has been hypothesized, for example, that glycyrrhizin may combine with insulin to cause increased electrolyte disturbances. One authority suggests that potential for interaction exists with any drugs with a narrow therapeutic index or mechanism of action dependent upon potassium levels (e.g., cardiac glycosides, loop diuretics, and potassium-sparing diuretics).

Glycyrrhetinic acid increases the half-life of hydrocortisone applied topically and potentiates the action of hydrocortisone in lung tissue. There are also several reports that oral administration of glycyrrhizin inhibits the metabolism of prednisone, thus increasing plasma concentrations.

DGL (deglycyrrhizinated licorice) has been reported to increase the bioavailability of nitrofurantoin by more than 50% if they are administered together; however, it also appears to decrease feelings of nausea associated with nitrofurantoin ingestion.

One study involving 32 participants has demonstrated that 3.5 g of licorice root extract given with 100 mg spironolactone daily to women with polycystic ovarian syndrome can decrease the diuretic side effects of spironolactone when compared to 100 mg spironolactone daily given alone.

Dosage Regimens

- **Powdered root:** 1–4 g daily in three divided doses.
- **Fluid extract (1:1):** 4–6 mL daily in three divided doses.
- **Solid (dry powdered) extract (4:1):** 250–500 mg daily in three divided doses.
- **Deglycyrrhizinated licorice tablets:** 380–1,140 mg (1 to 3 chewable tablets) three times daily.
- **Licorice extract:** 0.6–2 g daily.
- **Decoction:** Add 2–4 g (5 mL) herb to 120 mL boiling water and simmer for 5 minutes. Strain and drink this quantity three times daily after meals.
- **Lozenges and candies:** as an expectorant and cough suppressant (make sure they actually contain real licorice).

Note: The Commission E has approved the indication for ulcer treatment (200–600 mg of glycyrrhizin daily) for a maximum of 4 to 6 weeks.

Selected References

Martin MD, Sherman J, Van der Ven P, Burgess J. A controlled trial of a dissolving oral patch concerning glycyrrhiza (licorice) herbal extract for the treatment of aphthous ulcers. General Dentistry 2008;56(2):206–10.

Stewart PM, et al. Mineralcorticoid activity of liquorice: 11-beta-hydroxysteroid dehydrogenase deficiency comes of age. Lancet 1987; II:821–24.

Lobelia

Lobelia inflata L.

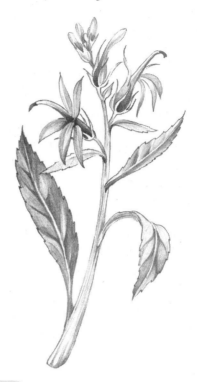

THUMBNAIL SKETCH

Common Uses
- Respiratory conditions (such as bronchial asthma and bronchitis)
- Tobacco addiction

Active Constituents
- Piperidine alkaloids (notably (-)- lobeline)

Adverse Effects
- Nausea, vomiting, diarrhea
- Coughing and dizziness
- Administration of high doses may result in more severe symptoms, such as convulsions, hypothermia, coma, and even death

Cautions/Contraindications
- Nicotine (situations where nicotine is contraindicated)
- Cardiovascular and respiratory disease
- Pregnancy and lactation

Drug Interactions
- None found

Doses
- *Dried herb:* 0.2–0.6 g three times daily
- *Liquid extract (1:1 in 50% alcohol):* 0.2–0.6 mL three times daily

Note: Given its potential for adverse effects, it is questionable whether lobelia is appropriate for self-medication.

Introduction

Family
- Campanulaceae

Synonyms
- Indian tobacco
- Wild tobacco
- Asthma weed
- Gagroot
- Emetic herb
- Vomit wort
- Puke weed

Medicinal Forms
- Dried leaves
- Liquid extract

Description

Lobelia is a hairy annual or biennial indigenous to the western parts of North America. It produces pale blue flowers and is often found in particularly acid soils. While *Lobelia inflata* L. is the plant most common to herbal practice in North America and Western Europe, other members of this genus have a medicinal reputation in many other traditional healing models. For example, in the Chinese pharmacopoeia, *L. chinensis* Lour. is specified.

Parts Used

The aerial parts are dried for use.

Traditional Use

Lobelia has a rather infamous medical history. It was used by First Nations peoples primarily for respiratory conditions and as an emetic. It later became popular among the early European settlers. Lobelia was also smoked in a similar fashion to tobacco, giving rise to one of the synonyms, Indian tobacco. The New England healer Samuel Thomson used it as one of the primary botanical medicines, naming it "Old No. 1." In fact, after one of his patients died from taking the herb, Thomson was charged with murder (and later acquitted). Many still consider lobelia to be a poison rather than a medicine.

Current Medicinal Use

As with its traditional use, lobelia is primarily used for respiratory conditions such as asthma and bronchitis. Lobeline (a constituent found in lobelia) products are often used in treating tobacco addictions because lobeline is chemically similar to nicotine.

Relevant Research

Preventative and Therapeutic Effects

Constituents

- Alkaloids: more than 14, notably of the piperidine type, including (-)-lobeline (main one at 0.36–2.25% dry weight), lobelanine, norlobelanine, lobelanidine, norlobelanidine, lelobanidine, lobinine, isolobinine.

- Miscellaneous: lobelacrin (a bitter glycoside), chelidonic acid, beta-amyrin palmitate, resins, gums.

Traditional Uses

Lobelia is considered to have expectorant, diaphoretic, emetic, antispasmodic, and sedative properties and to act as a respiratory stimulant. It is primarily used for conditions of the respiratory tract, notably bronchial asthma and bronchitis. Expectorant and decongestant registered drugs containing lobelia are available in Canada. External applications are used to relieve muscle spasm and tension. Indian tobacco is also used in the treatment of tobacco addition. Commercial cigarette-smoking deterrents containing lobelia herb are available in Canada and Europe, while the purified alkaloidal salts, lobeline hydrochloride or lobeline sulphate, are marketed for this purpose in several countries but not Canada. Its use as an emetic seems primarily to be an historical one.

> *Lobelia is primarily used for conditions of the respiratory tract, notably bronchial asthma and bronchitis.*

Miscellaneous Effects

The medicinal action of lobelia appears to be primarily due to lobeline's nicotinic properties. The exact action of lobeline at the nicotine receptor site appears complex and novel. Lobeline is known to cause stimulation of the central nervous system, followed by severe respiratory depression. Administration in a number of animal studies has resulted in bronchoconstriction, while bronchodilation was also reported in guinea pigs. A proposed explanation for these differing results is that guinea pigs are particularly sensitive to adrenergic bronchodilating agents Bronchodilation resulting from adrenal stimulation has also been suggested.

Animal studies suggest that lobeline acts as a cardiovascular stimulant, causing sympathetically mediated hypertension, as well as parasympathetically mediated bradycardia. Lobeline has also been shown to inhibit intestinal motility in dogs. Vomiting, commonly seen with lobeline use, is centrally mediated. An antidepressant action has been seen in mice following administration of beta-amyrin palmitate extracted from *Lobelia inflata* L.

> *A number of human clinical trials of lobeline, either alone or combined with other substances, have reported that it is effective in the treatment of tobacco addition.*

Lobeline has been reported to improve memory in rodents and the performance of rats in sustained memory attention tasks.

A number of human clinical trials of lobeline, either alone or combined with other substances, have reported that it is effective in the treatment of tobacco addition. A recent study reported that lobelane (another compound found in lobelia) could decrease methamphetamine self-administration in rats in a dose-dependent relationship.

No clinical trials could be found in which the action of the herb lobelia, rather than the alkaloid lobeline, was investigated.

Adverse Effects

Adverse effects are similar to those of nicotine and include nausea, vomiting, diarrhea, coughing, and dizziness. Administration of high doses may result in more severe symptoms, such as convulsions, hypothermia, coma, and even death. Many practitioners comment that the plant's emetic properties limit the potential for serious side effects. One authority does not recommend use of the crude herb due to the lack of standardized product and relatively high risk-to-benefit ratio.

A case of death following inhalation of an herbal asthma product containing lobeline (together with stramonium) in a 48-year-old asthmatic female has been documented. Stramonium (*Datura stramonium* L., Solanaceae) is a plant rich in alkaloids with a very high potential for toxicity.

Cautions/Contraindications

Lobelia should be used with caution in cases of cardiovascular disease, respiratory conditions, and where nicotine is contraindicated. It should also be considered contraindicated in pregnancy and lactation.

Drug Interactions

No clinical cases of drug interactions could be found. Given the pharmacological action of lobeline, this herb should be used cautiously with conventional medication in general.

Dosage Regimens
- Dried herb: 0.2–0.6 g three times daily.
- Liquid extract (1:1 in 50% alcohol): 0.2–0.6 mL three times daily.

Note: Given its potential for adverse effects, it is questionable whether lobelia is appropriate for self-medication.

Selected References

Felpin F-X, Lebreton S. History, chemistry and biology of alkaloids from *Lobelia inflata*. Tetrahedron 2004;60(45):10,127–153.

Neugebauer N, Harrod S, Stairs D, et al. Lobelane descreases methamphetamine self-administration in rats. European Journal of Pharmacology 2007;571(1):33–38.

Ma Huang

Ephedra sinica Stapf.

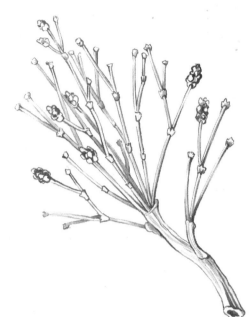

THUMBNAIL SKETCH

Common Uses
- Respiratory tract diseases (including asthma and bronchitis)
- Weight loss

Active Constituents
- Alkaloids (including ephedrine and pseudoephedrine)

Adverse Effects
- Dizziness and headache
- Insomnia
- Decreased appetite and gastrointestinal distress
- Tachycardia, sweating, hypertension
- Psychosis
- Stroke, seizures, and death

Cautions/Contraindications
- Heart disease, hypertension, thyroid disease, diabetes, prostate conditions, anxiety, glaucoma
- Impaired cerebral circulation, pheochromocytoma, thyrotoxicosis
- Pregnancy and breastfeeding

Drug Interactions
- Similar precautions should be applied as for conventional medicines containing ephedrine and pseudoephedrine, including antihypertensives and antidepressants

Doses
- *Dried herb:* Maximum 8 mg of ephedrine every 6 hours up to a maximum of 24 mg daily for no more than 7 days

Note: It is highly questionable whether ma huang products containing appreciable amounts of alkaloids are appropriate for self-medication. Consultation with an appropriately trained health-care professional is advised.

Introduction

Family
- Ephedraceae

Synonyms
- Ephedra
- Chinese ephedra
- Herba ephedrae
- Cao mahuang

Medicinal Forms
- Dried stems
- Tincture

Description

Many members of the genus *Ephedra* are reputed to have medicinal properties. This monograph will concentrate primarily on ma huang, which is the one most often encountered in North America. Other members of this genus with medicinal applications include *Ephedra intermedia* Shrenk ex C.A. Mey. (intermediate ephedra), *Ephedra equisetina* Bunge (Mongolian ephedra), *Ephedra geradiana* Wallich ex Stapf. (Pakistani ephedra), and *Ephedra nevadensis* S. Wats. (Mormon tea).

Ma huang is a fragrant perennial shrub growing to 50 centimeters (20 inches) with long stems and tiny leaves, native to many parts of Asia. It is one of the smallest members of the genus, with greenish herbaceous stems producing small, white, flower-like cones.

Parts Used

Usually the aerial parts of the plant, including the stems, are used medicinally.

Traditional Use

Ma huang has a long medicinal history in traditional Chinese medicine (TCM), where it is used for a number of conditions, most notably of the respiratory system, including asthma, colds, and coughs. This herb — or more correctly one of the alkaloids found in it, ephedrine — was probably the first traditional Chinese herbal product to receive acceptance in the West. Ephedrine was first synthesized in the 1920s and has been used widely in cold and allergy remedies. *Ephedra* species native to North America, such as *Ephedra nevadensis* S. Wats., do not contain any alkaloids.

Current Medicinal Use

While ephedrine has been shown to be effective in promoting weight loss, the potential for serious adverse effects makes it questionable whether ma huang has a legitimate use unless taken under the guidance of an appropriately trained health-care professional.

Relevant Research

Preventative and Therapeutic Effects

Constituents
- Alkaloids of the protoalkaloid class: include: (-)- ephedrine (L-ephedrine, major portion), (+)-pseudoephedrine, (+)-norpseudoephedrine, and (-)-norephedrine.

- Tannins: catechin, gallic acid, condensed tannins.

- Miscellaneous, including: ephedrans (glycans), ephedradine, volatile oil, flavonoid glycosides.

Roots
• Macrocyclic spermine alkaloids (e.g. ephedradine), L-tyrosine betaine (maokonine).

Note: The alkaloid content may vary from 0.5% to 2.5% (dry weight), 30% to 90% of which is ephedrine, depending on the species. *E. sinica* contains approximately 1.3% alkaloids, with ephedrine making up 60% of this amount.

Traditional Uses
Ma huang is considered an herb of particular importance in many Asian healing models. Ma huang is considered particularly useful in the treatment of respiratory conditions associated with fever, asthma, allergic rhinitis, and bronchitis. It is also considered to be a stimulant and hypertensive agent. Ma huang is often included in weight-loss formulas because of its stimulant action.

Medicinal Action
The alkaloids, especially ephedrine and pseudoephedrine, are the main constituents responsible for this plant's medicinal action. Ephedrine acts primarily in the periphery as an indirect adrenomimetic agent, causing an increased release of norepinephrine. While it has a longer duration of action than norepinephrine, its peripheral action is limited because its effects decrease over time. It is less potent than norepinephrine but is effective after oral administration.

Ephedrine and pseudoephedrine are known to cross the blood-brain barrier, resulting in a stimulant action. Administration of ephedrine results in direct bronchodilation. Pseudoephedrine appears to work in a similar manner but is generally considered less potent than ephedrine.

Localized anti-inflammatory properties have been demonstrated for both ephedrine and pseudoephedrine in a number of animal models.

Respiratory System Activity
Traditionally, ma huang has primarily been used for the treatment of asthma, bronchitis, and conditions of the upper respiratory tract. Ephedrine has bronchodilating properties, causing prolonged relaxation of the smooth muscles of the bronchioles upon oral administration. Constriction of the blood vessels in the mucosa of the respiratory system results in decreased mucus production, providing a decongestant action. The presence of the "drying" astringent tannins and aromatic volatile oils may also be playing a part in the treatment of bronchial asthma and bronchitis. While ephedrine was once used to treat asthma, the fact that its action is selective to beta-2 adrenoreceptors is a significant disadvantage. It has now been superseded by more selective agents, such as salbutamol and albuterol, that have fewer adverse effects.

> *Traditionally, ma huang has primarily been used for the treatment of asthma, bronchitis, and conditions of the upper respiratory tract.*

Cardiovascular Effects
One randomized, double-blind crossover trial involving 8 participants observed the effects of administering 150 mg caffeine and ma huang standardized to 20 mg ephedra alkaloids simultaneously in capsule form, compared to a placebo. The authors reported a significant increase in heart rate, blood pressure, and resting energy expenditure, which was highest between 90 and 180 minutes.

Administration of ephedrine results in vasoconstriction, as well as increased systolic and diastolic blood pressure, force of cardiac contraction, and cardiac output. Pseudoephedrine appears to have a weaker hypertensive action than ephedrine. A number of medical herbalists comment that the hypertensive action of plant extracts seems to be less pronounced than those seen with ephedrine alone.

Paradoxically, intravenous administration of mahuangen (the roots of ma huang) has been reported to cause vasodilation in a number of animal models. A variable effect on blood pressure may be observed, depending on the relative concentrations of hypotensive ephedradines (ganglionic blocking agents) versus hypertensive maokonine, due to phytochemical differences between the various ephedra species.

Effect on Obesity

A number of clinical studies have shown that supplementation with ephedrine, normally combined with other agents, such as caffeine, can result in weight loss in both animals and humans. However, the use of ephedrine-containing products, especially those containing caffeine, has been associated with serious adverse effects, including death, and thus it is not recommended for use in weight-loss protocols.

> *A number of clinical studies have shown that supplementation with ephedrine, normally combined with other agents, such as caffeine, can result in weight loss in both animals and humans.*

Ephedrine appears to act as a thermogenic agent, increasing the ability of the body to produce heat from food. It has been suggested that this action is influenced by adrenoreceptor stimulation and that ephedrine can influence all the receptor subtypes. The increased action of ephedrine-methylxanthine and ephedrine-aspirin combinations over ephedrine alone could be due to inhibition of feedback mechanisms. The thermogenic action appears to be more pronounced with chronic administration. Ephedrine also appears to reduce appetite. The ephedrine-caffeine combination seems to be protective against reducing high-density lipoprotein (HDL) cholesterol during weight loss.

While ma huang may be of use in the treatment of obesity, there is no reason to believe that it will offer any preferential benefits over ephedrine alone. Obesity is not generally considered a traditional indication for ma huang, and there is no significant empirical evidence to support its use. Claims for use of ephedra-containing products as stimulants or diet aids for weight loss are not allowed by Health Canada, for example, because of the safety concerns associated with this use (see Adverse Effects and Cautions/Contraindications for more detail).

> *Claims for use of ephedra-containing products as stimulants or diet aids for weight loss are not allowed by Health Canada because of the safety concerns associated with this use.*

Effect on Athletic Performance

A review article concluded that there is very little evidence to support the use of ephedrine or pseudoephedrine to improve sporting performance. While some athletes may take ephedrine to reduce body fat and promote muscle mass, there is no evidence to support this indication in individuals who are not overweight. Products containing ephedrine or pseudoephedrine are prohibited by a number of sporting authorities.

Most of the evidence purported to support the use of ma huang for the indications described above comes from work carried out using ephedrine or pseudoephedrine alone and not the herb ma huang.

Adverse Effects

Numerous concerns have been voiced regarding the increased popularity of "natural" commercial products containing ma huang, or ephedra. These products include sports supplements, diet aids, and products intended to induce euphoria and increase sensory acuity. While consumption does provide central nervous system stimulation, high amounts can lead to hallucinations, paranoia, psychosis, and even death. In many of these cases, the products ingested were labeled "ma huang," but the products were not actually tested to verify their contents. It is likely that at least some of the adverse events were associated products to which synthetic ephedrine was added. In addition, ma huang products that contain caffeine are much more likely to be associated with adverse effects.

A number of deaths have resulted from consumption of ma huang products in the United States. A review designed to evaluate possible cardiovascular effects associated with ma huang found 926 cases of possible ma huang toxicity that were reported to the US Food and Drug Administration (FDA) from 1995 to 1997. The authors concluded that: "(1) Ma huang use is temporally related to stroke, myocardial infarction, and sudden death; (2) underlying heart or vascular disease is not a prerequisite for ma huang–related adverse events; and (3) the cardiovascular toxic effects associated with ma huang were not limited to massive doses. Although the pathogensis of the cardiotoxic effects of ma huang remains incompletely defined, available observational and circumstantial evidence indicates that use of the substance may be associated with serious medical complications." In one case, a healthy 23-year-old male died of "patchy myocardial necrosis" after taking a commercial product containing ma huang and caffeine for approximately 6 weeks. The individual appears to have followed the instructions appearing on the product label.

Products intended for weight loss containing ma huang have been implicated in cases of both mania and psychosis. Other adverse effects seen following consumption of ephedrine products include dizziness, headache, decreased appetite, gastrointestinal distress, irregular heart beat, tachycardia (increased heart rate), sweating, insomnia, hypertension (increased blood pressure), stroke, and seizures.

> *A number of deaths have resulted from consumption of ma huang products in the United States.*

Several cases of liver toxicity have also been reported to be associated with use of ma huang supplements. Acute hepatitis potentially resulting from administration of ma huang has been reported. In one case, symptoms of hepatotoxicity were identified after ingestion of an unspecified amount of ma huang supplement; however, the authors of the case report suggest that the symptoms were possibly caused by an adulterant in the product rather than the ma huang itself. A second case of acute hepatitis in a 36-year-old woman who was taking 36 mg ma huang daily as a dietary supplement has been reported. In both of these cases, health was restored to normal after discontinuation of the supplement.

Two additional cases of hepatotoxicity resulting in liver transplant possibly caused by ma huang have also been reported. One involved a 57-year-old woman who had been taking two Chinese herbal products, called Qialbai Biya Pain and *Cordyceps sinensis*, the former of which contains ma huang (dosage not reported), as well as other herbs. These products were taken for a total of 7 days, and symptoms of nausea, anorexia, abdominal pain, and jaundice were still present at 14 days. The second report summarizes 10 case studies in which patients were using a variety of weight-loss products containing ma huang, two of which resulted in liver transplants and one of which resulted in death.

> *Several cases of liver toxicity have also been reported to be associated with use of ma huang supplements.*

Concerns have also been expressed that prolonged administration of products containing ma huang may result in a "weakening" of the adrenal gland. Subsequently, some practitioners may combine it with "adrenal tonics," such as licorice.

Health Canada has warned consumers not to use products containing ma huang unless the product label carries a drug identification number (DIN) or natural product number (NPN) and the consumer strictly follows the dosage directions and precautions. Products that combine ma haung and caffeine are not allowed for sale in Canada due to concerns about their safety.

Drug Interactions

Concomitant administration with stimulants, including caffeine, and any centrally acting medication, such as antidepressants and antihypertensives, should be avoided. It would seem prudent to apply the restrictions associated with ephedrine to ma huang. The action of ephedrine is known to be affected by antacids and agents that alter the pH (acidity) of the urine. Ephedrine is also known to interact with corticosteroids and theophylline.

The German Commission E monograph on this herb further warns of possible interactions with cardiac glycosides or halothane, resulting in disturbance of heart rhythm; guanetjidine, resulting in enhancement of the sympathomimetic effect; monoamine oxidase inhibitors, resulting in greatly increased sympathomimetic action of the ephedrine; and secale alkaloid derivatives or oxytocin, resulting in development of hypertension.

Cautions/Contraindications

Products containing ephedrine should not be taken by people suffering from heart disease, hypertension (high blood pressure), thyroid disease, diabetes, conditions associated with enlarged prostate, anxiety, glaucoma, impaired circulation of the cerebrum, pheochromocytoma, or thyrotoxicosis. Because ephedrine has uterostimulant properties, ma huang should be avoided in pregnancy and lactation.

Dosage Regimens

* Dried herb: FDA guidelines suggest a maximum dose of 8 mg of ephedrine every 6 hours up to 24 mg per day for no more than 7 days.

Note: Given the above concerns, it is highly questionable whether ma huang products containing appreciable amounts of alkaloids are appropriate for self-medication. Consultation with an appropriately trained health-care professional is advisable.

Selected References

Boozer CN, Daly PA, Homel P, Solomon JL, Blanchard D, Nasser JA, et al. Herbal ephedra/caffeine for weight loss: A 6-month randomized safety and efficacy trial. International Journal of Obesity & Related Metabolic Disorders 2002;26(5):593–604.

Breum L, Pedersen JK, Ahlstrom F, Frimodt-Moller J. Comparison of an ephedrine/caffeine combination and dexfenfluramine in the treatment of obesity. A double-blind multi-centre trial in general practice. International Journal of Obesity & Related Metabolic Disorders 1994;18(2):99–103.

Neff GW, Reddy KR, Durazo FA, Meyer D, Marrero R, Kaplowitz N. Severe hepatotoxicity associated with the use of weight loss diet supplements containing ma huang or usnic acid. (Letter to the Editor). Journal of Hepatology 2004;41:1061–67.

Samenuk D, Link MS, Homoud MK, Contreras R, Theohardes TC, Wang PJ, et al. Adverse cardiovascular events temporally associated with ma huang, an herbal source of ephedrine. Mayo Clinical Proceedings 2002;77(1):12–16.

Meadowsweet

Filipendula ulmaria (L.) Maxim

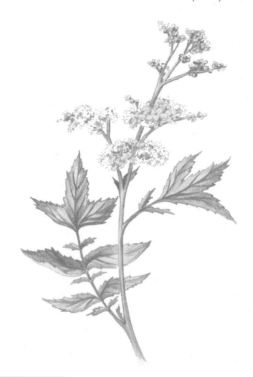

THUMBNAIL SKETCH

Common Uses
- Digestive upset (including ulceration, dyspepsia, and hyperacidity)
- Rheumatic conditions and pain

Active Constituents
- Salicylate-rich volatile oil
- Flavonoids
- Tannins

Adverse Effects
- None noted

Cautions/Contraindications
- Salicylates (classic ones applicable to salicylates, e.g., aspirin, in general)

Drug Interactions
- Salicylates (classic ones applicable to salicylates, e.g., aspirin, in general)

Doses
- *Dried herb:* 4–6 g three times daily
- *Fluid extract (1:1 in 25% alcohol):* 1.5–6 mL three times daily
- *Tincture (1:5 in 45% alcohol):* 2–4 mL three times daily

Introduction

Family
- Rosaceae

Synonyms
- Filipendula
- Queen of the meadows
- *Spiraea ulmaria* L.
- Bridewort

Medicinal Forms
- Dried herb
- Fluid extract
- Tincture

Description
Meadowsweet is a perennial native to Europe, growing 1.5 meters (5 feet) tall with a thick, pink aromatic root and elongated stems leading to creamy white flowers that have a distinctive sweet almond scent. The English herbalist Gerard described the aroma produced by this plant as follows: "For the smell thereof makes the heart merry, delighteth the senses; neither doth it cause headache, or loathsomeness to meat, as some other sweet smelling herbs do." The term "spiraea," used in a former binomial name, comes from the fact that the fruits have a twisted appearance. Established growths of meadowsweet often completely dominate the marshy areas in which they grow, making another common name, "queen of the meadow," very appropriate.

Parts Used
The aerial parts of the plant (fresh flowering tops and leaves) are used medicinally.

Traditional Use
Salicylic acid was first extracted from the flowering buds of this medicinal herb. The term "aspirin" (acetylsalicylic acid) means "from spiraea." Meadowsweet was traditionally used to reduce inflammation and relieve pain, especially arthritis pain. It was also used as a remedy for indigestion and diarrhea, even in children.

Current Medicinal Use
As with its traditional uses, meadowsweet products are primarily used as an analgesic in treating arthritic pain and for digestive upset and hyperacidity.

Relevant Research

Preventative and Therapeutic Effects
Constituents
- Volatile oils: salicylates (including salicylaldehyde, gaultherin, salicin, and salicylic acid), vanillin, benzaldehyde.
- Flavonoids: rutin, hyperoside, spireoside, kaempferol.
- Miscellaneous: hydrolyzable tannins, coumarins, mucilage, ascorbic acid.

Common Uses
Meadowsweet is considered by many herbalists to be an important medicinal herb for the management of conditions of the digestive system. It is reputed to have a soothing and healing action and is frequently used to treat such conditions as hyperacidity, indigestion, peptic ulcer disease, nausea, and pediatric diarrhea.

The other primary use of meadowsweet is as an analgesic and anti-inflammatory. It has been suggested that it is useful in the management of pain and rheumatic conditions. It may also act as an antipyretic. While these properties are generally considered to be due to the presence of salicylates in the volatile oil portion, these applications easily predate the identification of these components.

> Meadowsweet is reputed to have a soothing and healing action and is frequently used to treat such conditions as hyperacidity, indigestion, peptic ulcer disease, nausea, and pediatric diarrhea.

Miscellaneous Effects

Various extracts of meadowsweet have been reported to lower vascular permeability, increase bronchial tone in cats, increase the bronchospasm induced by histamine in guinea pigs, increase tonus in test tube studies of guinea pig intestine and rabbit uterus, decrease rectal temperature, and potentiate narcotic action. In addition, an anti-ulcer action has been noted in various animal models, especially with aqueous extracts of the flowers. In contrast, the ulcerogenic nature of histamine was potentiated by an extract of meadowsweet in the guinea pig.

Extracts of meadowsweet have also been shown to possess bactericidal and bacterostatic properties. The flowers and seeds have been shown to exert an anticoagulant and fibrinolytic effect in both test tube and animal studies. Topical administration of a decoction made from meadowsweet flowers has been shown to decrease the frequency of experimentally induced squamous cell carcinoma of the cervix and vagina in mice. Application of an ointment was shown to increase regression of cervical dysplasia in 32 patients.

Adverse Effects

No instances of adverse reactions could be found for this herb.

Cautions/Contraindications

Given the lack of objective information, the presence of salicylates, and the fact that meadowsweet effects uterine smooth muscle in vitro, it has been suggested that meadowsweet should be avoided during pregnancy and lactation. While no clinical examples could be found, it has been argued that the classic precautions applicable to salicylates in general are applicable to products containing meadowsweet. Consequently, it should be used with caution in individuals sensitive to aspirin and people with asthma, gout, diabetes, hemophilia, active peptic ulcer disease, hypoprothrombinemia, or kidney or liver disease. Although salicylates are generally considered contraindicated in patients with active peptic ulcer disease, it is important to balance this caution with the empirical uses mentioned previously.

Drug Interactions

While no clinical examples could be found, there is every reason to believe that classic drug interactions with salicylates in general (e.g., concomitant oral anticoagulants) are relevant here.

Dosage Regimens

- Dried herb: 4–6 g three times daily.
- Fluid extract (1:1 in 25% alcohol): 1.5–6 mL three times daily.
- Tincture (1:5 in 45% alcohol): 2–4 mL three times daily.

Note: Meadowsweet is often combined with other "digestive" herbs, such as chamomile, licorice, marshmallow, and peppermint. Many herbal painkillers also contain meadowsweet, often combined with black or white willow bark.

Selected References

"*Filipendualae Ulmariae* Herba Medowsweet" in European Scientific Cooperative (ESCOP). ESCOP Monographs. The Scientific Foundation for Herbal Medicinal Products, 2nd edition. New York: Thieme, 2003:157–61.

Hikino H, Kiso Y. Natural products for liver diseases. Economic and Medicinal Plant Research 1988; 2:39–72.

Milk Thistle

Silybum marianum (L.) Gaertner

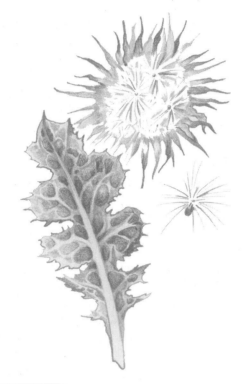

Introduction

Family
- Asteraceae (also known as Compositae)

Synonyms
- Bull thistle
- *Cardui mariae fructus*
- *Cardui mariae herba*
- *Cardum marianum* L.
- *Carduus marianus* L.
- *Cnicus marianus*
- Emetic root
- Fructus Silybi mariae
- Fruit de chardon Marie
- Heal thistle
- Holy thistle
- Isosilibinin
- Lady's thistle
- Legalon
- Marian thistle
- Mariana mariana
- Mariendistel
- Marienkrörner
- Mary thistle
- Mediterranean milk thistle
- Mild thistle
- Milk ipecac
- Our Lady's thistle
- Pig leaves
- Royal thistle
- Silidianin
- *Silybi* mariae fructus
- Snake milk
- Sow thistle
- St. Mary's thistle
- Variegated thistle
- Wild artichoke

Medicinal Forms
- Standardized extract
- Dried herb
- Teas
- Tincture

Description
Although milk thistle originally grew wild throughout much of Europe, it is now naturalized to the east coast of North America, California, and South America. This biennial grows up to 1 meter (40 inches) in height, with spiny leaves that are marked with white along the veins. The plant is crowned with a bright pink to red flower head that produces numerous small seeds. Milk thistle is sometimes confused with blessed thistle (*Cnicus benedictus* L., Asteraceae). Although they are members of the same botanical family, their medicinal actions are quite different.

Parts Used
The flower heads, fruit, and seeds are used medicinally.

Traditional Use
The specific name "marianum" refers to the legend that the leaves have a white mottling because a drop of the Virgin Mary's milk landed on them. In keeping with this legend, milk thistle has traditionally been used as a galactogogue (i.e., to stimulate milk production in lactating women). Fresh milk thistle flower heads were boiled and eaten like artichokes as a spring tonic. The herb has also been used in treating jaundice and other liver-related conditions. Milk thistle has been used medicinally for several thousand years. Both the Greeks and the Romans noted its hepatoprotective effects; however, current interest in this product did not begin until the late 1960s, when silymarin, a combination of flavonolignans believed to be responsible for the hepatic activity, was first isolated from the ripe seeds.

Current Medicinal Use
Milk thistle is primarily used for its hepatoprotective properties, but recent reviews of the clinical trials for this indication have been generally negative. Most reviews comment on the poor quality of the studies conducted to date.

Relevant Research

Preventative and Therapeutic Uses

Constituents

Fruit

- Flavolignans: 1.5% to 3% silymarin (a mixture containing silybin, silichristin, silidianin, and traces of other constituents). Silybin (aka silibinin) makes up 50% of the silymarin and is thought to be the most biologically active constituent of the herb.

- Flavinoids: quercetin, taxifolin, dehydrokaempferol.

- Lipids: linoleic acid, oleic acid, palmitic acid.

- Sterols: cholesterol, campesterol, stigmasterol.

- Other: sugars, mucilages, amines, saponins.

Leaves

- Flavinoids: apigenin; luteolin and kaempferol and their glycosides.

- Other: beta-sitosterol and its glucoside; triterpene acetate.

Liver Protective Activity

Currently, milk thistle is known primarily for its purported ability to protect the liver from damage and to restore its function following damage. However, five reviews of milk thistle's use in liver disease concluded that silymarin, the key active compound in milk thistle, does not reduce mortality, improve liver histology, or improve biochemical parameters of liver function in patients with liver disease (all types included). The most recent, a 2008 Cochrane Collaboration review of 13 randomized clinical trials including 915 patients, concluded that the overall methodological quality of the trials was poor and that milk thistle had no significant effect on mortality, complications of liver disease, or liver histology. A 2005 systemic review and meta-analysis of nine studies reported that milk thistle did not significantly help patients with alcohol-related liver diseases.

Although the complete mechanism of action is unknown, many studies have investigated the antioxidant and free radical–antagonizing actions of milk thistle. This is thought to be the key mechanism of action when used to treat liver disease. In vitro and in vivo studies show that silymarin influences the expression and activity of the superoxide dismutase (SOD) enzyme in erythrocytes and lymphocytes of alcoholic cirrhosis patients. Other suggested actions include increased protein synthesis, stabilized immunologic response, and alteration and increased stability of cellular membranes.

Because there are so many different types of liver disease, the evidence for liver cirrhosis, hepatitis (alcohol-induced, viral, B, and C), and liver damage from exposure to toxins individually is discussed here.

> *Currently, milk thistle is known primarily for its purported ability to protect the liver from damage and to restore its function following damage.*

Cirrhosis

A 2001 meta-analysis that investigated the effect of milk thistle on patients with liver cirrhosis from all causes by pooling data from five studies chosen to reflect the variety of patient settings and increase the external validity of the analysis concluded that use of silymarin (a compound found in milk thistle) significantly reduced liver-related mortality by 7% ($p < 0.01$) in patients with liver cirrhosis but produced a non-significant reduction of total mortality.

There are two (one weakly positive and one negative) double-blind, randomized controlled trials (RCTs) that investigate the effects of milk thistle on patients suffering from liver cirrhosis caused by alcohol use.

Overall, the evidence for alcoholic liver cirrhosis is weaker than for liver cirrhosis in general. It must be noted that the study populations were small, but clinical benefits in treating the disease did not occur in most studies. Further research is needed for this subset of liver cirrhosis.

Hepatitis

A 2007 systematic review of six clinical trials investigating the efficacy of silymarin in patients with viral hepatitis concluded that treatment with silymarin does not affect viral load or improve liver histology, but it likely decreases serum transaminases in patients with chronic viral hepatitis. However, it is unknown whether transaminase levels have any clinical significance. A 2005 systematic review reported similar findings.

In a small study of children with hepatitis A, no conclusions could be drawn about the efficacy of silymarin since all patients showed improvement. In another poor-quality double-blind, randomized controlled trial, patients with acute hepatitis A and B were either given silymarin 120 mg (N=28) or a placebo (N=29) three times daily for 3 weeks. The number of patients with hepatitis A is unknown, and no subgroup analysis was performed. Bilirubin and AST levels were normalized in significantly more patients in the silymarin group, but no significant differences were seen in ALT and AP levels between the silymarin group and the control group.

> *Silymarin is possibly ineffective in treating hepatitis C patients, although more high-quality randomized controlled trials assessing patients with hepatitis C are needed to confirm this finding.*

There have been two additional human clinical studies looking at silymarin use in patients with hepatitis B and several studies that included patients with hepatitis B among many other conditions. The current evidence is generally negative, but more trials with only hepatitis B patients are needed to draw conclusions about the efficacy of silymarin in treating this indication.

There have been five clinical studies looking at silymarin use in patients with hepatitis C. In one positive randomized controlled trial, there was an improvement in an aminotranferase level. However, in four negative clinical trials, there were no significant differences in aminotransferase levels, quality of life, or psychological well-being, and thus it was concluded that silymarin was not as effective as traditional therapy for hepatitis C. Several additional studies included patients with hepatitis C among many other conditions. Since no subgroup analysis was done with only the hepatitis C patients in these studies, no conclusions could be made regarding the efficacy of silymarin for this indication. Silymarin is possibly ineffective in treating hepatitis C patients, although more high-quality randomized controlled trials assessing patients with hepatitis C are needed to confirm this finding.

Protection of Liver from Chemical Toxins

Milk thistle has been used to treat liver damage from environmental, medication, and mushroom toxins. Although many studies have shown evidence of promising results, the poor study descriptions make it difficult to draw conclusions. Additional randomized controlled trials with larger numbers of participants are needed to confirm these preliminary findings.

Miscellaneous Effects

Cancer Prevention

A number of animal and in vitro studies suggest that silymarin from milk thistle may have anticancer effects, especially against skin and prostate cancer. In addition, there has been one case study documenting silymarin use in a male with liver cancer. Due to the lack of human trials, further research is required to assess the efficacy for this indication.

Hyperlipidemia (High Cholesterol)

There have been two positive human studies that have assessed the efficacy of milk thistle in treating patients with hyperlipidemia. A-lipoprotein levels were significantly decreased compared to baseline in one study, while silybin, a component of milk thistle, reduced biliary cholesterol concentration in humans and rats in the other. Due to the lack of randomized controlled trials, small sample sizes, and inconsistent clinical parameters and outcome measures reported in the trials, further research is required to assess the efficacy for this indication.

Diabetes

One randomized, double-blind, placebo-controlled trial investigated the effect of adding milk thistle seed extract containing 200 mg silymarin or a placebo to conventional medication treatment in 51 patients diagnosed with type 2 diabetes. The study concluded that milk thistle improved the glycemic profile, compared to the placebo. Additional studies are needed to confirm these preliminary findings.

Milk thistle may cause hypoglycemia in patients with type 1 diabetes with alcoholic cirrhosis. There was a significant decrease ($p < 0.01$) in fasting glucose levels, mean daily blood glucose levels, daily glucosuria, and HbA1c levels in insulin-treated diabetics with alcoholic cirrhosis after only 4 months of therapy. Patients used silymarin 600 mg daily for 12 months in total.

Adverse Effects

Milk thistle is relatively well tolerated. There are a number of case studies reporting hypersensitivity and anaphylactic reactions in patients who have ingested milk thistle. Other adverse effects that have been reported in small numbers of patients in clinical trials include arthralgia (joint pain); fatigue; gastrointestinal complaints; headache; hypoglycemia in patients with pre-existing diabetes; impotence; pruritis (itching); and urticaria (hives).

Cautions/Contraindications

Since milk thistle belongs to the plant family Asteraceae/Compositae, it is best to avoid the use of milk thistle if a known allergy already exists to species of this family. Milk thistle may cause hypoglycemia in diabetes patients. Pregnant or nursing mothers should use milk thistle with caution due to lack of evidence that it is safe.

Drug Interactions

Patients should be cautioned against taking medications metabolized through the hepatic (liver) cytochrome P450 enzymes in addition to milk thistle. Silybin, the active ingredient of silymarin, may inhibit CYP 3A4 and CYP 2C9, and influence the metabolism of other medications. However, it should be noted that several human studies, including a randomized controlled trial, have shown that silymarin does not significantly reduce the levels of indinavir or irinotecan, both of which are CYP3A4 substrates.

Other theoretical interactions that have not yet been reported in humans, but appear possible based on animal and in vitro studies include:

- **Hypoglycemic agents:** Dose adjustments may be necessary for insulin and other hypoglycemic agents if taken with milk thistle.

- **Penicillin:** A retrospective analysis of 205 cases of clinical poisoning from the mushroom *Amanita phalloides* from 1971 to 1980 found that the combination of penicillin with silymarin was associated with increased survival compared to penicillin alone.

- **Psychotropic drugs (e.g., butyrophenones, phenothiazines, phenytoin):** Patients taking butyrophenones or phenothiazines in combination with silymarin at submaximal doses found a decrease in psychotropic drug-induced lipoperoxidative hepatic damage.

Significance in comparison to controls was not given. A human case report also found that silymarin reduced the hepatotoxic effects of phenytoin.

- **Chemotherapy agents (e.g., doxorubicin, carboplatin, cisplatin, methotrexate):** Silybin synergizes with doxorubicin, carboplatin, and cisplatin for increased growth inhibition of prostate carcinoma DU145 cells. Silymarin also prevented glutathione depletion in human hepatocyte cultures with methotrexate-induced damage (in vitro). The clinical significance of these preclinical findings is not clear.

- **Cyclosporine A:** Intraperitoneal administration of silybin in rats showed it may protect the exocrine pancreas from cyclosporine A toxicity by preventing the pancreatic secretions from decreasing.

- **Estrogens:** Inhibition of beta-glucuronidase by silymarin may increase the clearance of estrogen.

- **Halothane:** When silybin was given to mice (dosage form unknown), triglyceride and malic enzyme increases induced by halothane were prevented.

Dosage Regimens

- **Dried herb:** 12–15 g daily, unless otherwise directed or prescribed.
- **Standardized extract (70% silymarin):** 200 mg three times daily. Extracts standardized for at least 70% silymarin are usually equivalent to 200–400 mg silymarin, calculated as silybin.
- **Teas:** silymarin is not very water soluble; thus, this herb should not be taken as a "tea."

Selected References

Bantle JP, Wylie-Rosett J, Albright AL, Apovian CM, Clark NG, Franz MJ, Hoogwerf BJ, Lichtenstei A, Mayer-Davis E, Mooradian AD, Wheeler ML. Nutrition recommendations and interventions for diabetes. A position statement of the American Diabetes Association. Diabetes Care 2007;30 (Supp 1):S48–S65.

Rambaldi A, Bradley P, Iaquino G, Gluud C. Milk thistle for alcoholic and/or hepatitis B or C liver diseases — a systemic Cochrane Hepato-biliary Group review with meta-analyses of randomized clinical trials. American Journal of Gastroenterology 2005;100:2583–91.

Rambaldi A, Jacobs B, Iaquino G, Gluud C. Milk thistle for alcoholic and/or hepatitis B or C liver diseases (review). Cochrane Database of Systematic Reviews 2007;4.

Saller R, Meier R, Brignoli R. The use of silymarin in the treatment of liver diseases. Drugs 2001;61(14):2035–63.

Nettle

Urtica dioica L., U. urens L.

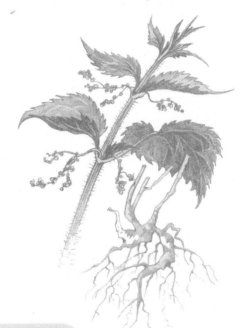

THUMBNAIL SKETCH

Common Uses
Leaf
- Rheumatism and gout
- Hay fever
- Nutritive supplement

Root
- Micturition disorders (associated with benign prostatic hyperplasia)

Active Constituents
Leaf
- Flavonoids
- Amines
- Carboxylic acids (in stinging hairs)

Root
- Sterols
- Lectins

Adverse Effects
- Skin irritation
- Gastric distress

Cautions/Contraindications
- Pregnancy (safety not established)

Drug Interactions
- Root should be used with caution in cases of concomitant administration with conventional antihypertensive, diabetes, and diuretic medication

Doses
Aerial Parts
- *Dried herb (normally as an infusion):* 3–6 g three times daily
- *Liquid extract (1:1 in 25% alcohol):* 3–4 mL three times daily
- *Tincture (1:5 in 45% alcohol):* 2–6 mL three times daily

Root
- *Dried root:* 4–6 g daily
- *Liquid extract (1:1 in 45% ethanol):* 1.5–7.5 mL daily
- *Tincture (1:5 in 40% ethanol):* 5 mL daily

Introduction

Family
- Urticaceae

Synonyms
- Stinging nettle
- Urtica
- Common nettle (*Urtica dioica* L.)
- Small nettle (*Urtica urens* L.)

Medicinal Forms
Leaves
- Dried leaves
- Liquid extract
- Tincture

Root
- Dried root
- Liquid extract
- Tincture

Description
Nettle is a perennial standing up to 1.5 meters (60 inches) in height, with lanced leaves and green and yellow flowers. Different members of the genus *Urtica* grow naturally throughout most of Europe and North America.

Parts Used
The aerial parts and the roots (rhizomes) of two species, *U. dioica* L. and *U. urens* L., are used medicinally.

Traditional Use
Nettle has been used in cleansing tonics, teas, and soups for detoxification, skin conditions, and allergies. While it has enjoyed a long medicinal history in many different models of traditional herbalism, nettle is considered by many members of the public to be a noxious weed, causing a characteristic pruritic rash on contact with the skin. Stinging nettle is also a common homeopathic remedy.

Current Medicinal Use
The use of the nettle depends on the part of the plant used. Products made from the leaf are primarily used to treat arthritic conditions, such as gout, and hay fever. A growing amount of scientific research suggests that nettle root, either alone or with other herbal medicines, may be useful in treating benign prostatic hypertrophy (enlargement of the prostate gland).

Relevant Research

Preventative and Therapeutic Effects

Constituents
Leaf
- Amines: histamine, choline, acetylcholine, serotonin, etc. (especially in stinging hairs).
- Flavonoids: include isoquercetin, rutin, kaempferol, quercetin.
- Minerals: include calcium, potassium, iron, silicon.
- Acids: include silicic acid, malic acid, carbonic acid, formic acid.
- Miscellaneous: sitosterol, glycoprotein, chlorophyll (high levels), tannins.

Root
- Lectins: Urtica dioica agglutinin, separated into 6 isolectins.
- Sterols (and their glucosides): include 3-beta-sitosterol, sitosterol-3-D-glucoside.
- Miscellaneous: include lignans, various fatty acids, scopoletin.

Common Uses
In the traditional herbal medicine paradigm, nettle leaves are considered very nutritive, and consequently they are often used in situations of convalescence and recuperation. They are also used to aid milk production in nursing mothers. In addition, nettle is used

for its astringent properties in the treatment of bleeding conditions, such as wounds, hemorrhoids, and uterine hemorrhage.

Benign Prostatic Hyperplasia

Stinging nettle root has become one of the major herbs used in the management of benign prostatic hyperplasia, especially in Europe. It can be taken alone but is more commonly administered with other phytomedicines used in the management of benign prostatic hyperplasia, such as *Serenoa repens* (saw palmetto) and *Prunus africana* (African pygeum). The European Scientific Cooperative on Phytotherapy lists the symptomatic treatment of micturition disorders (increased frequency of urination at night or during the day, painful urination, and urine retention) in benign prostatic hyperplasia as one of the indications for stinging nettle root.

A number of clinical trials have demonstrated the therapeutic benefit of nettle root in the management of benign prostatic hyperplasia. A review conducted in 2007 identified 34 clinical studies in which a total of 40,000 men have been treated for benign prostatic hyperplasia with a variety of nettle root preparations. Duration of treatment ranged from a few weeks to 4 years. The authors noted that most of these trials were uncontrolled with an open-label design. Only six studies were randomized controlled studies. Based on the available evidence, they concluded that nettle treatments may have some short-term effectiveness, although trials with more rigorous structure need to be conducted to produce conclusive results.

A randomized, double-blind clinical trial not included in the review described above compared the effects of a combination product containing extracts of saw palmetto and nettle root (PRO 160/120) or finasteride. The results of the study indicated that PRO 160/120 was equally as effective as finasteride, regardless of prostate volume, and that patients tolerated PRO 160/120 better. Since saw palmetto has been found to be as effective as finasteride in other studies, it is difficult to determine how much the nettle contributed to the effects noted in this trial.

Preparations made primarily from the roots of *Urtica dioica* L. have been shown in vitro and in vivo to affect many aspects of prostate physiology thought to be implicated in benign prostatic hyperplasia. These include inhibition of sex hormone–binding globulin to human prostatic tissue, possible suppression of prostate cell metabolism and growth, and weak inhibition of aromatase activity.

> *Stinging nettle root has become one of the major herbs used in the management of benign prostatic hyperplasia, especially in Europe.*

Musculoskeletal Conditions

Oral preparations made from nettle leaf have long been used in the management of various arthritic conditions, including rheumatism and gout. It has been suggested that the nettle leaf could have a diuretic effect, resulting in an increased elimination of "toxins," such as uric acid. The localized irritation resulting from topical application of the stinging leaves of this plant is also reputed to be beneficial.

The three clinical trials that have investigated the use of nettle for musculoskeletal complaints are described below. An open-label, randomized pilot study of 40 patients suffering from acute arthritis compared the effectiveness of stewed stinging nettle leaves (50 g daily) plus diclofenac (50 mg daily) to a larger daily dose of diclofenac (200 mg). Both treatments were administered for 14 days. The drug-herb combination was found to be as effective as the higher dose of drug in decreasing elevated acute phase protein concentrations and relieving the clinical arthritic symptoms. The authors concluded that the action of diclofenac was potentiated by nettle leaves. Although this may seem promising, it was only a pilot study, and some criticism has been made regarding the design of the research.

A randomized, placebo-controlled, double-blind crossover trial in 27 patients with osteoarthritic pain at the base of the thumb or index finger investigated the effects of daily topical application of stinging nettle leaf. The placebo used in this trial was white deadnettle leaf. After 1 week of treatment, score reductions on both the pain visual analog scale and a disability health assessment questionnaire were significantly greater in the nettle group than in the placebo group.

> Oral preparations made from nettle leaf have long been used in the management of various arthritic conditions, including rheumatism and gout.

Finally, a pilot study investigating the use of nettle in patients with chronic knee pain has also been conducted. This patient-blinded trial randomized 42 participants to experience treatment with either *Urtica dioica* (the stinging nettle treatment group) or *Urtica galeopsifolia* (the control group). *Urtica galeopsifolia* appears identical to the treatment plant, but being a different species is not thought to have the same medicinal effects. Participants were given a plant, taught how to care for it, and instructed to press the leaves on the affected area once daily for 1 week. The authors reported a decrease in pain in both groups and noted that upon examination after the study, the control species appeared to have stinging hairs on it and was therefore not an appropriate inactive control.

In vitro trials have demonstrated that a hydroalcoholic preparation of the leaves of stinging nettle possesses anti-inflammatory properties. The mechanism of action proposed is that it influences the synthesis of leukotrienes and cyclo-oxygenase-derived prostaglandins. It was also reported to decrease the production of a number of related inflammatory cytokines in whole human blood.

Effect on Hay Fever

In a double-blind randomized study, the anti-allergic action of a freeze-dried preparation of nettle was compared to a placebo. The study was carried out during the peak season for allergic rhinitis (hay fever). A total of 98 volunteers were assigned to the treatment (300 mg capsules of freeze-dried *Urtica dioica*) or the placebo group and were advised to take 2 capsules at the onset of the symptoms of allergic rhinitis. Assessment was made by comparing diary symptoms and global response at a follow-up appointment after 1 week of therapy. Stinging nettle was rated higher than the placebo according to the global assessment and slightly higher according to patient diary ratings.

Miscellaneous Effects

In vitro trials have demonstrated that nettle leaves increase rate of urination, lower blood pressure, increase blood sugar, and can act as a central nervous system depressant and produce analgesic effects. The implication of these findings to clinical practice has not yet been elucidated. In an open study, administration of 15 mL of nettle herb juice was shown to significantly increase the volume of urine excreted by 32 patients suffering from myocardial or chronic venous insufficiency. Another trial using blood samples of participants with type 2 diabetes has suggested that nettle extract may decrease platelet aggregation (blood clotting) in these individuals.

Adverse Effects

Adverse effects following oral consumption of products containing nettle seem rare. Instances of scanty urination, skin irritation, and gastric distress have been noted. One case report has described unilateral breast enlargement in a man after 1 month of consuming 500 mL of nettle tea daily and induction of lactation in a woman after drinking large amounts of nettle tea for 1 month. Symptoms were relieved 1 month after these patients had stopped consuming nettle in both cases. A case of herbal misuse has been reported in which severe tongue swelling and pain resulted after a woman tried to suck sap from a fresh nettle leaf.

Cautions/Contraindications

No safety details exist regarding the use of this herb in pregnancy or during breast-feeding. Significant contraction of pregnant mouse uterine muscle has been reported in vitro.

Drug Interactions

No specific cases of drug interactions could be found. Given the information contained in in vitro and in vivo studies, caution is advisable when administering this herb at the same time as conventional antihypertensive (blood pressure), diabetes, and diuretic medications.

Dosage Regimens
Aerial Parts
- Dried herb (normally as an infusion): 3–6 g three times daily.
- Liquid extract (1:1 in 25% alcohol): 3–4 mL three times daily.
- Tincture (1:5 in 45% alcohol): 2–6 mL three times daily.

Root
- Dried root: 4–6 g daily.
- Liquid extract (1:1 in 45% ethanol): 1.5–7.5 mL daily.
- Tincture (1:5 in 40% ethanol): 5 mL daily.

Selected References

Chrubasik JE, Roufogalis BD, Wagner H, Chrubasik S. A comprehensive review on the stinging nettle effect and efficacy profiles. Part II: Urticae radix. Phytomedicine 2007;14:568–79.

Randall C, Dickens A, White A, Sanders H, Fox M, Campbell J. Nettle sting for chronic knee pain: A randomised controlled pilot study. Complementary Therapies in Medicine 2008;16:66–72.

Oregano

Origanum vulgare

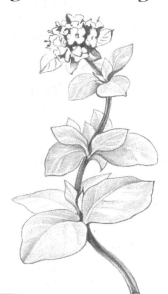

Introduction

Family
- Lamiaceae

Synonyms
- Dostenkraut
- European oregano
- Mediterranean oregano
- Mountain mint
- Oil of oregano
- Oregano oil
- *Origani vulgaris herba*
- Origano
- Wild marjoram
- Winter marjoram
- Wintersweet
- Za'atar

Description
This perennial herb, native to the Mediterranean but now grown in a number of climes, is a low-growing, fast-spreading groundcover that bears attractive white to purplish flowers and showy bracts in summer. Leaves can vary from green to gray-green and hairy to smooth. The leaves and flowers are commonly used as a preservative and for cooking, and it is sometimes called the pizza herb.

Parts Used
Leaves, stems, and flowers are the parts used medicinally.

Traditional Use
In the past, oregano has been used to treat gastrointestinal disorders, menstrual problems, and respiratory conditions.

Current Medicinal Use
The most common modern indication for oregano is for the treatment of infections; however, there is no good evidence from clinical studies in humans to support this use.

Medicinal Forms
- Droplets (orally)
- Aqueous extract (dried powdered leaves with distilled water)
- Enriched tea and juice
- Unsweetened oregano tea as a gargle or mouthwash
- Dried leaves as a bath additive

Relevant Research

Preventative and Therapeutic Effects

Constituents
- **Acids:** aristolochic acid I and II, raffinose acid, oleanolic acid, ursolic acids, caffeic acid, rosmarinic acid, lithospermic acid.
- Triterpenoids.
- Flavonoids.
- Hydroquinones.
- Tannins.
- Phenolic glycosides.

Volatile oil
- Carvacrol, gamma-terpinene, p-cymeme, alpha-pinene, myrcene, thymol, linalool, terpinene-4-ol, caryophyllene, germacren D, sabinene.

Leaves
- Flavones, flavanones, dihydroflavonols, flavonols.

Antimicrobial Action
It has been suggested that oregano's antibacterial activity may be due to the phenolic components thymol and carvacrol, which appear to inhibit bacteria at relatively low concentrations. The exact mechanism of action is still unclear and requires further investigation. One study suggested that fungicidal

activity was a result of direct damage to the cytoplasmic membrane by carvacrol and p-cymene.

Antihyperglycemic Activity

Another study suggested that antihyperglycemic activity occurs via inhibition of amylase by phenolic antioxidants in oregano extract. Four major phenolics in oregano (rosmarinic acid, quercetin, protochatechuic acid, and p-coumaric acid) may potentially inhibit the activity of porcine pancreatic amylase, which is responsible for the breakdown of starch into glucose. Flavonoids in oregano extracts may also act separately or synergistically to cause hypoglycemic effects. Lithospermic acid was found to be the most active compound in the inhibition of aldose reductase, the first enzyme of the polyol pathway implicated in the secondary complications of diabetes. The exact mechanism of action is still unclear and requires further investigation.

Antibacterial Effects

Several in vivo and in vitro studies have reported that oil of oregano acts against a range of bacteria, including *Shigella sonne* and *Shigella flexneri* in mice, *Helicobacter pylori*, and *Pseudomonas aeruginosa*. Further studies are needed to verify the efficacy of oregano in treatment and prevention of bacterial infections in humans.

Antifungal Effects

Several in vivo and in vitro studies have reported that oil of oregano has antifungal activity for a range of fungi, including *Candida albicans* and *Trichophyton mentagrophytes*. Further studies are needed to verify the efficacy of oregano in treatment and prevention of fungal infections in humans.

Antiparasitic Effects

One human study investigated the effect of oregano oil in the treatment of parasitic infections. Thirteen adult patients who initially tested positive for enteric parasites (eight cases for *Blastocystis hominis*, four for *Entamoeba hartmanni*, and one for *Endomalix nana*) were orally administered 4 drops of emulsified oregano oil (200 mg) three times daily with meals. No other dietary changes or therapeutic interventions were employed. After 6 weeks of supplementation, parasites were completely eradicated in 10 patients and 7 out of 8 patients who had originally tested positive for *Blastocystis hominis* reported an improvement in gastrointestinal symptoms, such as bloating, gastrointestinal cramping, alternating diarrhea, constipation, and fatigue. Further evidence is required to confirm oregano as an effective antiparasitic agent.

Anticancer Effects

There are no human trials of oregano as an anticancer agent. However, one test tube study found that several isolated components of oregano, including aristolochic acid I and II and ursolic acid, can possibly exert an effect against leukemia and other types of cancer. Another in vitro study suggested that the antimutagenic and anticarcinogenic properties can be attributed to the rosmarinic acid in oregano. Oregano contains a high polyphenol content and has strong antioxidant properties, suggesting that it may delay or inhibit peroxidative reactions, which are generally associated with many degenerative physiopathologic events such as cancer. Additional evidence is required to confirm which active ingredients demonstrate anticancer activity and whether there is any clinical use for oregano in those diagnosed with cancer.

> *Additional evidence is required to confirm which active ingredients demonstrate anticancer activity and whether there is any clinical use for oregano in those diagnosed with cancer.*

Effect on Diabetes

There are no studies of oregano's effects in people diagnosed with diabetes, but two animal studies have examined the antihyperglycemic activity of oregano. The first study looked at the effect of oregano leaves and found a significant decrease in blood glucose levels, without any change in the basal plasma insulin concentration, in diabetic rats. The second study looked at the relationship between various combinations of essential oils and insulin sensitivity. The essential oil combinations were composed of varying amounts of pumpkinseed oil, extra-virgin olive oil, oregano, cinnamon, fenugreek, cumin, fennel, myrtle, allspice, and ginger. Lower circulating glucose levels and systolic blood pressure was noted in rats in response to each of the three combinations. However, because this study tested combination products, it is difficult to make any conclusions regarding the antihyperglycemic effect of oregano. Quality randomized controlled trials using oregano alone as the active ingredient are needed to confirm these findings.

Adverse Effects

Long-term exposure of gastrointestinal mucosa to concentrated, non-emulsified oregano oil can cause localized irritation. Oregano is generally not recommended for long-term use.

One study identified four individual cases of abortion after ingestion of an over-the-counter herbal product, Carachipita, containing pennyroyal, yerba de la perdiz, oregano, and guaycuru. Given the number of ingredients involved, time elapsed, ingestion of other plant mixtures, and association with other pharmaceutical products the patients may have been taking, it is difficult to determine the role, if any, that oregano played in these cases.

One animal study found that oregano essential oil significantly increased the rate and incidence of cell death in mouse preimplantation embryos. In addition, there have been a number of cases of allergic reactions to foods containing oregano. Symptoms have included eczematous skin reaction and upper respiratory difficulties.

Further research on the effect of oregano alone on human is required to draw any conclusions; however, caution is warranted in the meantime.

Cautions/Contraindications

Oregano belongs to the Lamiaeceae family and can show cross-sensitivity reactions when taken by those with known allergic reactions to plants of this family, such as basil, hyssop, lavender, marjoram, mint, sage, and thyme.

Oregano is not recommended for use during pregnancy and/or breastfeeding due to lack of sufficient safety data. Several cases of abortion associated with a combination product containing oregano have been reported (see Adverse Effects).

Drug Interactions

There are no clinically documented drug interactions. However, oregano may theoretically interact with

- **Anticoagulants:** Oregano has been suggested to have antithrombin effects, so it may theoretically potentiate the action of anticoagulant drugs.

- **Antihyperglycemics:** It has been found that oregano can possibly alter circulating glucose levels, so it may theoretically potentiate the action of antihyperglycemic drugs.

- **Hormones:** Oregano has been reported to contain estrogenic properties, so it may theoretically potentiate the action of exogenous sources of hormones (e.g., hormone replacement therapy, oral contraceptives).

Dosage Regimens

Note: There is no clinical evidence to support specific therapeutic doses of oregano, but the following oral and topical doses have been recommended. There is insufficient evidence to recommend use in children.

Oral

- Emulsified oregano oil: 200 mg three times daily orally.
- Tea: 250 mL boiling water poured over 5 mL oregano leaf and allowed to steep for 10 minutes before straining. The tea may be sweetened with honey.

Topical

- Gargle and mouthwash: unsweetened oregano tea.
- Bath additive: 1 L water poured over 100 g dried leaf and allowed to steep for 10 minutes before straining.

Selected Reference

Force M, Sparks WS, Ronzio RA. Inhibition of enteric parasites by emulsified oil of oregano in vivo. Phytotherapy Research 2000;14:213–14.

Passionflower

Passiflora incarnata L.

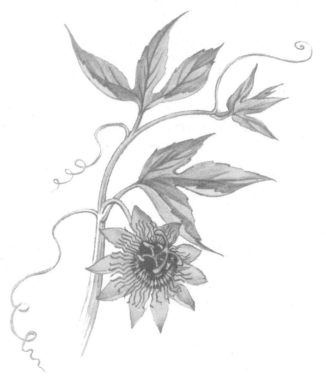

THUMBNAIL SKETCH

Common Uses
- Anxiety

Active Constituents
- Flavonoids
- Alkaloids

Adverse Effects
- Sedation
- Allergic reaction (rare)
- Gastrointestinal effects (rare)

Cautions/Contraindications
- Pregnancy and breastfeeding

Drug Interactions
- Potential exists for interactions with concomitant administration of centrally acting medications

Doses
- *Dried herb:* 0.25–1 g three times daily
- *Liquid extract (1:1 in 25% alcohol):* 0.5–2 mL three times daily
- *Tincture (1:8 in 45% alcohol):* 0.5–4 mL three times daily

Introduction

Family
- Passifloraceae

Synonyms
- Apricot vine
- Corona de cristo
- EUP
- Fleischfarbige
- Fleur de la passion
- Flor de passion
- Granadilla
- Grenadille
- Holy Trinity flower
- *Krishan-Kamala*
- Madre selva
- Maracoc
- Maracock
- Maracuja
- May apple
- Maycock
- Maypops
- Molly-pop
- Naturest
- Old field apricot
- Passiflora
- Passion vine
- Passionsblume
- Pop-apple
- Prem-pushpi
- Purple passionflower
- Water lemon
- White sarsaparilla
- Wild passionflower

Medicinal Forms
- Dried herb
- Liquid extract

Description
Passionflower is a perennial climbing vine growing up to 9 meters (30 feet) that is native to the southern United States. The vine has clusters of three leaves, purple to red flowers, and oblong fruit. Other members of the genus *Passiflora* are found throughout North, South, and Central America. The name arises from the plant's intricate and elaborate flower, which blooms for a maximum of 48 hours. The flower parts are thought to represent the elements of Christ's Passion. For example, the fringe-like crown is said to represent the crown of thorns, while the five anthers represent the five stigmata. *Passio* means "suffering" and *incarnata* means "incarnate."

Parts Used
The part used medicinally is the leaf.

Traditional Use
Passionflower was used in many traditional healing models in America. For example, the Aztecs prized it as a sedative. Modern phytotherapy has expanded these historical uses. While many species of *Passiflora* produce edible fruits, the ones commonly available are not from *P. incarnata* but rather *P. edulis* Sims. A number of references note that passionflower is rarely given as a single remedy but rather is combined with other phytomedicines determined by the indication. Because the constituents responsible for the reputed therapeutic action of passionflower have yet to be conclusively determined, one authority has advised against the use of standardized extracts.

Current Medicinal Use
Passionflower products are now used primarily to treat conditions associated with nervous tension, restlessness, irritability, and insomnia.

Relevant Research

Preventative and Therapeutic Effects

Constituents

- Alkaloids: harmaline, harmalol, harman, harmine, harmol (indole alkaloids based on the ß-carboline ring system).

- Carbohydrates: D-fructose, D-glucose, raffinose, sucrose.

- C-glycosyl flavonoids: 2-glucosylapigenin, 2"-O-glucosyl-6-C-glucosylapigenin, 6-ß-D-glucopyranosyl-8-ß-D-ribopyranosyl apigenin, isoorientin, isoorientin-2"-O-glucopyranoside, isoschaftoside, isoscoparin-2"-O-glucoside, isovitexin, isovitexin-2"-O-glucopyranoside, orientin, schaftoside, swertisin, vitexin.

- Essential oils: contain 2-hydroxy benzoic acid methyl ester (1.3%), 2-phenylethyl alcohol (1.2%), ß-bergamotol (1.7%), α-ionone (2.6%), benzyl alcohol (4.1%), carvone (8.1%), eugenol (1.8%), hexanol (1.4%), isoeugenol (1.6%), linalool (3.2%), phytol (1.9%), trans-anethol (2.6%).

- Flavonoids: 6-ß-D-allopyranosyl-8-ß-xylopyranosyl-apigenin, apigenin, chrysin, kaempferol, luteolin, quercetin.

- Other: 21 amino acids, ß-pinene, ß-benzo-pyrone derivative maltol, cyanogenic glycoside gynocardin, cumene, limonene, prezizanene, zizaene, zizanene.

Common Uses

Passionflower is reputed to have hypnotic, sedative, anodyne (analgesic), and antispasmodic properties. The French and Swiss herbal pharmacopoeia indicate that it is useful in the management of mild heart conditions. It is thought to be particularly useful in individuals who are weak or exhausted from overwork, illness, or age. A number of references mention its use in conditions of hysteria and convulsions.

Effect on Anxiety

Five clinical trials investigated the anxiolytic effects of passionflower. Only one high-quality randomized, double-blind, active-controlled pilot study (reporting positive results) used passionflower as a single ingredient. The remaining trials used combination products containing passionflower. The multiple ingredients studied make it impossible to determine the specific role of passionflower.

One high-quality randomized, double-blind, active-controlled pilot study with 36 individuals compared the efficacy of passionflower extract (details not provided) with oxazepam in treating general anxiety disorder diagnosed using *DSM-IV* criteria. Subjects were randomly assigned to a group of 18 receiving a passionflower extract (45 drops daily) plus a placebo tablet or another group of 18 receiving oxazepam tablets (30 mg daily) plus placebo drops over 4 weeks. Four subjects, two from each group, dropped out of the trial due to non-compliance. The authors found that both the passionflower extract and oxazepam were effective in treating generalized anxiety disorder, as measured using the Hamilton Anxiety Scale (HAS or HAMA). While no significant difference was observed between the two groups, oxazepam showed a more rapid onset of action compared to passionflower. Subjects receiving oxazepam also reported a higher degree of impairment in job performance, compared to the group receiving passionflower. Based on these preliminary results, a larger-scale trial is justified.

> *The authors found that both the passionflower extract and oxazepam were effective in treating generalized anxiety disorder, as measured using the Hamilton Anxiety Scale (HAS or HAMA).*

Researchers have proposed many different theories about the bioactive constituents responsible for passionflower's anxiolytic effects. Harmala alkaloids have been suggested to be the main bioactive constituents, due to their monoamine oxidase (MAO) enzyme-inhibiting properties. The flavonoids maltol (ß-benzo-pyrone derivative) and chrysin, a partial agonist to benzodiazepine receptors, have also been hypothesized to play a role in central nervous system (CNS) depression by passionflower. In contrast, one pharmacological study reported that neither the harmala alkaloids nor the flavonoids are likely the active compounds. Newer studies have attributed the plant's anxiolytic and sedative activity to the benzodiazepine and GABA receptor-mediated systems in the body and to a benzoflavone (BZF) moiety extracted from the plant's leaves. To date, there is no clear scientific consensus on the mechanism of passionflower's anxiolytic effects.

Opiate Withdrawal (Adjunct Treatment)

One randomized, double-blind, controlled trial involving 65 opiate addicts meeting the *DSM-IV* criteria for opioid dependence reported positive results for the use of passionflower as an adjunct treatment in the management of opiate withdrawal. Thirty subjects completed the trial and were evenly but randomly assigned to treatment with clonidine tablets plus passionflower extract (details not reported) versus clonidine tablets plus placebo drops over a 14-day trial. The fixed daily dose was 60 drops of passionflower extract or placebo and a maximum daily dose of 0.8 mg of clonidine, given in three divided doses. The authors concluded that both therapies were equally effective in treating the *physical* withdrawal symptoms; however, passionflower plus clonidine therapy was significantly better in managing *mental* symptoms compared to the clonidine plus placebo therapy. While the passionflower extract may be an effective adjuvant in the management of opiate withdrawal, the study is limited by a small sample size and a lack of details about baseline patient characteristics or the extract tested in the study. Further research is needed.

A benzoflavone compound isolated from the methanol extract of aerial parts of passionflower has been identified as the main bioactive component responsible for reducing symptoms of opiate withdrawal. It is postulated that this compound inhibits the enzyme aromatase, thereby preventing the metabolic conversion of testosterone to estrogens and increasing the levels of free testosterone. Another hypothesis is that the benzoflavone compound increases testosterone levels by eliminating a negative feedback loop that otherwise reduces testosterone levels due to chronic treatment with other substances, such as morphine, nicotine, cannabinoids, and alcohol. It is believed that increased levels of free testosterone account for a reduction in opiate and ethanol withdrawal symptoms. Chronic and acute administrations of a benzoflavone compound from passionflower leaves have also been reported to prevent the expression of alcohol withdrawal effects in mice.

> *Further research is required to determine the mechanism by which passionflower may alter exercise capacity in patients with dyspnoea and congestive heart failure.*

Congestive Heart Failure

Forty subjects completed a randomized, double-blind, placebo-controlled trial examining the effects of a hawthorn-passionflower extract on the exercise capacity of patients with dyspnoea and congestive heart failure. The authors reported mixed results, and the use of a combination product makes it impossible to determine the specific role that passionflower played in the study's outcomes. Further research is required before any conclusions can be made about passionflower's effectiveness for this indication.

The mechanism by which passionflower may alter exercise capacity in patients with dyspnea and congestive heart failure remains to be elucidated. However, the cardiovascular actions of three harmala alkaloids (harmine, harmaline, harmalol) found in passionflower leaves have been studied. All three alkaloids decreased heart rate and increased pulse pressure, peak aortic flow, and myocardial contractile force. Harmine also reduced systemic arterial blood pressure and total peripheral resistance, while harmaline-evoked decreases were often followed by secondary increases, and harmalol produced inconsistent results. Further research is required to determine the mechanism by which passionflower may alter exercise capacity in patients with dyspnoea and congestive heart failure.

Miscellaneous Effects

The methanol extract of passionflower leaves demonstrated dose-dependent analgesic activity, experimentally induced convulsions, an anti-inflammatory effect, and sedative effects in mice. While passionflower has traditionally been used for its analgesic, anticonvulsant, anti-inflammatory, and sedative effects, further research is required before any conclusions can be drawn about passionflower's effectiveness for these indications.

In addition, an in vitro assay reported that passionflower demonstrated cancer chemopreventive activity, which is not a traditional use. To date, no clinical trials have been conducted to assess the cancer chemopreventive effects of passionflower.

Adverse Effects

Case reports of allergic reactions, cardiovascular effects, and gastrointestinal upset, as well as drowsiness and fatigue, have been reported. As with all case reports, it is difficult to determine whether passionflower actually caused the problems described below.

A hypersensitivity reaction (vasculitis and urticaria) was reported in a 77-year-old man with rheumatoid arthritis. His symptoms resolved within a week after discontinuing a passionflower product (Naturest). Occupational asthma and rhinitis were also reported in a 30-year-old man preparing passionflower products. However, it is not clear what, if any, role passionflower played in these events.

A 34-year-old woman developed severe nausea, vomiting, drowsiness, and fatigue, along with episodes of non-sustained ventricular tachycardia and a prolonged QT interval, after taking Sedacalm, an extract of passionflower equivalent to 500 mg of the "active ingredients" per tablet. No other ingredients were reported. She had taken 3 tablets on one day, followed by 4 tablets on the second day. Her condition resolved after a week of hospitalization with supportive care following discontinuation of Sedacalm.

A brief Norwegian report states that five patients were hospitalized for mental status changes (drowsiness and confusion) after consuming Relaxir, which contained an extract from passionflower fruit and other unreported ingredients. It is not clear what, if any, role passionflower played in these events.

Animal studies have demonstrated that constituents of passionflower may stimulate uterine contractions. However, no human cases have been reported.

> *Passionflower is contraindicated during pregnancy. In addition, there is currently no evidence supporting its safety in breastfeeding.*

Cautions/Contraindications

Passionflower is not recommended for use in patients with known allergies or hypersensitivity to members of the Passifloraceae family. Cases of allergic reactions have been reported in people using passionflower products. Due to its potentially sedating effects, passionflower should be avoided prior to driving or operating heavy machinery.

Animal studies have reported that some constituents of passionflower can stimulate uterine contractions. Therefore, passionflower is contraindicated during pregnancy. In addition, there is currently no evidence supporting its safety in breastfeeding.

Drug Interactions

There are no clinical cases of passionflower interacting with any medications. However, based on animal and in vitro data, a number of interactions are theoretically possible, including

- **Anticoagulants and antiplatelet agents:** Passionflower contains coumarin derivatives and may theoretically increase the risk of bleeding in patients receiving anticoagulants or antiplatelet agents.

- **Monoamine oxidase inhibitors (MAOIs):** Small levels of harmala alkaloids, which are thought to inhibit monoamine oxidase (MAO), have been isolated from passionflower. Therefore, it may theoretically potentiate the effects of MAOIs. However, the levels of harmala alkaloids in passionflower leaves may be too low to be clinically relevant.

- **Sedatives:** Theoretically, passionflower may potentiate the central nervous system depressant effects of alcohol or other sedative or hypnotic drugs, including benzodiazepines, barbiturates, and opiates. This is based on a mechanism of benzodiazepine receptor affinity demonstrated in animal studies. Animal studies have reported synergistic sedative effects between passionflower and kava (*Piper methysticum* L.), an herb with anti-anxiety properties.

Dosage Regimens

- Dried herb (tea): 0.25–1 g three times daily.
- Liquid extract (1:1 in 25% alcohol): 0.5–2 mL three times daily.
- Tincture (1:8 in 45% alcohol): 0.5–4 mL three times daily.

- Children's dose: There is no evidence currently available concerning use of passionflower in children, but many experts recommend that children 3 to 12 years old be given *P. incarnata* only under medical supervision, with dosing proportioned by weight to adult doses (based on a 60 kg adult).

Selected References

Akhondzadeh S, Kashani L, Mobaseri M, Hosseini S, Nikzad S, Khani M. Passionflower in the treatment of opiates withdrawal: A double-blind randomized controlled trial. Journal of Clinical Pharmacy and Therapeutics 2001;26:369–73.

Akhondzadeh S, Naghavi HR, Vazirian M, Shayeganpour A, Rashidi H, Khani M. Passionflower in the treatment of generalized anxiety: A pilot double-blind randomized controlled trial with oxazepam. Journal of Clinical Pharmacy and Therapeutics 2001;26:363–67.

Peppermint
Mentha x *piperita* L.

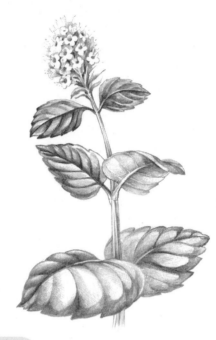

THUMBNAIL SKETCH

Common Uses
- Irritable bowel disease
- Spastic colon
- Colonoscopy and barium enema
- Gastritis (inflammation of the stomach)
- Dyspepsia (indigestion)

Active Constituents
- Menthol (and its derivatives)

Adverse Effects
- Heartburn, esophageal reflux, contact irritation when used as flavoring agent in oral products (rare)

Cautions/Contraindications
- Infants and young children
- Achlorhydria (lack of hydrochloric acid from gastric juice)

Drug Interactions
- None known

Doses
- *Enteric-coated peppermint oil capsules:* 1–3 capsules three times daily away from meals
- *Tincture (1:5 in 45% ethanol):* 2–3 mL three times daily away from meals
- *Tea:* 1.5 g of recently dried leaves taken on an empty stomach three to four times daily to relieve upset stomach

Introduction

Family
- Laminaceae (also known as Labiatae)

Synonyms
- *M. x piperita* L. *var vulgaris* Sole (black mint)
- *M. x piperita* L. *var officinalis* Sole (white mint)

Medicinal Forms
- Enteric-coated tablets (peppermint oil)
- Dried herb
- Tincture

Description

Peppermint (*Mentha* x *piperita* L.), once thought to be a unique species, is now considered a hybrid of two other members of the mint family: water mint (*Mentha aquatica* L.) and spearmint (*Mentha spicata* L.). Although it is native to Europe, peppermint is now an important aromatic and medicinal crop throughout North American temperate zones, especially in the states of Indiana, Wisconsin, Oregon, Washington, and Idaho. This perennial grows to a height of approximately 1 meter (40 inches), spreads by surface runners, and has pink to purple flowers. In addition, it has a square stem characteristic of all members of the mint family.

Parts Used

The leaf, as an infusion and as an essential oil, is the part used medicinally.

Traditional Use

Both the peppermint leaf, often taken as a tea, and the essential oil, which is distilled from the leaves, have a long history of medicinal use. Peppermint is considered a carminative. Peppermint leaf tea has been used for indigestion, nausea, diarrhea, colds, headache, and cramps. The most common use of peppermint oil today is as a flavoring agent in a variety of oral products, including toothpastes, chewing gum, and after-dinner mints. This review will primarily deal with the use of peppermint when taken orally or applied topically and not on its use as an aromatherapy agent.

Current Medicinal Use

Peppermint is now primarily used for its digestive actions in the treatment of such conditions as irritable bowel syndrome and indigestion. It is also used in the management of nausea.

Relevant Research

Preventative and Therapeutic Effects

Constituents
- Volatile oil: (-)-menthol and its esters (acetate and isovalerate), (+)- and (-)-menthone, (+)-isomenthone, (+)-neomethone, (+)-menthofuran, eucalyptol, (-)-limonene.

- Miscellaneous: flavonoids, phytol, tocopherols, carotenoids, betain, choline, azulenes, rosmarinic acid, tannins.

Note: 1-Menthol makes up 29% to 48% of the essential oil but is considered a distinctly different agent, not to be confused with the volatile oil of peppermint. Although menthol can be obtained from peppermint oil, the high price of peppermint oil makes this use very uncommon. Today, menthol is usually produced synthetically by the hydrogenation of thymol. Synthetic menthol differs from that produced from peppermint in that it is racemic.

Common Uses

Peppermint is reputed to have antispasmodic, carminative, anti-emetic, diaphoretic, hepatic, and antiseptic properties. As with all carminatives, oral consumption is considered useful in the treatment of many digestive disorders, especially nausea, vomiting, bloating, nervous bowel, and indigestion. Peppermint is also commonly used to treat colds and flus.

Gastrointestinal Effects

According to a 1990 study of a variety of over-the-counter (OTC) products conducted by the Food and Drug Administration (FDA) in the United States, there is not sufficient evidence to demonstrate that peppermint oil is effective as a digestive aid. However, this conclusion was based solely on evidence submitted by the manufacturers of the OTC products being reviewed, and one authority strongly criticizes this review. In contrast, the German Commission E's review of the scientific literature has concluded that there is sufficient evidence to demonstrate that peppermint and its volatile oil are effective spasmolytics, and that they promote gastric secretions and the flow of bile.

Several studies have found that, for peppermint oil to effectively alleviate the symptoms of a variety of bowel conditions, including irritable bowel and spastic colon, the oil must reach the colon in its original (i.e., unmetabolized) state. Thus, most peppermint oil products sold for this purpose in Canada are enteric-coated. Gelatin-coated capsules release the peppermint oil in the stomach, where it is metabolized before reaching the colon.

Irritable Bowel Syndrome

Irritable bowel presents with abdominal pain, feelings of distention, and "variations in bowel habits." Three meta-analyses and reviews have concluded that enteric-coated peppermint oil capsules are effective at relieving these symptoms.

One study, published in 2005, identified 16 clinical trials investigating 180–200 mg enteric-coated peppermint oil in patients diagnosed with irritable bowel syndrome or recurrent abdominal pain in 651 children. Eight double-blind, placebo-controlled studies indicated that enteric-coated peppermint oil, given at 180–200 mg three times daily over 2 to 4 weeks, showed significant effects over a placebo. Three double-blind crossover studies testing peppermint oil against conventional smooth muscle relaxants (mebeverine, hyoscyamine, and alverine) showed equivalent efficacy between treatments. The authors concluded that peppermint oil may be effective in alleviating general symptoms of irritable bowel syndrome in patients with non-serious constipation or diarrhea.

> *Irritable bowel presents with abdominal pain, feelings of distention, and "variations in bowel habits." Three meta-analyses and reviews have concluded that enteric-coated peppermint oil capsules are effective at relieving these symptoms.*

A review published in 2006 included an additional randomized, double-blind, placebo-controlled trial investigating 42 children, all over 8 years of age, with irritable bowel syndrome. Enteric-coated peppermint oil capsules (Colpermin, consisting of 187 mg of peppermint oil per dose) were found to reduce the severity of pain after a 2-week treatment period. Patients weighing more than 45 kg received 2 peppermint oil or placebo capsules daily and those weighing between 30 and 45 kg received 1 capsule three times daily.

One additional trial was published later. This prospective, double-blind, placebo-controlled, randomized 4-week trial, conducted in 2007, included 57 patients with irritable bowel syndrome and found that 2 capsules of peppermint oil (Mintoil, containing 225 mg peppermint oil per capsule), administered twice daily, resulted in significant reduction in irritable bowel syndrome symptoms.

Overall, there is good evidence that enteric-coated peppermint oil capsules are beneficial for managing symptoms of irritable bowel syndrome.

Antispasmodic

Several in vitro (test tube) studies have demonstrated peppermint oil's ability to relax smooth muscle via a blockade of the calcium channel transport mechanism. Two reviews also presented human evidence that peppermint oil exerts a spamolytic effect on the smooth vasculature of the intestinal tract. One research team reported that colon spasms during endoscopy were relieved within 30 seconds when diluted suspension of peppermint oil was injected along the biopsy channel of the colonoscope in 20 patients. This clinical observation was confirmed by a study that investigated patients undergoing colonscopy (409 in a treated group, 36 in a control group) and found that administration of 0.8% peppermint oil solution into the lumen of the large intestine significantly reduced the spasmolytic effect in 88.5% of the treated patients, compared with a reduction of 33.3% in the control group.

Several clinical studies have noted that the addition of peppermint to barium enema suspension decreased the incidence of spasm during double-contrast barium enema examination. One double-blind study involving 141 patients found that peppermint oil (added to barium sulphate suspension) was effective at relieving colonic muscle spasm during examination. The authors suggested that this simple, safe, and inexpensive technique could decrease the need for intravenous spasmolytic agents during barium enema procedures.

A more recent study reported that orally administered peppermint oil reduced spasm of the esophagus, lower stomach, and duodenal bulb, as well as inhibiting barium flow to the distal duodenum and improving double-contrast barium meal quality.

> *Several clinical studies have noted that the addition of peppermint to barium enema suspension decreased the incidence of spasm during double-contrast barium enema examination.*

Miscellaneous Gastrointestinal Effects

One double-blind, placebo-controlled, crossover study with six patients found that peppermint oil decreases colonic motility in humans. Another double-blind, placebo-controlled, multi-center trial with 45 patients found that a peppermint oil (90 mg) and caraway oil (50 mg) combination significantly reduced the symptoms of non-ulcer dyspepsia (indigestion) after 4 weeks of treatment. Promising results were reported from another 4-week randomized controlled trial comparing a peppermint oil (90 mg) and caraway oil (50 mg) combination with cisapride (30 mg daily) in 120 outpatients with functional dyspepsia (indigestion). In this case, both treatment regimens were found to be equally effective and well tolerated.

Antimicrobial Activity

Antibacterial Effects

In vitro testing indicates that peppermint inhibits the growth of a variety of bacteria, including *S. aureus*, *B. brevis*, *B. circulans*, *Citrobacter* species, *E. coli*, *Klebsiella* species, *S. typhi*, *S. typhimurium*, *S. boydii*, *S. flexneri*, and *V. cholerae*. In addition, peppermint oil was found to be ineffective against *Pseudomonas aeruginosa*. The clinical significance of these findings is unknown.

Antifungal Effects

Peppermint is reported to inhibit the growth in vitro of a variety of fungi, including *C. albicans*, *C. neoformans*, *S. schenkii*, *A. citrii*, *A. fumigatus*, *A. oryzae*, *F. oxysporum*, *F. solani*, *H. compactum*, *M. phaseolina*, *S. rolfsii*, and *T. mentagrophytes*. The clinical significance of these findings is unknown.

Antiviral Effects

Peppermint is reported to have activity against herpes simplex virus and Newcastle disease in vitro. The clinical significance of this is unknown.

Miscellaneous Effects

A randomized, double-blind 14-day trial involving 216 breastfeeding mothers who each gave birth to only one child compared the effect of peppermint gel, modified lanolin, and neutral ointment in the prevention of nipple crack. Participants were seen for a maximum of four follow-up visits within 14 days and a final visit at week 6. Peppermint gel was found to be more effective than the other two treatments and was suggested as a prophylaxis for nipple crack at the initiation of breastfeeding.

Peppermint oil has traditionally been used externally for a wide range of indications, including headaches. One double-blind, placebo-controlled, randomized crossover clinical trial with 32 patients reports that a combination of peppermint oil (10 g), eucalyptus oil (5 g), and ethanol (ad 100 g) significantly increased cognitive performance, as well as producing mental and pericranial muscle relaxation. In addition, peppermint oil (10 g) in combination with ethanol (ad 100 g) produced a significant analgesic effect.

Adverse Effects

Regular consumption of peppermint leaf tea is considered safe; however, excessive use of the volatile oil (more than 0.3 g, or 12 drops) may cause problems. Clinical trials of enteric-coated peppermint oil capsules for a variety of gastrointestinal complaints report few side effects. Heartburn and esophageal reflux can occur if the peppermint oil is accidentally released in the stomach. In addition, a burning sensation during defecation — thought to be due to unabsorbed menthol reaching the rectum — has occasionally been observed when peppermint oil is taken in high doses. Reducing the dose reduces this adverse effect.

There have also been several reports of contact sensitivity to the peppermint in a variety oral products, including toothpaste. Symptoms include a burning sensation in the mouth, recurrent oral ulceration, stomatitis (inflammation of the mouth), glossitis (inflammation of the tongue), gingivitis (inflammation of the gum), and perioral dermatitis (inflammation of the skin around the mouth).

> *Regular consumption of peppermint leaf tea is considered safe; however, excessive use of the volatile oil (more than 0.3 g, or 12 drops) may cause problems.*

One case report describes veno-occlusive (liver) disease in an 18-month-old boy who had regularly consumed a tea believed to contain peppermint and coltsfoot (*Tussilago farfara* L., Asteraceae) for the previous 12 months. Analysis of the tea revealed that the tea contained *Adenosyles alliariae* (Gouan) Kern., Asteraceae, rather than the reported coltsfoot. The peppermint was not thought to play any role in the toxicity of the product.

There has been a report of a 49-year-old woman who presented with difficulty in breathing, as well as drooling and fever 12 hours after ingestion of 40 drops of pure non-heated peppermint oil for treatment of a common cold (1–2 drops each time). Other symptoms included respiratory function disorder, excess salivation, rapid heart rate, multiple burns in the mouth and throat, and swelling around and inside the mouth. After injection of steroids and antibiotics into the veins and a trans-nasal awake intubation for 24 hours, swelling, burn signs, and other symptoms gradually resolved over the next 2 weeks. Since the patient did not experience any form of an allergic reaction upon previous administration of peppermint oil, it was suggested that a chemical reaction led to damage to the oral mucosa.

There has been another case report of an 18-year-old woman in her 28th week of pregnancy suffering from acute lung injury following injection of 5 mL peppermint oil into the veins as an attempt to commit suicide. Acute lung injury was most likely the result of direct toxicity and increase in the permeability of blood vessels in the lungs.

Cautions/Contraindications

Peppermint should generally be given between meals, and it should not be taken by patients with achlorhydria (i.e., patients with no hydrochloric acid in gastric juices). Generally, peppermint (tea and topical application to nostrils) should be avoided in young children or infants because the menthol may cause a choking sensation. In addition, oral consumption of peppermint oil should be avoided in situations of glucose-6 phosphate dehydrogenase deficiency because menthol may be implicated in this condition.

Drug Interactions

No known drug interactions have been reported with medicinal peppermint supplements. However, cardiac fibrillation has been reported in patients whose condition was controlled with quinidine following the use of mentholated cigarettes or consumption of peppermint candy.

Dosage Regimens

- Enteric-coated peppermint oil capsules (0.2 mL peppermint oil per capsule): 1–2 capsules three times daily away from meals.
- Tincture (1:5 in 45% ethanol): 2–3 mL three times daily away from meals.
- Tea: Mix 160 mL boiling water with 1.5 g recently dried leaves and steep for 5 to 10 minutes. This amount is taken on an empty stomach three to four times daily to relieve upset stomach.

Selected References

Grigoleit HG, Grigoleit P. Gastrointestinal clinical pharmacology of peppermint oil. Phytomedicine 2005;12:607–11.

Grigoleit HG, Grigoleit P. Peppermint oil in irritable bowel syndrome. Phytomedicine 2005;12:601–6.

McKay DL, Blumberg JB. A review of the bioactivity and potential health benefits of peppermint tea (*Mentha piperita* L.). Phytotherapy Research 2006;20:619–33.

Red Clover

Trifolium pratense L.

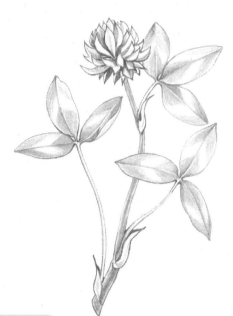

THUMBNAIL SKETCH

Common Uses
- Menopausal symptoms
- Osteoporsis
- Cardiovascular disease (especially hypercholecterolemia)
- Prostate conditions
- Breast cancer prevention

Active Constituents
- Isoflavones (e.g., genistein, daidzein, biochanin A, and formononetin)

Adverse Effects
- Generally well tolerated
- Headaches and mild increases in liver enzymes reported

Cautions/Contraindications
- Pregnancy and breastfeeding

Drug Interactions
- No clinically documented interactions
- Anticoagulants (theoretical)
- Hormone replacement therapy (theoretical)
- Oral contraceptives (theoretical)

Doses
General
- *Dried flower head:* 4 g or by infusion three times daily
- *Liquid extract (1:1 in 25% alcohol):* 1.5–3 mL three times daily

Specific
- *Menopausal symptoms:* 40–80 mg isoflavones from red clover daily
- *Hypercholesterolemia:* 28.5–85.5 mg isoflavones from red clover daily
- *Osteoporosis:* 40 mg isoflavones from red clover daily
- *Prostate conditions:* 40 mg isoflavones from red clover daily

Introduction

Family
- Leguminosae

Synonyms
- Ackerklee
- Bee bread
- Cow clover
- Meadow clover
- Purple clover
- Rotklee
- Trefoil
- Trefle des pres
- Wild clover

Medicinal Forms
- Liquid extract
- Tincture
- Tablets and capsules
- In most cases, forms standardized for isoflavone content are recommended

Description
Red clover is a legume commonly used as feed for grazing cattle and other animals. It is a perennial that grows wild in meadows throughout Europe and Asia and has been naturalized to grow in North America.

Parts Used
The red flower heads at the end of the branched stems are usually dried for therapeutic use.

Traditional Use
Red clover has been traditional used for respiratory disorders by folk healers in China and Russia. North American Native healers used it to treat coughs and types of cancer. It has also been reported to be used to treat skin conditions, such as psoriasis, and to speed wound healing.

Current Medicinal Use
Red clover is currently most often used for symptoms associated with menopause. There is also interest in its purported ability to prevent cancer and to treat cardiovascular symptoms.

Relevant Research

Preventative and Therapeutic Effects

Constituents
- Carbohydrates: arabinose, glucose, glucuronic acid, rhamnose, xylose (following hydrolysis of saponin), galactoglucomannan.
- Coumarins: coumarin, medicagol.
- Isoflavonoids: biochanin A, daidzein, formononetin, genistein, pratensin, trifoside, calycosine galactoside, pectolinarin.
- Flavonoids: isorhamnetin, kaempferol, quercetin.
- Saponins: soyasapogenols B-F.

Isoflavone Action
The isoflavones, a class of phytoestrogens in red clover, are believed to be responsible for its therapeutic action. The mechanism of action of isoflavones (e.g., genistein, daidzein, biochanin A, and formononetin) is not fully understood. Proposed mechanisms from various in vitro and in vivo studies include estrogenic, antiproliferative, and antioxidant properties. The isoflavones exhibit weak estrogenic activity ($1/1000$ times weaker than estradiol) and behave like estradiol when it is in low concentration. There are many proposed mechanisms, and it is uncertain which best explain red clover's in vivo effects. Isoflavones in red clover are

known to influence the metabolism of steroids and the transfer of hormones; bind weakly to both alpha- and beta-estrogen receptors; and differ from estradiol in that they may bind preferentially to a beta-estrogen receptor (beta-ER) as opposed to alpha-ER. Beta-ER is found in the vasculature, brain, bone, and heart, while alpha-ER is found in the ovaries, breast, and uterus. In addition, red clover was also found to exhibit anti-androgen and antiprogestin activity.

> *The isoflavones, a class of phytoestrogens in red clover, are believed to be responsible for its therapeutic action.*

Cardiovascular Effects

There are many proposed mechanisms by which isoflavones may reduce the risk of cardiovascular disease. The main mechanisms are hypocholesterolemic, antiplatelet, and antithrombotic. Isoflavones may have effect on plasma lipid levels by increasing bile acid turnover and removal of low-density lipoprotein (LDL) cholesterol; by altering hepatic metabolism through heightened removal of very low-density lipoprotein (VLDL) and high-density lipoprotein (HDL); by up-regulation of LDL receptors; and by inhibition of endogenous cholesterol synthesis.

Isoflavones, specifically genistein and daizein, are also known to reduce platelet aggregation (i.e., antithrombotic and anticollagen) during the process of atherosclerosis, blocking the biochemical signaling that initiates this action. It has been proposed that genistein may be capable of inhibiting specific signaling pathways, such as INCAM-1, VCAM-1, and tyrosine kinase, or inhibiting the binding of thromboxane A2 to its receptors, resulting in decreased platelet aggregation. In addition, isoflavones have been shown in studies to improve systemic arterial compliance, induce endothelium-independent relaxation of coronary arteries via calcium

antagonism in the animal model, and induce the synthesis of nitric oxide (an arteriole vasodilator) in vitro.

Bone Remodeling

Specifically with respect to bone remodeling, isoflavones prevent urinary calcium loss, have beneficial effects on osteoblasts and osteoclasts, may affect the secretion of calcitonin (a hormone that suppresses bone resorption) and induce apoptosis perhaps through an estrogen receptor-mediated pathway.

Hormone Effects

Isoflavones derived from red clover have shown estrogenic and anti-androgenic effects, which may explain its effects on the prostate with in vivo models, suggesting that isoflavones increase the production of beta-estrogen receptors and down-regulate androgen receptors (AR) in the prostates of male rats. Through an increased sensitivity of AR, it can be expected that a decrease of circulating testosterone would occur as a result of negative feedback from luteinizing hormone. However, the opposite was found to be true. Studies have shown that an increase in testosterone occurs in conjunction with a decrease in the levels of dihydroxytestosterone (DHT), the active form of testosterone that increases the size of the prostate and increases the risk of prostate cancer, a phenomenon that would not occur under normal conditions. It is hypothesized that isoflavones (genistein and biochanin A) reduce the incidence of prostate cancer by the inhibition of 5-alpha reductase, the enzyme that converts testosterone to DHT, leading to apoptosis of cells in the prostate.

Antitumor Effects

There is evidence to support that, as an antitumor agent, isoflavones inhibit tyrosine kinase (an enzyme involved in cell proliferation) and DNA topoisomerase activity, and suppress angiogenesis. As an antioxidant (protection of cell from chemical damage, such as in the case of heart disease or cancer), phytoestrogens inhibit oxidation of LDL, inhibit hydrogen peroxide, and increase catalases and superoxide dismutase, glutathione peroxidase, and reductase. Other effects include a reduction in the synthesis of prostaglandin E2, thromboxane B2, and inhibitory activity of cyclo-oxygenase-2.

Prevention of Cardiovascular Disease

There have been four positive and four negative published randomized controlled trials on the use of red clover for indicators associated with cardiovascular disease in menopausal women. In five of these trials, positive results for some indicators of cardiovascular disease were observed as secondary outcome measures. There are also three trials that measured many outcomes and observed both positive and negative (inconclusive) results.

In most trials, healthy pre- or postmenopausal women were used to assess the efficacy of red clover, which makes it difficult to identify its effects on women with existing cardiovascular problems. The majority of these trials are short term, making it impossible to assess whether red clover taken as a prophylactic prevents cardiovascular disease in the long term. To test the use of red clover for the treatment of cardiovascular disease, future studies on subjects with high cholesterol, high blood pressure, or other elevated indicators of cardiovascular disease are necessary. At present, it is uncertain whether red clover taken preventatively or as a treatment for CVD is effective.

> *There have been four positive and four negative published randomized controlled trials on the use of red clover for indicators associated with cardiovascular disease in menopausal women.*

Improvement of Cognitive Function

There has been one published randomized, double-blind, placebo-controlled crossover trial on the use of red clover for cognitive function in menopausal women. Women who had been postmenopausal for at least 5 years who complained of memory difficulties were given either 2 tablets of red clover extract (Rimostil), each containing 25 mg formononetin, 2.5 mg biochanin, and less than 1 mg genistein and daidzein per tablet (N=14), or placebo (N=14) for 6 months. There were no statistically significant differences between the two groups when corrections were made for the potential of chance findings due to multiple comparisons. The authors conclude that isoflavone supplementation does not appear to have major short-term effects on cognitive function.

Prevention of Osteoporosis

There have been two positive randomized, double-blind studies of the effect of red clover on bone metabolism as a marker for osteoporosis. A third randomized, double-blind study did not report significant results. Overall, there appears to be a positive relationship between red clover and bone metabolism in menopausal and postmenopausal women; however, more trials are necessary to confirm this relationship.

Treatment of Premenstrual Breast Pain

There has been one published randomized, placebo-controlled trial of the use of red clover for the treatment of cyclical mastalgia (premenstrual breast pain), suggesting that 40 mg (but not 80 mg) of isoflavones derived from red clover taken twice daily for 3 months significantly reduces premenstrual breast pain compared to baseline. Given the mixed results from this study, further trials are necessary to confirm the effects of red clover for cyclical mastalgia. In addition, this study was funded and co-authored by Novogen, the manufacturer of the red clover product used in this trial.

Effect on Menopause Symptoms

There have been five positive randomized, double-blind, placebo-controlled studies and one open-label observational study, as well as three randomized, double-blind, placebo-controlled negative studies investigating the effect of red clover as a single agent for hot flashes and other related menopause symptoms. In addition, there have been three positive studies on combination treatment products containing red clover. In the positive studies, hot flashes were significantly reduced in the isoflavone group compared to baseline or a placebo. In the negative studies, either there were no significant decreases in hot flashes in the red clover group compared to the placebo or isoflavone therapy proved to be no more effective than the placebo for the treatment of hot flashes and other menopausal symptoms. Overall, the evidence suggests that red clover products may be helpful in the management of hot flashes and other symptoms related to menopause; however, further research is necessary before a firm conclusion can be drawn.

> *Overall, the evidence suggests that red clover products may be helpful in the management of hot flashes and other symptoms related to menopause; however, further research is necessary before a firm conclusion can be drawn.*

Cancer Prevention

Prostate Cancer

There have been two positive studies (one open-label matched control design and one open-label uncontrolled design) and one negative open-label uncontrolled study on the effect of red clover for prostate cancer prevention. The positive studies reported increases in apoptosis in prostate tissue and decreases in mean prostate-specific antigen values compared to baseline. The negative study reported that red clover has no sig- nificant effect on plasma testosterone, dihy- drotestosterone (DHT), androstenedione, dehydroepiandrosterone, androsterone, and epiandrosterone, suggesting it would not be useful in preventing prostate cancer.

There was also one case study of a 66-year-old male taking phytoestrogen (160 mg Promensil red clover isoflavones) daily for 1 week before radical prostatectomy for moderately high-grade adenocarcinoma that appeared to result in prominent apop- tosis of the resected tumor. Further research is needed before definitive conclusions can be drawn about red clover's use in the pre- vention of prostate cancer.

Breast Cancer

High concentrations of insulin growth factor (IGF) and high patterns of breast density may be associated with an increased risk of breast cancer after menopause. One randomized controlled trial and one high-quality trial assessed the effects of red clover on IGF and breast density respectively. Red clover did not have a beneficial effect on either parameter. One combination supplement of red clover and kudzu appeared to decrease the ratio of 2-hydroxyestrone to 16-alpha-hydroxys- terone, another risk factor of breast cancer. Although there is not enough evidence to be conclusive, it appears that red clover is not likely effective in the prevention of breast cancer during or after menopause.

Endometrial Cancer

In a randomized, double-blind, placebo- controlled, high-quality study, a red clover extract was assessed to determine if it has an effect on reducing the risk of endometrial cancer associated with the onset of menopause. A group of perimenopausal women in their late reproductive years were randomly selected to receive either 1 tablet of isoflavone extract (50 mg) derived from red clover (N=12) or a placebo (N=10) for 3 months. The primary outcome measure was the effect of red clover on the Ki-67 antigen proliferative marker in endometrial biopsies. Baseline measurements indicated no significant differences between the treatment and placebo groups. After the 3-month treatment phase, there was no significant change in the Ki-67 proliferation index after treatment with red clover compared to the placebo. The authors concluded that, based on this small study, there is no evidence to conclude that red clover has an antiproliferative effect on the endometrium.

> *Although there is not enough evidence to be conclusive, it appears that red clover is not likely effective in the prevention of breast cancer during or after menopause.*

Adverse Effects

In seven clinical trials that included adverse events in the results, six trials reported no adverse effects in the red clover treatment group or no difference between the treatment and the placebo group. Headaches were reported in several trials, but it is not clear whether these were caused by red clover. One study reported a significant increase in liver transaminase levels to the high normal range in 15 out of 17 patients during the course of the therapy, while 2 patients had transaminase levels elevated above the normal ranges. In view of the infrequent reporting of this event, it is not possible to conclude with certainty that the rise in liver enzyme levels was caused by red clover consumption. Psoriasis and thrush have also been reported in one subject each in clinical trials of red clover.

Theoretically, because red clover contains isoflavones, which are a class of phytoestrogens, any adverse effects associated with estrogen, such as breast tenderness, endometrial hyperplasia, menstrual changes, and weight gain, are possible. That being said, none of these have been reported in clinical trials of red clover.

Red clover contains coumarins and coumarin derivatives, and may theoretically interfere with platelet aggregation, increasing the risk of bleeding. There are currently no case reports or evidence from research to support this effect.

Cautions/Contraindications

Red clover should not be given to children under the age of 2 until its effect on the reproductive tract in children is determined. Red clover is not recommended during pregnancy and breastfeeding because of its estrogenic effects.

Drug Interactions

There are no clinically documented interactions between red clover and any medications. However, there are a number of theoretically possible interactions, including

- **Anticoagulant and antiplatelet drugs:** Red clover contains coumarin and coumarin derivatives, and may theoretically enhance the effects of anticoagulant and antiplatelet agents, such as heparin or warfarin.

- **Drugs metabolized via cytochrome P450:** In one in vitro study, red clover was found to inhibit the cytochrome P450 enzyme CYP 3A4. Drugs metabolized by this enzyme may accumulate or fail to be effective when taken with red clover.

- **Hormone replacement therapy drugs (HRT):** Red clover contains isoflavones, a class of phytoestrogens that mimic natural estrogens or estradiol and may enhance or block estrogen receptors. Simultaneous use of red clover with HRTs (for example tamoxifen or raloxifene) may enhance or inhibit the estrogenic effects.

- **Non-steroidal anti-inflammatory drugs (NSAIDs):** Red clover contains coumarin and coumarin derivatives, and may theoretically enhance the effects of NSAIDs, such as aspirin.

- **Oral contraceptive pill (OCP):** Red clover contains isoflavones, a class of phytoestrogens that mimic natural estrogens or estradiol and may enhance or block estrogen receptors. Simultaneous use of red clover with OCPs may enhance or inhibit the estrogenic effects.

Dosage Regimens
General
- Dried flower head: 4 g or by infusion three times daily.
- Liquid extract (1:1 in 25% alcohol): 1.5–3 mL three times daily.
- Tincture (1:10 in 45% alcohol): 1–2 mL three times daily.

Specific
- Menopausal symptoms : 40–80 mg isoflavones from red clover daily.
- Hypercholesterolemia : 28.5–85.5 mg isoflavones from red clover daily.
- Osteoporosis : 40 mg isoflavones from red clover daily.
- Prostate conditions : 40 mg isoflavones from red clover daily.

Standardized formulations
- Promensil: each tablet is standardized to contain 40 mg isoflavones from red clover: 4 mg genistein, 3.5 mg daidzein, 24.5 mg biochanin A, and 8 mg formononetin.
- Rimostil: each tablet is standardized to contain 57 mg isoflavones from red clover.
- Trinovin: each tablet is standardized to contain 40 mg isoflavones from red clover.

Note: Not recommended for children.

Selected References

Blakesmith S, Lyons-Wall P, George C, Joannou G, Petocz P, Samman S. Effects of supplementation with purified red clover (*Trifolium pratense*) isoflavones on plasma lipids and insulin resistance in healthy premenopausal women. British Journal of Nutrition 2003; 89:467–74.

Hidalgo L, Chedraui P, Morocho N, Ross S, San Miguel G. The effect of red clover isoflavones on menopausal symptoms, lipids, and vaginal cytology in menopausal women: A randomized, double-blind, placebo-controlled study. Gynecological Endocrinology 2005;21(5): 257–64.

Van de Weijer P, Barentsen R. Isoflavones from red clover (Promensil) significantly reduce menopausal hot flash symptoms compared with placebo. Maturitas 2002;42:187–93.

Red Raspberry

Rubus idaeus L.

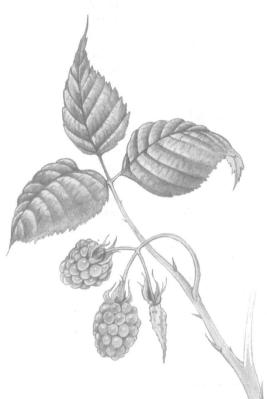

THUMBNAIL SKETCH

Common Uses
- Pregnancy aid
- Diarrhea

Active Constituents
- Tannins

Adverse Effects
- None known

Cautions/Contraindications
- Pregnancy (concerns given lack of evidence)

Drug Interactions
- None known

Doses
- *Dried leaf:* 4–8 g taken as an infusion three times daily
- *Liquid extract (1:1 in 25% ethanol):* 4–8 mL three times daily

Introduction

Family
- Rosaceae

Synonyms
- Raspberry
- Framboisier
- Wild raspberry
- Rubus
- Hindberry

Medicinal Forms
- Dried leaves
- Liquid extract

Description
Red raspberry is a deciduous shrub, native to Europe and Asia but now widespread in North America, growing wild and cultivated primarily for its fruit. The plant grows 2 meters (5 to 6 feet) tall, with prickly woody stems, small green leaves, and red berries.

Parts Used
Many fruit berries are used for their medicinal properties. In this case, the leaves rather than the berries are the part of the plant used therapeutically.

Traditional Use
The very astringent tannins in the red raspberry leaf have a drying effect and have long been taken as an infusion or tea for a number of reasons. Red raspberry leaf has a long history of use in women's health, most particularly during pregnancy. It has long been claimed that raspberry leaf tea is used to "cleanse and purify the blood."

Current Medicinal Use
Red raspberry is an herbal medicine steeped in tradition but with little modern evidence to support its use. Because of the lack of clear scientific evidence, the German Commission E has suggested that no therapeutic use can be recommended for red raspberry at this time. Nevertheless, under the supervision of an appropriately trained health-care practitioner, red raspberry is often used to aid pregnancy. The nutritious value of the berries should also not be forgotten, as they are rich in many vitamins and minerals.

Relevant Research

Preventative and Therapeutic Effects

Constituents
- Tannins: gallotannins, elagitannins.
- Miscellaneous: flavonoids (rutin), polypepetides.

Common Uses
Red raspberry leaf is considered by many herbalists to be particularly useful as a *partus praeparator*, preparing the uterus for childbirth and aiding delivery. Red raspberry is arguably the most commonly used herbal medicine for childbirth and is recommended by a number of health-care professionals, including midwives, medical herbalists, and naturopaths. It is also often recommended in cases of morning sickness and as a general tonic in women's health. Due to the drying effect of the tannins, leaves are also used as a mouthwash in tonsillitis, to treat diarrhea, skin conditions and abrasions, and urinary tract infections, and even as an eye lotion in cases of conjunctivitis. Red raspberry leaf is also considered to useful for diabetes.

Extracts of red raspberry leaf have been shown to inhibit the contraction of rat uterus muscle and increase regularity of contractions in human uterine tissue. The actions appeared to be more pronounced in tissue taken from pregnant women rather than women who were not expecting. A published abstract makes mention of one Australian double-blind, randomized, placebo-controlled trial. While precise details of the study could not be found, it was suggested that when 1.2 g of raspberry leaf herb was taken twice daily from 32 weeks of gestation to commencement of labor, the second stage of labor was shortened and there was a lower rate of forceps delivery. While these results are promising, more research is needed before a definitive conclusion can be reached.

> *Red raspberry is arguably the most commonly used herbal medicine for childbirth and is recommended by a number of health-care professionals, including midwives, medical herbalists, and naturopaths.*

Adverse Effects
Red raspberry leaves appear to be quite safe in most cases. There are been no reported cases of significant adverse effects in the literature.

Cautions/Contraindications
The main controversy regarding red raspberry leaf is its use in pregnancy. The lack of any scientific studies to show that it is safe, together with the fact that it has been shown to act on uterine tissue, has led many to suggest that red raspberry leaf should not be taken in pregnancy. This goes against the recommendations of many complementary health-care providers, which are based on historical use of the product. In light of the lack of scientific evidence from clinical trials of both the safety and efficacy of red raspberry, many feel that the recommendation that it be used by pregnant women is inappropriate and may in fact be the most significant risk associated with this particular herbal medicine.

Drug Interactions
No drug interactions could be found for red raspberry leaf. Theoretically, the high tannin concentration may decrease the absorption of certain minerals, notably calcium and magnesium.

Dosage Regimens
- Dried leaf: 4–8 g taken as an infusion three times daily.
- Liquid extract (1:1 in 25% ethanol): 4–8 mL three times daily.

Selected References

Wilkinson J. What do we know about herbal morning sickness treatments? A literature review. Midwifery 2000;16(3):224–28.

Yarnell E. Botanical medicine in pregnancy and lactation. Alternative and Complementary Therapies 1997 April:93–101.

Saw Palmetto
Serenoa repens (Bartram) Small

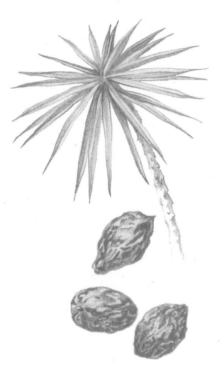

THUMBNAIL SKETCH

Common Uses
- Benign prostatic hyperplasia (BPH), or enlargement of the prostate gland

Active Constituents
- Fatty acids and sterols

Adverse Effects
- Gastrointestinal upset (rare)

Cautions/Contraindications
- Pregnancy and breastfeeding (safety not established)

Drug Interactions
- Hormonal therapy (theoretical)

Doses
- *Dried berries:* 0.5–1 g taken as a tea three times daily
- *Liquid extract:* 0.6–1.5 mL daily
- *Liposterolic extract:* 160 mg twice daily or 320 mg once daily

Introduction

Family
- Arecaceae (also known as Palmae)

Synonyms
- *Serenoa serrulata* (Michx.) Nichols.
- *Sabal serrulata* (Michx.) Nutall ex. Schultes & Schultes
- Sabal

Medicinal Forms
- Dried fruit berries
- Liquid extract

Description
The only surviving species of *Seronoa* is *Seronoa repens*, which can be found growing along the Atlantic coast of North America. The shrub grows up to 3 meters (10 feet) in height, with fan-shaped crowns of palm-like leaves bearing white flowers and dark red to deep purple oblong berries.

Parts Used
The dried berries are used medicinally.

Traditional Use
Historically, the ripe fruit was partially dried and used for a variety of conditions of the bladder, urethra, and prostate. It was called the plant catheter. This herb was considered primarily a "male" remedy and was used to "improve flagging reproductive function," as well as "debility and senility in men." Saw palmetto was also a food source for early settlers in North America.

Current Medicinal Use
Today, saw palmetto is best known for it use as a treatment for benign prostatic hyperplasia (BPH). Several excellent reviews have been written on this topic.

Relevant Research

Preventative and Therapeutic Effects

Constituents
- Fatty acids: lauric acid, linoleic acid, linolenic acid, capric acid, caproic acid, palmitic acid, oleic acid, caprylic acid, myristic acid, stearic acid.
- Phytosterols: beta-sitosterol, stigmasterol, campesterol.
- Alcohols: docosanol, hexacosanol, octacosanol, triacontanol.
- Miscellaneous: carotenes, lipase, tannins.

Benign Prostatic Hyperplasia (BPH)
A number of clinical studies on the effect of saw palmetto on benign prostatic hyperplasia have been completed to date, including open trials; double-blind, placebo-controlled trials; and double-blind trials comparing saw palmetto with other treatments. The majority of human clinical trials tested 160 mg of a liposterolic extract containing 85% to 95% fatty acids and sterols twice daily. This is equivalent to approximately 10 g of crude berries twice daily.

Four systematic reviews and meta-analyses have concluded that saw palmetto use is associated with a significant improvement in peak flow rate and reduction in nocturia (excessive urination at night) in men diagnosed with benign prostatic hyperplasia, compared with a placebo. One Cochrane review, which included 21 studies with a total of 3,139 men, concluded that, compared with finasteride, saw palmetto has been shown to produce similar improvement in urinary tract symptoms and urinary flow and has been associated with fewer adverse effects in clinical trials.

In addition, several clinical trials have concluded that saw palmetto is equally as effective as tamsulosin (an alpha blocker). For example, in a large (N=811) randomized, double-blind comparison study, saw palmetto (Permixon, 320 mg daily) was found to be equivalent to tamsulosin in the treatment of symptoms of benign prostatic hyperplasia over a 12-month period. Two years later, 124 patients from this study with severe lower urinary tract symptoms were evaluated in another 12-month study, and saw palmetto (Permixon, 320 mg daily) was found to be slightly superior to tamsulosin after 3 months and for up to 12 months of treatment. An open-label, 6-month, three-arm study in 2007 including 320 mg saw palmetto per day (N=20), tamsulosin 0.4 mg/day (N=20), and a combination of saw palmetto and tamsulosin (N=20) found that saw palmetto and tamsulosin are equally effective alone, and combined therapy does not provide additional benefits. Several herbal blends containing saw palmetto have also been reported to be effective in the management of BPH symptoms.

Four systematic reviews and meta-analyses have concluded that saw palmetto use is associated with a significant improvement in peak flow rate and reduction in nocturia (excessive urination at night) in men diagnosed with benign prostatic hyperplasia.

However, a recent review indicated that newer studies of better methodological quality put earlier conclusions about the documented effect into question. Two double-blind, placebo-controlled, randomized trials published after the 2002 Cochrane review compared the effect of saw palmetto extract with a placebo for treatment of benign prostatic hyperplasia. The 12-week trial of 100 patients found that 320 mg saw palmetto provided some improvement in symptoms of benign prostatic hyperplasia, but the beneficial effect was insignificant. A 1-year trial including 225 patients found that 320 mg (160 mg twice a day) saw palmetto showed no significant differences compared to the placebo and did not improve symptoms of benign prostatic hyperplasia. Currently, these negative trials do not outweigh the positive evidence, but more research is needed to draw a conclusion in this ongoing debate.

Anti-BPH Activity

Most saw palmetto products are composed of "liposterolic extracts" (i.e., containing the fatty acids and sterols) of the fruit. There are three primary mechanisms by which these extracts appear to work against benign prostatic hyperplasia:

1. **Androgen receptor blockade:** Dihydrotestosterone is an active androgen (more active than testosterone), which has been implicated as a causative factor benign prostatic hyperplasia.

2. **5a-reductase inhibition:** 5a-reductase catalyzes the metabolism of testosterone to dihydrotestosterone. One recent study does not support this hypothesis; however, the researchers used half the usual dose of saw palmetto (80 mg twice daily) in their experiments. Several recent in vitro studies that support this hypothesis suggest that the inhibition of saw palmetto extract is non-competitive in nature.

3. **Disruption of the arachidonic cascade:** Saw palmetto is reported to inhibit both the cyclo-oxygenase and lipoxygenase pathways, which is believed to result in an anti-inflammatory effect that will provide added relief for the symptoms of benign prostatic hyperplasia.

In addition, saw palmetto has a phyto-estrogenic effect — it appears to compete with endogenous estrogen for receptor sites. One research team suggests that this may play a key role in its ability to decrease the symptoms of benign prostatic hyperplasia. It does not appear to affect plasma levels of testosterone, follicle-stimulating hormone, or luteinizing hormone. One study in rats demonstrated that saw palmetto extract was able to inhibit experimental estradiol- and testosterone-induced prostate enlargement.

Miscellaneous Effects

A randomized, double-blind, placebo-controlled pilot study with 26 patients reported that a product containing 200 mg saw palmetto (standardized for 85% to 95% liposterolic content) and 50 mg beta-sitosterol that was taken once or twice daily appeared to significantly improve andro-genetic alopecia (receding hairline and/or hair loss). The authors argue that these results justify the investigation of this combination product in larger clinical trials. Although no human clinical trials were available for review, saw palmetto has also been reported to be useful in the treatment of hirsutism (excessive hairiness).

Adverse Effects

Clinical trials report that saw palmetto is well-tolerated; however, the Food and Drug lists saw palmetto as an herb of unknown safety. There has been one case report of acute hepatitis and pancreatitis (inflammation of the liver and pancreas) after ingestion of saw palmetto. Symptoms resolved when saw palmetto was discontinued, but reemerged when it was used again. Gastrointestinal upset, due probably to the fatty nature of the extracts, is rare, but possible.

Cautions/Contraindications

Safety has not been established in pregnancy and breastfeeding.

Drug Interactions

Theoretically, because of its anti-androgen and estrogenic activity, saw palmetto may interact with existing hormonal therapy, including hormone replacement therapy (HRT) and contraceptive pills.

Dosage Regimens

- Dried berries: 0.5–1 g taken as a tea three times daily.
- Liquid extract: 0.6–1.5 mL daily.
- Liposterolic extract: 160 mg twice daily or 320 mg once daily.

Selected References

Bent S, Kane C, Shinohara K, Neuhaus J, Hudes ES, Goldberg H, et al. Saw palmetto for benign prostatic hyperplasia. The New England Journal of Medicine 2006 Feb 9; 354(6):557–66.

Boyle P, Robertson C, Lowe F, Roehrborn C. Updated meta-analysis of clinical trials of *Serenoa repens* extract in the treatment of symptomatic benign prostatic hyperplasia. British Journal of Urology International, Apr 2004;93(6):751–56.

Wilt T, Ishani A, MacDonald R. *Serenoa repens* for benign prostatic hyperplasia. Cochrane Database of Systematic Reviews 2002(3).

Scullcap

Scutellaria lateriflora L.

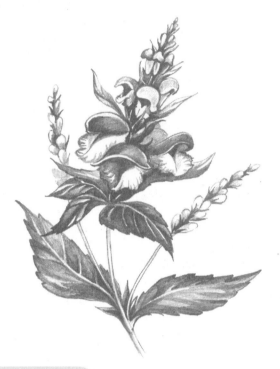

Introduction

Description

Many different species of the genus *Scutellaria* are used medicinally, although most texts identify *lateriflora* as the most common species. In addition, *Scutellaria baicalensis* Georgi (Baikal scullcap, or huang-qin) is a major medicinal herb used in traditional Chinese medicine. *Scutellaria lateriflora* is native to North America, where it still grows wild, reaching 60 centimeters (2 feet), with a straight stem and pink to blue flowers. The dried seed husks look like skullcaps. *Scutellaria baicalensis* is a perennial native to China, Japan, and Russia, with a fibrous root and erect stems growing up to 120 centimeters (4 feet), topped with purple flowers.

Parts Used

In the Western tradition, the aerial parts of *Scutellaria lateriflora* are used medicinally, whereas the roots of *Scutellaria baicalensis* (Baikal scullcap) are used in the traditional Chinese medical model.

Traditional Use

The Native peoples of North America used *Scutellaria lateriflora* for ailments associated with menstruation and breast pain. In the 19th century, herbalists used it to treat hysteria, epilepsy, convulsions, schizophrenia, and even rabies. In traditional Chinese medicine, *Scutellaria baicalensis* was used to treat fevers, colds, coughs, diarrhea, and dysentery.

Current Medicinal Use

Based on traditional evidence, scullcap is now primarily used to treat conditions of nervous tension and exhaustion, such as insomnia and anxiety.

Relevant Research

Preventative and Therapeutic Effects

Constituents

Since there is a lack of information specifically relating to *Scutellaria lateriflora* L., the information provided here refers to a number of species contained in the *Scutellaria* genus.

- Flavonoids: include apigenin, luteolin, scutellarin (baicalein, wogonin, baicalin are found in *S. baicalensis* Georgi).

- Volatile oils: primarily monoterpenes and sesquiterpenes.

- Iridoids: catalpol is found in both *S. lateriflora* and *S. galericulata* L.

- Miscellaneous: include tannins and resin.

Common Uses

Scutellaria lateriflora L. is reputed to have sedative, nervine, antispasmodic, and anti-convulsant properties. Oral consumption is considered useful in the treatment of conditions related to nervous tension and exhaustion. It is often used in patients with hysteria, spasms, or convulsions.

Miscellaneous Effects

Little or no clinical information could be found about the pharmacology of *Scutellaria lateriflora* L., with most of the available work referring to *Scutellaria baicalensis* Georgi. Extracts of *Scutellaria baicalensis* Georgi and its constituents have been shown in vivo and in vitro to inhibit lipid peroxidation, possess antibacterial and antiviral properties, influence arachidonate metabolism, influence the breakdown and synthesis of fats, decrease the release of histamine from rat mast cells, and decrease serum lipid levels. Given the different species and the fact that the aerial parts rather than the root are used in Western herbalism, it is unknown how applicable the above information is to scullcap products used medicinally in North America.

Adverse Effects

Large doses of scullcap can cause giddiness, confusion, drowsiness, and convulsions. In addition, herbal products containing scullcap as one of the ingredients have been implicated in a number of cases of liver toxicity, which has resulted in the removal of a number of herbal scullcap preparations from the market in the United Kingdom. Instances of liver toxicity may have been due to adulteration or substitution of scullcap with any of several species of germander (*Teucrium canadense* L., *T. chamaedrys* L., etc.).

> *Herbal products containing scullcap as one of the ingredients have been implicated in a number of cases of liver toxicity, which has resulted in the removal of a number of herbal scullcap preparations from the market in the United Kingdom.*

There is one case report of a 53-year-old Japanese man with recurrent interstitial pneumonia that appears to have been induced by scullcap (species not specified) contained in a traditional herbal medicine.

Cautions/Contraindications

Given the lack of information and the cases of possible liver toxicity mentioned above, products containing scullcap should not be used in pregnancy or while breastfeeding.

Drug Interactions

While no clinical examples could be found, given the reputed sedative action of scullcap, it should be used with caution in patients taking conventional centrally acting medications.

Dosage Regimens

- Dried herb: 0.5–2 g up to four times daily.
- Liquid extract (1:1 in 25% alcohol): 0.5–2 mL up to four times daily.
- Tincture (1:8 in 25% alcohol): 2–4 mL up to four times daily.

Selected References

Kimura Y, Okuda H, Taira Z, Shoji N, Takemoto T, Arichi S. Studies on *Scutellaria* radix; Part IX: New component inhibiting lipid peroxidation in rat liver. Planta Medica 1984; 50:290–95.

Kubo M, Kimura Y, Odani T, Tani T, Namba K. Studies on *Scutellaria* radix; Part II: The antibacterial substance. Planta Medica 1981; 43:194–201.

Kubo M, Matsuda H, Kimura Y, Okuda H, Arichi S. Studies on *Scutellaria* radix; Part X: Inhibitory effects of various flavanoids on histamine release from rat peritoneal mast cells in vitro. Chemical & Pharmaceutical Bulletin 1984; 32(12):5051–54.

Slippery Elm

Ulmus rubra Muhl.

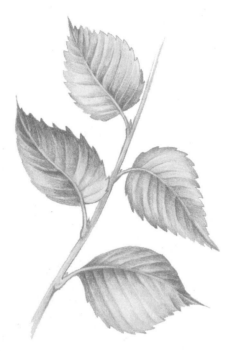

Common Uses

Internal
- Mucous membrane irritations (including gastritis peptic ulcer disease)
- Coughs, sore throats
- Diarrhea

Topical
- Sores, ulcers, and abscesses

Active Constituents
- Mucilage
- Tannins

Adverse Effects
- None known

Cautions/Contraindications
- Bark may be abortifacient (producing abortion)

Drug Interactions
- None known

Doses
- *Liquid extract (1:1 in 60% alcohol):* 5 mL three times daily
- *Decoction of powdered bark (1:8):* 4–16 mL three times daily
- *Lozenges:* Many proprietary lozenges containing slippery elm may be found on the North American market

Introduction

Family
- Ulmaceae

Synonyms
- *Ulmus fulva* Michx.
- Red elm
- Moose elm
- Indian elm
- American elm

Medicinal Forms
- Liquid extract
- Decoction of powdered bark
- Lozenges

Description
Slippery elm is a deciduous tree standing 15 to 20 meters (50 to 65 feet) in height that is native to the United States and Canada. The leaves are yellow to olive in color, and the fruit is winged and round. The bark has a brownish yellow outer surface and an inner yellow-white color, with a distinctive fenugreek-like odor. Commercial harvesting of the bark often results in the death of the tree.

Parts Used
The part used medicinally is the inner part of the bark.

Traditional Use
Slippery elm gained favor among the First Nations peoples. When the bark is mixed with water, it produces a thick, viscid mucilage that was used in conditions where the mucous membranes were inflamed and irritated, both externally and internally. It was also applied externally to sores, wounds, and abscesses. It was also often used as a food during convalescence because it is nutritious and easy to digest.

Current Medicinal Use
Based primarily on traditional evidence, slippery elm is used to treat inflammation of the mucosa membranes, notably in cases of gastritis, peptic ulcers, and diarrhea. Slippery elm is often available as lozenges to treat sore throats. In addition, the herb may also be used externally to sooth sores, ulcers, and abscesses.

Relevant Research

Preventative and Therapeutic Effects

Constituents
- Carbohydrates: complex mucilage containing a number of sugars.
- Miscellaneous: tannins, sesquiterpenes, calcium oxalate.

Common Uses
Slippery elm is reputed to have demulcent, nutrient, emollient, astringent, and antitussive (cough suppressant) properties. Oral consumption is considered useful in the treatment of any condition presenting with inflamed mucous membranes, including gastritis, peptic ulcer disease, enteritis, and colitis. Due to their astringent action, slippery elm products are also used within the herbal tradition to treat diarrhea and food poisoning. In addition, slippery elm is often taken as a lozenge for the relief of coughs and minor throat irritation. External application, usually as a poultice (a soft moist mass that is heated, medicated, and spread on cloth over the skin), is used for ulcers, boils, wounds, and abscesses.

No information on the pharmacology of slippery elm in particular could be found.

Research on other plant species has shown that mucilage has a demulcent action and that tannins have astringent properties.

> *Oral consumption is considered useful in the treatment of any condition presenting with inflamed mucous membranes, including gastritis, peptic ulcer disease, enteritis, and colitis.*

Adverse Effects

No adverse effects could be found on the use of this medicinal herb.

Cautions/Contraindications

Products prepared from the whole bark were traditionally used to induce abortion. However, it appears that the same caution is not applicable to powdered slippery elm.

Drug Interactions

None could be found.

Dosage Regimens

- Liquid extract (1:1 in 60% alcohol): 5 mL three times daily.
- Decoction of powdered bark (1:8): 4–16 mL three times daily. The decoction should be made in the following manner: Use 1 part of the powdered bark to 8 parts of water. Mix the powder in a little water initially to ensure it will mix. Bring to a boil and simmer gently for 10 to 15 minutes. Drink half a cup three times a day.
- Lozenges: Many proprietary lozenges containing slippery elm may be found on the North American market.

Note: Slippery elm is often mixed with other demulcents, notably marshmallow (*Althaea officinalis* L., Malvaceae).

Selected References

Slippery Elm, in B LaGow (editor). PDR for Herbal Medicines, 3rd ed. Montvale, NJ: Thomson PDR, 2004:736–38.

Slippery Elm, in CE Ulbricht and EM Basch (editors). Natural Standard Herb and Supplement Reference. Evidence-Based Clinical Reviews. St. Louis, MO: Elsevier Mosby, 2005:675–78.

St. John's Wort
(Hypericum perforatum L.)

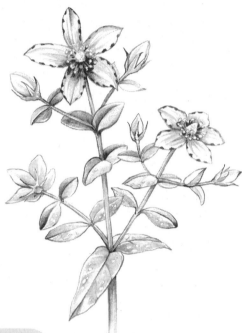

THUMBNAIL SKETCH

Common Uses
- Depression (mild to moderate)

Active Constituents
- Hypericin
- Isohypericin
- Protohypericin
- Flavonoids
- Hyperforin
- Adhyperforin

Adverse Effects
- Photosensitivity (skin reactions when exposed to sunlight)
- Gastrointestinal upset
- Dizziness
- Sedation
- Hypomania

Cautions/Contraindications
- Pregnancy and breastfeeding

Drug Interactions
- Combined oral contraceptives, cyclosporine, digoxin, general anesthesia, inidinivir, nefazadone, paroxetine, phenprocoumon, sertraline, theophylline, trazadone, warfarin, drugs causing photosensitivity

Dose
- *Standardized extract (standardized to 0.3% hypericin and/or 2% to 5% hyperforin): 350–1,800 mg daily in divided doses*
- *Dried herb: 2–4 g three times daily*

Introduction

Family
- Clusiaceae (also known as Guttiferae, sometimes placed in Hypericaceae)

Synonyms
- Hypericum
- Millepertuis
- Amber
- Goatweed
- Johnswort
- Klamath weed
- Tipton weed

Medicinal Forms
- Dried flowers
- Standardized extract

Description
St. John's wort is a shrub-like perennial plant that reaches a height of 60 centimeters (2 feet). The leaves grow from cylindrical or oval stems in an irregular, oblong shape and produce a red sap when crushed. The underside of the leaves is distinguished by pinpricks and black spots. The five-petal yellow flowers bloom in the summer months. The plant has a turpentine-like odor and a bitter, acidic flavor. It is indigenous to all of Europe and Asia but is now also found in North America, where it is listed as a noxious weed in many provinces and states due to its invasion of rangeland and photosensitization of livestock. This makes it necessary to take special precautions when the herb is being cultivated.

Parts Used
The flower tops and petals are used medicinally.

Traditional Use
St. John's wort has been recognized in the West as having medicinal properties since the classical period. The name itself has been associated with a colorful mythology involving Saint John the Baptist, and there are varied customs that use the plant as a talisman to ward off misfortune. It was mentioned in the texts of Hippocrates, Pliny, and Galen as helpful for wound healing and pain and as a diuretic. The use of this herb continued though the Renaissance and Victorian eras, when it was also used as a treatment for emotional and nervous complaints.

Current Medicinal Use
Both traditional and modern scientific evidence support the use of St. John's wort products in the treatment of mild to moderate depression.

Relevant Research

Preventative and Therapeutic Effects

Constituents
- **Anthraquinone derivatives:** hypericin, isohypericin, protohypericin, psuedohypericin.
- **Flavonoids:** quercetin, hyperoside, quercitrin, isoquercitrin, rutin, campherol, luteolin, I3-II8-biapigenin.
- **Prenylated phloroglucinols:** hyperforin, adhyperforin.
- Procyanidines.
- Phenols.
- Phloroglucinols.
- Tannins.
- Volatile oils.
- Xanthones.
- Miscellaneous organic acids, hydrocarbons, and alcohols.

Hyperforin and Hypericin

Extracts of St. John's wort contain many constituents that vary depending on the variety or genotype. All the main active compounds have yet to be identified definitively; however, studies suggest that the major constituent responsible for the antidepressant effects is hyperforin. Hyperforin exerts a similar potency as standard antidepressants by enhancing intracellular $Na+$ ion concentrations and non-competitively inhibiting synaptic reuptake of monoamines, serotonin, dopamine, noradrenaline, and the amino acid neurotransmitters gamma-aminobutyric acid (GABA) and glutamate. Hyperforin is also capable of stimulating IL-8 expression in human intestinal epithelia cells and primary hepatocytes, both of which participate in immune and inflammatory responses.

Additional constituents in St. John's wort, such as hypericin, may also play a role in its antidepressant action. The red-pigmented hypericins were found to be absorbed in a dose-dependent manner within 2 hours, to be widely distributed, and to have a plasma half-life of approximately 24 hours, allowing steady-state concentrations to be reached within days of thrice-daily dosing. Approximately 14% to 21% of the compounds were estimated to be systemically available. In vitro experiments localize hypericin primarily in the cytoplasmic membrane and cytoplasm, with smaller amounts in the nucleus.

Antidepressant Effects

Although there is considerable evidence that St. John's wort has some antidepressant effects, clinical recommendations about its use must be tempered at present by the lack of long-term human data and studies in severe depression, uncertainty about the mechanism of action and interaction with other medications, and concerns about standardization and regulation of the content of commercial products in North America.

Extracts of St. John's wort have reported affinities for a variety of neurotransmitter receptors, including adenosine, GABAA (gamma-aminobutyric acid A), GABAB, 5HT1 (5-hydroxytryptamine, or serotonin), central benzodiazepine, forskolin, inositol triphosphate, and the monoamine oxidase A and B enzymes. Based on the concentrations normally attained after oral administration, however, only GABA binding appears possible in vivo. Non-clinical studies have found evidence for inhibition of serotonin uptake, decreased serotonin receptor expression, inhibition of benzodiazepine binding, changes on animal behavioral tests of antidepressant activity, increased excretion of adrenergic metabolites, modulation of cytokine expression, and inhibition of monoamine oxidase. Changes in behavioral test outcomes of animal studies caused by St. John's wort extracts are similar to those documented with other antidepressants.

> *Although there is considerable evidence that St. John's wort has some antidepressant effects, clinical recommendations about its use must be tempered at present.*

Mild to Moderate Depression

In humans, there is evidence of efficacy in mild to moderate depression. While the majority of reviews are positive, they are not universally so. For example, several reviews have concluded that there is currently insufficient evidence to establish whether St. John's wort is as effective as conventional antidepressants. A 2005 Cochrane Collaboration review of St. John's wort for depression assessed 37 double-blind, randomized clinical trials, including 26 comparisons with a placebo (3,320 patients) and 14 comparisons with conventional synthetic antidepressants (2,283 patients). The outcomes of placebo-controlled trials were mixed, while the outcomes of trials comparing hypericum extracts and standard antidepressants suggested comparable beneficial effects. The authors emphasized that the quality of St. John's wort preparations can differ considerably, resulting in variable efficacy of St. John's wort extracts in different patient populations.

Overall, St. John's wort extracts improved symptoms more than a placebo and similar to synthetic antidepressants in adults with mild to moderate depression. In addition, fewer adverse effects were observed with hypericum extracts compared to standard antidepressants or SSRIs (selective serotonin reuptake inhibitors).

Compared to randomized controlled trials, observational studies may be more useful when investigating rare adverse effects and long-term outcomes. Another 2005 systematic review assessed 16 large-scale observational studies including a total of 34,804 patients and concluded that St. John's wort extracts are well tolerated and seem to be effective in routine treatment of mild to moderate depressive disorders.

St. John's wort extracts have been compared directly with several tricyclic antidepressants and found to be equally as effective as imipramine, maprotiline, and amitriptyline. However, these studies have been heavily criticized due to the small numbers of patients and the low doses of conventional tricyclic antidepressants to which the St. John's wort was compared.

St. John's wort has also been compared with selective serotonin reuptake inhibitor (SSRI) antidepressants. A systematic review of studies comparing St. John's wort extracts and fluoxetine in the management of subthreshold and mild depression concluded that there was no relevant difference in efficacy, based on the studies reviewed. The authors cautioned, however, that the St. John's wort products tested in the studies differed widely and that there was wide methodological variability in the studies reviewed, making it impossible to conduct a meta-analysis of the data.

Several additional studies have also reported that St. John's wort is as effective as fluoxetine and is associated with fewer

> *Overall, St. John's wort extracts improved symptoms more than a placebo and similar to synthetic antidepressants in adults with mild to moderate depression. In addition, fewer adverse effects were observed.*

adverse effects when used in the treatment of mild to moderate depression. A 4-week randomized, double-blind trial with 163 patients, which was completed later, reported that a St. John's wort extract containing 900 mg hypericum (LI 160), 20 mg fluoxetine, and a placebo are equally ineffective in short-term treatment of mild to moderate depression, but a similar 12-week trial with 135 patients at the same dose regimen found that St. John's wort was significantly more effective than fluoxetine and showed a trend toward superiority over a placebo. A Canadian study that compared the efficacy of St. John's wort (300 mg standardized for 0.3% hypericin given three times daily) and sertraline (50 mg daily) over a 12-week period concluded that there were no important differences between the two treatments and that significantly more adverse effects were reported by individuals taking sertraline. This finding is further supported by another American comparison trial.

Severe Depression

One systematic review in 2000 concluded that St. John's wort does not appear to be effective in the management of severe depression. A randomized, double-blind, placebo-controlled trial published after this review also reported that St. John's wort (standardized 900 mg/day for at least 4 weeks, increased to 1,200 mg/day if necessary for the second 4 weeks) was not effective (compared to a placebo) in treating 200 patients diagnosed with severe major depression, defined as Hamilton Depression Scale (HDS or HAMD) scores of 20 or more. The publication of this study generated significant debate.

The findings of this study are supported by another randomized, double-blind, controlled study with 340 patients that compared St. John's wort (250 mg twice daily of extract LI 160) to a placebo and fluoxetine (20 mg daily) in patients with severe depression (defined as Hamilton Depression Scale scores of 20 or more) over an 8-week period. In this study, neither treatment (St. John's wort nor fluoxetine) was found to be significantly better than the placebo on the two primary outcome measures of the trial (change in HDS total score and rates of full response). This study also stimulated much discussion. There were concerns, for example, that the trial had a low assay sensitivity for a number of reasons, including that there may have been a relatively large number of treatment-resistant participants, an inadequate assessment of the blinding, and use of an inclusion criteria of 20 or more on the Hamilton Depression Scale, which is higher than in many earlier trials.

> *St. John's wort does not appear to be effective in the management of severe depression.*

In contrast to the studies described above, a randomized, double-blind trial comparing 1,800 mg daily of St John's wort extract LI 160 to 150 mg daily of imipramine in 209 severely depressed patients from 20 psychiatric centers reported that both were equally effective (on the Hamilton Depression Scale) over the 6-week treatment period. Another randomized, double-blind 6-week trial comparing 900 mg daily of St. John's wort extract WS 5570 to 20 mg daily of paroxetine in 251 adult outpatients with acute major depression (score ≥ 22 on the HDS) reported that St. John's wort extract WS 5570 was at least as effective as paroxetine and was better tolerated in the treatment of moderate to severe major depression. In non-responsive patients, the doses were increased to 1,800 mg hypericum or 40 mg

paroxetine daily after 2 weeks, and a substantial decrease in the depression score was observed following the dose increase in both groups.

Antiretroviral Effects

Relatively recent investigations into the potential antiretroviral activity of St. John's wort have paralleled the search for other effective treatments for HIV infection and AIDS. Antibacterial and antifungal effects of some constituents have been demonstrated in vitro (in test tubes). Antiviral activity against Sindbis, human poliovirus 1, and herpes simplex virus 1 has been found in vitro. Murine cytomegalovirus and human immunodefficiency virus 1 (HIV-1) were also inactivated in vitro. Light was found to potentiate the antiviral effects both on isolated virions and on virally infected cells. No damage to the cultured cells was observed. Although the mechanism of the antiviral effects are not known, researchers have found evidence of the ability of the hypericins to inhibit protein kinase C. A more detailed review of the potential mechanisms is available.

The best data on the antiretroviral activity of hypericins come from a trio of papers from the *Proceedings of the National Academy of Sciences (PNAS)*. One paper reported in vitro and in vivo antiretroviral activity with little toxicity. The same group found increased survival in retrovirus-infected animals treated with hypericin and pseudohypericin. These compounds were thought to affect retrovirus assembly and to inactivate mature viral particles. Another paper reported that both hypericin and rose bengal (another pigmented compound) were able to photoinactivate enveloped viruses (human stomatitis and HIV) at nanomolecular concentrations. Fusion or hemolysis (breakdown of red blood cells) was inhibited in cells infected by these, as well as by Sendai and influenza viruses. In cells induced to express the HIV gp120 protein, sycytium formation with CD4+ cells was photoinhibited.

It is not clear whether these kinds of antiretroviral activities will be clinically significant in humans.

> *Relatively recent investigations into the potential antiretroviral activity of St. John's wort have paralleled the search for other effective treatments for HIV infection and AIDS.*

Miscellaneous Effects

Somatization Disorder

One randomized, double-blind, placebo-controlled 6-week study involving 151 patients reported that St. John's wort (600 mg daily of LI 160 extract) was significantly more effective than a placebo in treating the symptoms of somatization disorder, independent of depressive symptomatology. The findings of this study are supported by another randomized, double-blind, placebo-controlled 6-week study with 173 patients that found that daily administration of 600 mg of St. John's wort extract LI 160 is effective and safe in the treatment of somatoform disorders.

Polyneuropathy

One randomized, double-blind, placebo-controlled, crossover study with 47 patients reported that St. John's wort (3 tablets, each containing 900 mcg total hypericin, given daily) over 5 weeks had no effect on pain associated with polyneuropathy.

Menopause Symptoms and Lipid Metabolism

One randomized, double-blind, placebo-controlled 12-week study involving 77 individuals reported that a black cohosh and St. John's wort combination product (Gynoplus 264 mg tablets, each containing 84 mg hypericum dried extract) was effective in alleviating menopausal symptoms and providing benefits to lipid metabolism.

Smoking Cessation

In an open-label, uncontrolled pilot study, 28 smokers who had consumed 10 or more cigarettes per day for at least 1 year were randomized to receive 300 mg St. John's wort extract once or twice daily for 1 week before and continued for 3 months after a target quit date. The authors concluded that St. John's wort extract, in combination with individual motivational and behavioral support, did not appear to aid smoking cessation.

Premenstrual Syndrome

A prospective open-label, uncontrolled observational study of St. John's wort for the treatment of premenstrual syndrome (300 mg hypericum extract per day, standardized for 900 mg hypericin and given for two complete menstrual cycles) found significant reductions in all outcome measures. Following this pilot study, a randomized, placebo-controlled, double-blind trial was conducted (600 mg hypericum extract, standardized for 1,800 mg hypericin and given for two complete menstrual cycles) and the result was not statistically significant. The authors found a trend for St. John's wort to be superior to the placebo, however, and the lack of statistical significance was likely because the effects were small but the variability in the outcome measures were high.

Obsessive-Compulsive Disorder

Although a 12-week open-label trial with a fixed dose of 450 mg of 0.3% hypericin twice daily found a significant improvement in 12 obsessive-compulsive disorder patients, a 12-week, randomized, double-blind, placebo-controlled trial involving 43 patients given a flexible dose schedule of 600 to 1,800 mg St. John's wort daily found no significant difference when compared to the placebo. These authors also reported in a 12-week randomized, placebo-controlled, double-blind trial (N=40) that a flexible dose of 600 to 1,800 mg per day had no significant effect on the treatment of social anxiety disorder.

Mouth Ulcers

A randomized, placebo-controlled, double-blind trial (N=30) evaluating the efficacy of St. John's wort extract on the management of recurrent mouth sores over three episodes reported that hypericum mouthwash (0.5%) may be beneficial in the reduction of pain and healing time of recurrent mouth ulcers.

Adverse Effects

In general, there are few side effects associated with St. John's wort when used for depression. St. John's wort is associated with fewer adverse effects than conventional antidepressants, but they may include photodermatitis (skin reactions to UV rays of the sun, though this adverse affect is very rare), gastrointestinal irritation, dizziness, dry mouth, nosebleeds, sedation, restlessness, constipation, serotonin syndrome–like symptoms, hair loss, an elevation in thyroid-stimulating hormone levels, sexual dysfunction (appears to be very rare), induction of mania or hypomania, and hypertensive crisis.

> *In general, there are few side effects associated with St. John's wort when used for depression. St. John's wort is associated with fewer adverse effects than conventional antidepressants.*

There has been one case report of a patient experiencing a first episode of psychosis after taking an extract of St. John's wort for the treatment of depression. One patient died from bone marrow necrosis while taking St. John's wort for depression; however, it is not clear if his death was in any way related to his use of St. John's wort. Characteristic EEG (electroencephalography, a measurement of electrical activity produced by the brain) and sleep changes seen with tricyclic antidepressants are not observed with St. John's wort, although there is some shortening of evoked potential latencies and enhancement of theta and beta-2 regions in the resting EEG.

Cautions/Contraindications

Prolonged or intense exposure to sunlight should be avoided by patients ingesting St. John's wort. St. John's wort should by used with caution by pregnant or lactating women due to the lack of available research establishing the herb's safety in these populations.

Drug Interactions

Several reviews of drug interactions with St. John's wort exist. Cases describing possible drug interactions between St. John's wort and the following drugs have been reported:

- Atorvastatin (resulting in increased serum level of LDL cholesterol and total cholesterol)
- Combined oral contraceptive (resulting in decreased hormone levels, break-through bleeding and pregnancy)
- Cyclosporine (resulting in decreased cyclosporine levels)
- Digoxin (resulting in decreased digoxin levels)
- General anesthesia (resulting in delayed emergence)
- Indinavir (resulting in decreased indinavir levels)
- Nefazodone (resulting in symptoms of serotonin syndrome)
- Paroxetine (resulting in symptoms of serotonin syndrome)
- Phenprocoumon
- Sertraline (resulting in symptoms of serotonin syndrome)
- Theophylline (resulting in decreased theophylline levels)
- Trazadone (resulting in symptoms of serotonin syndrome)
- Warfarin (resulting in decreased warfarin levels)

St. John's wort appears to induce cytochrome P450 enzymes, specifically CYP 1A2, CYP 3A2, and CYP3A4, thus enhancing the metabolism of these medications — and potentially others. St. John's wort has also been reported to reduce the expression of serotonin receptors. A 2-week washout period is recommended between usage of St. John's wort and a selective serotonin reuptake inhibitor (SSRI), such as paroxetine or fluoxetine. In addition, it probably actives P-glycoprotein, which can further increase the elimination of many drugs.

Until more information is available, the following drugs should also be used with caution in combination with St. John's wort:

- Anticonvulsants: carbamazepine, phenobarbitone, phenytoin.
- HIV protease inhibitors: indinavir, nelfinavir, ritonavir, saquinavir.
- HIV non-nucleoside reverse transcriptase inhibitors: elfavirenz, nevirapine.
- Monoamine oxidase onhibitors (MAOIs): phenelzine, tranylcypromine, isocarboxazid.
- Selective serotonin reuptake inhibitors (SSRIs): fluoxetine.
- Sympathomimetics: amphetamines, ephedrine (found in many cold and hay fever remedies), methyldopa, dopamine, levodopa, trytophan.
- Triptans: sumatriptan, naratriptan, rizatriptan, zolmitriptan.

Theoretically, St. John's wort may also have an additive effect with other drugs that cause photosensitization (e.g., piroxicam, tetracycline, and others).

Dosage Regimens

- Standardized extract (standardized to 0.3% hypericin and/or 2% to 5% hyperforin): 350–1,800 mg daily in divided doses.
- Dried herb: 2–4 g three times daily.

Selected References

Gaster B, Holroyd J. St John's wort for depression: A systematic review. Archives of Internal Medicine 2000;160(2):152–56.

Linde K, Knuppel L. Large-scale observational studies of hypericum extracts in patients with depressive disorders — a systematic review. Phytomedicine 2005;12:148–57.

Linde K, Mulrow CD, Berner M, Egger M. St. John's Wort for depression (review). The Cochrane Library 2005;2.

Miller LG. Drug interactions known or potentially associated with St. John's wort. Journal of Herbal Pharmacotherapy 2001;1(3):51–64.

Werneke U, Horn O, Taylor DM. How effective is St. John's wort? The evidence revisited. Journal of Clinical Psychiatry 2004 May; 65:611–17.

Tea Tree Oil

Melaleuca alternifolia
(Maiden & Betche) Cheel

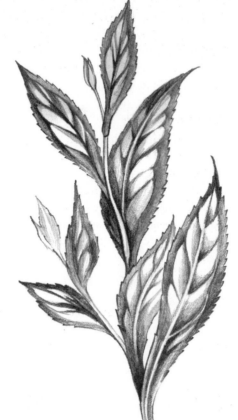

THUMBNAIL SKETCH

Common Uses
- Fungal infections

Active Constituents
- Terpinen-4-ol

Adverse Effects
- Skin irritation

Cautions/Contraindications
- Oral administration

Drug Interactions
- None found

Doses
- No guidelines could be found, but products should contain 30% or more terpinen-4-ol and less than 15% cineole

Introduction

Family
- Myrtaceae

Synonyms
- Melaleuca

Medicinal Forms
- Essential oil

Description
Tea tree is a member of the myrtle family and is found only in Southeastern Australia. The tree grows to a height of 6 meters (20 feet), with layered, paper-like bark, narrow, pointed leaves, and white to yellow, brush-shaped flowers.

Parts Used
The essential oil produced from steam distillation of the leaves is the part used medicinally.

Traditional Use
The indigenous people of Australia have long prized the aromatic leaves both for religious purposes and for medicinal use as an antiseptic and antifungal agent in treating skin, oral, and vaginal infections. Its name comes from the fact that a "tea" was made from it by the early European settlers. Due to increased popular demand, the commercial production of Australian tea tree oil increased in the early 1990s from 20 to 140 tonnes per annum. In addition to its medicinal applications, it is now used extensively in the cosmetic and skin-care industry.

Current Medicinal Use
Tea tree oil products are now primarily used as creams and gels in the treatment of fungal infections, such as athlete's foot and infections of the nail beds.

Relevant Research

Preventative and Therapeutic Effects
Constituents
- Volatile oil: contains various terpenes, including terpinen-4-ol, pinene, terpinene, cymene, cineole.

Common Uses
The essential oil is considered to be both an antiseptic and an antimicrobial. It is reputed to be useful in the management of many conditions, including acne, fungal infections (tinea pedis, or athlete's foot; onychomycosis, or fungal infection of the nail; ringworm), vaginal yeast infections, oral thrush, and a number of skin conditions.

Antimicrobial Effect
Tea tree oil has been reported to act against a number of bacteria, fungi, and yeasts, most notably *Candida* species, *Trichophyton rubrum*, and *Staphylococcus aureus* in vivo. It appears that *Staphylococcus aureus* is less susceptible to tea tree oil than *Candida albicans*. A small (N=30) pilot randomized controlled study compared a 4% tea tree oil nasal ointment and 5% tea tree oil body wash with the usual care (2% mupirocin nasal ointment and triclosan body wash) for the eradication of methicillin-resistant *Staphylococcus aureus* carriage. The authors report that "the tea tree oil combination appeared to perform better than the standard combination, although the

difference was not statistically significant due to the small number of patients." Additional research in this area appears warranted.

> *Tea tree oil has been reported to act against a number of bacteria, fungi, and yeasts, most notably* Candida species, Trichophyton rubrum, *and* Staphylococcus aureus *in vivo.*

Effect on Acne Vulgaris

In a clinical trial of 124 patients suffering from acne vulgaris, the effectiveness of a 5% tea tree oil gel was compared to that of a 5% benzoyl peroxide lotion after 3 months. While the tea tree oil product was considered effective, it had a longer onset of action and it was found to be less active on the inflamed lesions than the benzoyl peroxide product. However, the tea tree oil treatment resulted in an appreciably lower incidence of side effects, including skin dryness, pruritis (itchiness), and skin scaling, than the benzoyl peroxide.

Topical Fungal Infections

In a randomized, double-blind trial of 104 patients suffering from tinea pedis (athlete's foot), the effectiveness of a tea tree oil cream (10%) was compared to 1% tolnaftate cream or a placebo. Outcome measures included culture and clinical symptoms (skin scaling, inflammation, itching, and burning). While the tea tree oil was shown to be as effective as tolnaftate and superior to the placebo in causing relief of symptoms, it was no better than the placebo with respect to the culture samples. The study was carried out over a 5-week period.

A second randomized, double-blind, controlled study (N=158) compared the safety and efficacy of 25% and 50% tea tree oil applied twice daily for 4 weeks in the treatment of interdigital tinea pedis. The authors concluded that both 25% and 50% tea tree oil were effective but that 25% tea tree oil was associated with fewer complications and thus should be recommended.

Another randomized, multi-center controlled trial in 117 patients suffering from onychomycosis (a superficial fungal infection that destroys the entire nail) compared the effectiveness of tea tree oil (100%) to a conventional treatment of 1% clotrimazole cream over 6 months. Comparable improvement (cure, clinical assessment, and subjective improvement) was seen in both groups. The two preparations were also comparable in cost and shared the same incidence of adverse effects (7%). Another randomized, double-blind, placebo-controlled 16-week trial of a cream containing 5% tea tree oil and 2% butenafine hydrochloride in 60 outpatients with onychomycosis reported that 80% of those using the cream were cured, as compared to no cures in the placebo group.

> *Many "tea tree oil products" used in the cosmetic and toiletries industry contain only small amounts of active substance, and the medicinal efficacy is often questionable.*

A randomized, single-blind, placebo-controlled 4-week study in 126 patients with mild to moderate dandruff reported that 5% tea tree oil was more effective than the placebo and appeared to be well tolerated. Additional research is needed to confirm these findings.

Miscellaneous Effects

One placebo-controlled, investigator-blinded, randomized pilot study (N=20) investigated tea tree oil gel (6%) for the treatment of recurrent herpes labialis and reported that the tea tree oil gel appeared to have some benefit over the placebo with respect to decreased time to re-epitheliazation (growth of new skin) after treatment and reduction in median duration of culture positivity. None of the differences between the tea tree oil group and the placebo group reached statistical significance, but the authors argue that this is likely due to the small sample size in this pilot study and recommend a larger study to confirm these preliminary findings.

Adverse Effects

Tea tree oil is considered very mildly irritating on topical application but strongly irritant following oral administration. It is not considered to result in either sensitization or phototoxicity; however, it is recommended that care should be taken when using very concentrated tea tree oil products in children and fair-skinned individuals.

Cautions/Contraindications

Given the lack of guidelines available, tea tree oil should not be administered orally.

Drug Interactions

No cases of interactions between conventional therapy and tea tree oil could be found.

Selected References

Buck D, Midorf D, Addino J. Comparison of two topical preparations for the treatment of onychomycosis: *Melaleuca alternifolia* (tea tree) oil and clotrimazole. Journal of Family Practice 1994;38:601–5.

Satchell AC, Saurajen A, Bell C, Barnetson RS. Treatment of interdigital tinea pedis with 25% and 50% tea tree oil solution: A randomized, placebo-controlled, blinded study. Australian Journal of Dermatology 2002;43(3):175–78.

Dosage Regimens

No dosage guidelines for tea tree oil could be found. The Australian guidelines for terpinen-4-ol/cineole content should be considered when using a tea tree oil product therapeutically. In 1985, an Australian standard for oil of melaleuca was established, suggesting that the essential oil should contain 30% or more terpinen-4-ol and less than 15% cineole. One authority cautions, "It is important that the commercial product not be derived from other *Melaleuca* species, some of which contain high concentrations of cineole, a skin irritant that also reduces the antiseptic effectiveness of terpinen-4-ol."

Note: Preparations used in clinical trials range from 5% to 100%, but in general the concentrations of tea tree oil used in the clinical trials described are considerably lower than those often seen in clinical practice. Many "tea tree oil products" used in the cosmetic and toiletries industry contain only small amounts of active substance, and the medicinal efficacy is often questionable.

Thyme

Thymus vulgaris L.

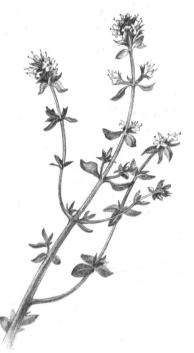

THUMBNAIL SKETCH

Common Uses
- Spasmodic respiratory conditions
- Dyspepsia (stomach pain)
- Parasites
- Fungal infections

Active Constituents
- Volatile oil (thymol and carvacrol)
- Flavonoids

Adverse Effects (Volatile Oil Portion)
Oral
- Nausea, vomiting, gastric distress
- Headache, dizziness, convulsions, coma
- Cardiac and respiratory collapse

Topical
- Skin irritations (moderate)

Cautions/Contraindications
- Pregnancy

Drug Interactions
- None known

Doses
Oral
- *Dried herb:* 1–4 g (often taken as an infusion)
- *Tincture (1:5 in 45% alcohol):* 2–6 mL three times daily
- *Tincture (1:10 in 70% alcohol):* 40 drops up to three times daily

Topical
- Thyme oil should be used only after dilution with a suitable carrier oil

Introduction

Family
- Lamiaceae (also know as Labiatae, or mint)

Synonyms
- Common thyme
- French thyme
- Garden thyme
- Rubbed thyme

Medicinal Forms
- Dried herb
- Liquid extract
- Tincture
- Oil

Description
Thyme is a shrub native to Mediterranean Europe but also cultivated throughout Northern and Central Europe and North America. It is an evergreen standing up to 45 centimeters (18 inches) in height, with multiple hairy stems arising from a single woody, fibrous root and mauve to pink flowers. Like other members of the mint family, it is rich in volatile oils, producing a characteristic aromatic scent.

Parts Used
The aerial parts are used medicinally as a dried herb or as an oil, which is extracted from the leaves and flowering tops by steam distillation. Two oils exist, the red oil and the white oil. The red oil is made by redistilling the white oil and has often been found to be adulterated. Many subspecies exist, and this can result in differences in the medicinal action and composition of the volatile oil, primarily due to differences in the proportion of phenols.

Traditional Use
Thyme has been a popular medicinal plant among British herbalists, praised by Nicholas Culpepper and used externally as an antiseptic and internally as a tonic for treating coughs and strengthening the respiratory system. The herb is also used widely for culinary purposes.

Current Medicinal Use
As with its traditional uses, thyme is primarily used now in cough mixtures for irritating spasmodic coughs and as an aid to digestion.

Relevant Research

Preventative and Therapeutic Effects

Constituents
- Volatile oils: contain monoterpenoids, predominately the phenols thymol and carvacrol, as well as unsubstituted cymene and terpinene and the alcohols alpha-terpineol, linalool, thujan-4-ol.

- Phenylpropanoids: include eugenol, caffeic acid, rosmarinic acid.

- Triterpenes: includeursolic acid, oleanolic acid.

- Miscellaneous: include flavonoids, dimethylbiphenyl, tannins.

Common Uses
Thyme is reputed to have many therapeutic actions, including carminative (relieves cramps and gas in the gastrointestinal tract), antimicrobial and antiseptic, expectorant (dissolves thick mucus to relieve respiratory symptoms), cough suppressant, and diaphoretic (increases sweating) actions. Oral consumption is considered useful in the treatment of conditions associated with spasm, including upper respiratory tract conditions (e.g., bronchitis, whooping cough, and asthma) and digestive upset. It is also used both orally and topically for a number of parasitic and fungal infections.

> *Oral consumption is considered useful in the treatment of conditions associated with spasm, including upper respiratory tract conditions (e.g., bronchitis, whooping cough, and asthma) and digestive upset.*

Miscellaneous Effects

Antispasmodic Effect

General antispasmodic activity and specific bronchospasmolytic action has been demonstrated in vitro. The flavonoid and phenolic components are thought to be responsible for this property, with calcium channel antagonism proposed as a mechanism of action.

Antibacterial and Antifungal Effects

The volatile oil has been shown to possess antibacterial and antifungal activity in vitro. The antibacterial action against *Staphylococcus aureus* was shown to be decreased by agents known to inhibit the action of the phenolic components. An aqueous extract of thyme has been reported to inhibit *Helicobacter pylori* in vitro.

Other Effects

Antimutagenic properties have been demonstrated in vitro. Thyme oil has also been shown to increase respiration and exert a hypotensive action in a number of animal models. Rosmarinic acid has also been shown to exert an anti-inflammatory action in both in vivo and in vitro models. Dimethylbiphenyl and a flavonoid, eriodictyol, have been shown to exert profound antioxidant action, possibly by inhibiting superoxide generation.

Adverse Effects

Thyme oil is considered a moderate skin irritant and a strong mucous membrane irritant. Adverse effects of the volatile oil include nausea, vomiting, digestive distress, headache, dizziness, sweating, convulsions, coma, and respiratory and/or cardiac collapse. Local irritation has resulted from the use of toothpaste containing thyme extracts. In addition, a case of occupational asthma was noted in an individual in contact with a number of aromatic herbs, including thyme. A sensitivity to thyme was confirmed later by skin prick test.

Cautions/Contraindications

Thyme is reputed to be a uterine stimulant and so should be used with caution in pregnancy, especially if given in high doses. Experimentally, cross-sensitivity with other members of the mint (Laminaceae) family has been noted.

Drug Interactions

No cases of drug interaction could be found.

Dosage Regimens
- Dried herb: 1–4 g (often taken as an infusion) or 0.5–1 g in children under 1 year of age several times a day.
- Tincture (1:5 in 45% alcohol): 2–6 mL three times daily.
- Tincture (1:10 in 70% alcohol): 40 drops up to three times daily.

Note: Thyme oil should be applied topically only after it has been diluted with a suitable carrier oil.

Selected Reference

European Scientific Cooperative on Phytomedicine. Thymi Herba/Thyme. Monographs (Fascicule 1). Exeter: 1996.

Turmeric

Curcuma longa Linn.

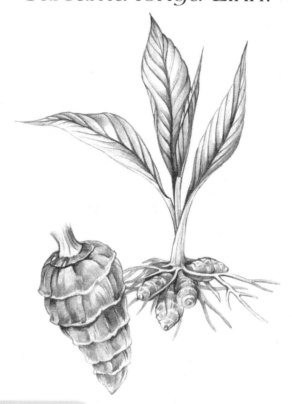

Common Uses
- Inflammation (e.g., arthritis)
- Liver disorders
- Gastrointestinal conditions

Active Constituents
- Curcumin

Adverse Effects
- Allergic reactions (rare)
- Gastrointestinal (rare and usually mild)

Cautions/Contraindications
- Bile duct blockage and gallstones
- Pregnancy and breastfeeding (safety not yet established)

Drug Interactions
- None reported in humans
- Anticoagulants and antiplatelet medications (theoretical)

Doses
- *Dried root:* 1.5–3 g three times daily
- *Curcumin:* 250–500 mg daily in divided doses

Introduction

Family
- Zingiberaceae

Synonyms
- *Curcuma domestica* Val.
- Curcuma
- Indian saffron

Medicinal Forms
- Dried root (rhizome)

Description
Turmeric is a perennial herb, native to Southern Asia and cultivated throughout the tropics, including many parts of the Caribbean. A member of the ginger family, this herb grows to 90 centimeters (3 feet) in height and produces large, oblong leaves that arise from a tuberous rhizome with a distinctive bright orange-yellow pulp.

Parts Used
The parts used medicinally are the primary and secondary rhizomes, which are usually cured (i.e., boiled, cleaned, and sun-dried) and polished.

Traditional Use
Turmeric has been used historically for both its flavor (e.g., it is a major ingredient in curry powder) and its color (e.g., it is used in the preparation of mustard). Turmeric is used medicinally in both traditional Chinese and Ayurvedic medicine for a variety of inflammatory conditions (arthritis and allergies), liver disorders (jaundice), flatulence, menstrual difficulties, bruises, and colic.

Current Medicinal Use
Turmeric products are primarily used today in the treatment of joint inflammation, such as arthritis and sports injuries. It is increasingly becoming popular in protecting the liver against environmental toxins.

Relevant Research

Preventative and Therapeutic Effects

Constituents
- Volatile oil: turmerone, zingiberene, bisabolane, guaiane, curlone, curcumin.
- Miscellaneous: sugars (including glucose, fructose, arabinose), resins, protein, vitamins, minerals.

Note: Curcumin is a phenylpropanoid derivative responsible for the characteristic yellow color, as well as the main pharmacological activity.

Curcumin
Curcumin is reported to be a potent anti-inflammatory component — its action is said to be comparable to hydrocortisone and phenylbutazone. Several hypotheses have been offered regarding its mechanism of action, including: (1) it has an indirect action via the adrenal cortex (2) it inhibits cortisone metabolism in the liver, thus increasing the amount of circulating cortisone; (3) it inhibits 5-lipoxygenase; and (4) it inhibits lipopolysaccharide (LPS)-induced production of tumor necrosis factor (TNF) and interleukin-1(IL-1) beta.

In addition, curcumin has been shown to have a variety of other direct effects, including inhibition of leukotriene formation and platelet aggregation, as well as increasing the breakdown of fibrin and promoting liver

> *Curcumin is reported to be a potent anti-inflammatory component – its action is said to be comparable to hydrocortisone and phenylbutazone.*

function in a variety of ways. Turmeric has also been reported to increase bile secretion and bile flow. It has also been shown to have a significant antioxidant activity.

Anti-Inflammatory Effects

Several experimental models have demonstrated the anti-inflammatory activity of the volatile oil component of turmeric, as well as curcumin and its analogs.

Rheumatoid Arthritis

Several clinical studies have reported curcumin's effectiveness in the treatment of rheumatoid arthritis. One study found that symptoms such as joint swelling, walking speed, and morning stiffness were improved to the same degree in patients taking either curcumin (1,200 mg daily) or phenylbutazone (300 mg daily). Another used the postoperative inflammation model for evaluating non-steroidal anti-inflammatory drugs (NSAIDs) and found 400 mg of curcumin to be as effective as 100 mg of phenylbutazone.

Gastrointestinal Effects

Turmeric has a long history of use in the management of ulcer conditions, though the evidence supporting its use is not consistently positive. Despite this, the German Commission E has approved turmeric as an effective cholagogue and digestive aid. In one study, in which turmeric was given at a dose of 250 mg three times daily, it relieved ulcer pain, but another randomized, double-blind, placebo-controlled trial of 130 patients newly diagnosed with duodenal ulcers reported no significant difference in the symptom relief of those receiving turmeric (6 g daily in three divided doses) when compared with

those taking a placebo after the 8-week study period.

A randomized double-blind study of 116 individuals with dyspepsia reported that turmeric (250 mg dried root containing 0.02 mL of volatile oil and 0.024 g of total curcuminoids) resulted in statistically significant clinical improvement compared to a placebo. Techniques used to measure symptom improvements were not described, and further research is needed to confirm these preliminary findings.

> *Turmeric has a long history of use in the management of ulcer conditions, though the evidence supporting its use is not consistently positive.*

Liver Effects

Historically, turmeric was used for a variety of liver conditions. Experimental evidence from animal studies confirms that it appears to increase bile flow and may play a role in protecting the liver from toxins. In addition, a related species, *Curcuma xanthorrhiza* Roxb., has been shown in animal experiments to provide protection from hepatotoxin-induced liver damage. However, a review of the literature did not find any human studies that investigated turmeric's efficacy for these indications.

Anticancer Effects

Animal studies suggest that curcumin may have an inhibitory effect on a variety of experimentally induced cancers, including carcinogen-induced cancers of the duodenum, colon, and forestomach in mice, Ehrlich ascites tumor in mice, carcinogen-induced skin tumor formation in mice, aflatoxin-induced hepatocarcinogenicity in rats, and carcinogen-induced cancer of the oral mucosa in hamsters. In vitro experiments have shown that curcumin may inhibit the growth of estragen-positive human breast

MCF-7 cells induced by a variety of carcinogens and that it is phototoxic to rat basophilic leukemia cells in the presence of oxygen. Researchers hypothesize that these effects are due in part to curcumin's antioxidant action (it appears to inhibit superoxide production). The clinical significance of these findings remains unknown.

Two case series, one assessing topical application of turmeric on the "foul smell" of cutaneous lesions associated with a variety of cancers and one investigating the effects of oral tumeric on urinary excretions of mutagens in "healthy" chronic cigarette smokers, reported beneficial results. However, the vague outcome measures and lack of control groups or blinding make these preliminary findings very difficult to interpret.

Anticholesterol Effects

Three case series provide preliminary evidence that orally ingested turmeric may lower serum low-density lipoprotein (LDL) and cholesterol levels. However, these were generally poorly described, and the absence of control groups, blinding, or randomization means additional research is needed to confirm these findings. Curcumin has also been reported to decrease cholesterol and lipid levels in animal studies.

Antimicrobial Effects

Several studies have reported that curcumin has the ability to inhibit the replication of human immunodeficiency virus (HIV). Researchers suggest that this activity is due in part to its inhibition of HIV-1 integrase. Clinical trials of curcumin in AIDS patients are reportedly scheduled. Turmeric has also been shown to have some nematocidal, antifungal, and antibacterial activity.

> *Several studies have reported that curcumin has the ability to inhibit the replication of human immunodeficiency virus (HIV).*

Miscellaneous Effects

A 12-week open-label clinical trial reported that 375 mg curcumin capsules taken three times daily alone (N=18) and in combination with antitubercular treatment (N=18) was effective in treating chronic anterior uveitis (inflammation of the eye) without any reported adverse effects. The efficacy and ability to prevent recurrences in a 3-year follow-up period were comparable to those reported in trials of corticosteroid therapy, presently the only standard treatment available for this disease. The authors suggest that the lack of adverse effects associated with curcurmin could be a significant advantage over corticosteroid therapy and recommend conducting a randomized, double-blind, clinical trial to confirm these preliminary findings.

Antioxidant properties have been reported in animal studies.

Adverse Effects

Very few adverse effects of turmeric or curcumin have been reported in clinical studies. In one clinical trial, a single patient reported itching at the site where the topical curcumin ointment was applied to the scalp. In another trial, a patient discontinued tumeric oil treatment after 3 days because of an allergic skin reaction. High doses of turmeric (e.g., 6 g daily) have been associated with gastrointestinal side effects, including epigastric burning, nausea, and diarrhea.

Cautions/Contraindications

Individuals with blockage of the common bile duct or gallstones should avoid consuming turmeric due to its reputed ability to increase bile flow. An animal study has demonstrated that the active constituents of turmeric are passed into breast milk. Safety in pregnancy and breastfeeding has not yet been established.

Drug Interactions

No known drug interactions have been reported in humans. However, based on animal and in vitro studies, turmeric may interact theoretically with anticoagulants and antiplatelet medications because turmeric has been found to inhibit platelet aggregation in animal studies and in vitro experiments.

Dosage Regimens
• Dried root: 1.5–3 g daily.

Note: The clinical trials reviewed used 400 mg curcumin three times daily.

Selected References

Satoskar RR, Shah SJ, Shenony SG. Evaluation of anti-inflammatory property of curcumin (di-feruloyl methane) in patients with post-operative inflammation. International Journal of Clinical Pharmacology Therapy and Toxicology 1986;24:651–54.

Thamlikitkul V, Bunyapraphatsara N, Dechatiwongse T, Theerapong S, Chantrakul C, Thanaveerasuwan T, et al. Randomized double-blind study of *Curcuma domestica* Val. for dyspepsia. Journal of the Medical Association of Thailand 1989;72(11):613–20.

Uva-Ursi

Arctostaphylos uva-ursi (L.) Spreng.

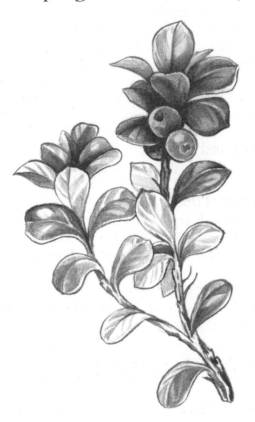

THUMBNAIL SKETCH

Common Uses
- Lower urinary tract infections (uncomplicated)

Active Constituents
- Phenolic glycosides (arbutin, methylarbutin)

Adverse Effects
- Nausea and vomiting
- Hydroquinone toxicity symptoms (large doses)

Cautions/Contraindications
- Pregnancy and breastfeeding
- Kidney disease

Drug Interactions
- None known

Doses
- *Dried leaves:* 1.5–4 g three times a day for a maximum of 2 weeks
- *Fluid extract (1:1 in 25% alcohol):* 1.5–4 mL three times a day for a maximum of 2 weeks

Introduction

Family
- Ericaceae

Synonyms
- Bearberry
- Common bearberry
- Beargrape
- Hogberry
- Rockberry
- Sandberry
- Mountain cranberry

Medicinal Forms
- Dried leaves
- Fluid extract

Description
Uva-ursi is a trailing evergreen shrub native to many regions of the Northern Hemisphere, including Canada. It produces small, leathery, oblong leaves and small, pale pink flowers. Bears are thought to like the sour red berries, giving rise to the popular name "bearberry." This also gave rise to its Latin binomial name, *Arctostaphylos*, meaning bearberry in Greek, and *uva-ursi*, meaning the same in Latin. The leaves, which are the part used medicinally, have an astringent and bitter taste.

Parts Used
The leaves are used medicinally.

Traditional Use
Uva-ursi has been considered one of the most effective herbal antiseptics for urinary tract (bladder and kidney) infections and cystitis. It has also been used to treat venereal diseases.

Current Medicinal Use
As with its traditional use, uva-ursi is still primarily used for uncomplicated urinary tract infections, such as cystitis.

Relevant Research

Preventative and Therapeutic Effects

Constituents
- Phenolic glycosides: arbutin (hydroquinone beta-glucoside), methylarbutin, piceoside, para-methoxyphenol.
- Flavonoids: include glycosides of quercetin, kaempferol, myricetin.
- Iridoids: monotropein, unedoside (root).
- Miscellaneous: include hydrolyzable tannins, ursolic acid, terpenoids, allantoin.

Common Uses
Uva-ursi is used primarily for its action as a urinary antiseptic, often in the management of uncomplicated infections of the lower urinary tract (e.g., cystitis, urethritis, and prostatitis). While it has been reported to be a diuretic, other research suggests that this is probably not the case. As a result of its astringent properties, uva-ursi has also been used in conditions of the lower digestive tract (e.g., diarrhea) and for enuresis. It is also reputed to be useful in bronchitis and urinary stones.

Antimicrobial Effect
The phenolic glycosides, especially arbutin, appear to be the primary active agents. However, the therapeutic effectiveness of uva-ursi is dependent on the conversion of these phenolic glycosides to a known antimicrobial agent, hydroquinone. Arbutin appears to be absorbed intact, undergoing hydrolysis in the urine to hydroquinone. It has been suggested that other agents in the whole extract may protect the arbutin from degradation in the gastrointestinal tract. Other researchers have argued that the conversion of arbutin to hydroquinone occurs

in the gastrointestinal tract, with the hydroquinone being transported as a conjugate systemically and free hydroquinone being liberated in the urine.

Antimicrobial properties have been demonstrated in vitro for uva-ursi against a number of organisms, including *Staphylococcus aureus*, *Bacillus subtilis*, *Escherichia coli*, and *Shigella* species.

> *Antimicrobial properties have been demonstrated in vitro for uva-ursi against a number of organisms, including* **Staphylococcus aureus, Bacillus subtilis, Escherichia coli,** *and* **Shigella** *species.*

Cystitis

One double-blind, placebo-controlled, randomized study evaluated the efficacy of uva-ursi in preventing episodes of cystitis (inflammation of the urinary bladder). The 57 women in the study received either UVA-E (composed of uva-ursi and dandelion extracts, additional details not available) or a placebo. All women had experienced at least three episodes of cystitis in the year preceding the trial. After 1 year, 23% of women in the placebo group had a cystitis episode, compared with 0% in the UVA-E group. The results were statistically significant (p = 0.05), and no adverse events were reported in either group. Although promising, further research is needed to confirm these preliminary findings. Since the product contained dandelion as well as uva-ursi, it is impossible to determine the specific role played by uva-ursi in the product's therapeutic effectiveness.

Adverse Effects

A case report describes how a healthy 56-year-old woman suffered from severe eye damage (bull's eye maculopathy) after ingesting uva-ursi tea regularly for 3 consecutive years to prevent bladder infections. The active ingredient, arbutoside, is known to stop the production of melanin by inhibiting an enzyme (tyrosine kinase) and is therefore found in many skin-lightening creams. Tyrosine kinase also governs the pigments in the retina of the eye, and its inhibition can result in vision loss.

Another case report describes how a 52-year-old woman with a pre-existing illness (hemoglobin SC disease) suffered from severe kidney damage (tubulointerstitial nephritis) after ingesting an herbal remedy called CKLS for 5 consecutive days. CKLS comprises aloe vera, chamomile, cascara segrada, chapparal, mullien, uva-ursi, fenugreek, cayenne, dandelion, and eucalyptus. The case report also alluded to the fact that uva-ursi has been associated with albuminaria, hematuria, and urine cast but does not provide a reference for this statement.

Consumption of large doses of uva-ursi has resulted in nausea and vomiting. In addition, hydroquinone is known to have a toxic potential resulting in tinnitus, nausea, vomiting, shortness of breath, cyanosis, convulsions, delirium, and collapse in doses far higher than that normally found in uva-ursi.

Cautions/Contraindications

Uva-ursi should be considered contraindicated in kidney disorders, pregnancy, and lactation. Due to the presence of hydroquinone and the large amount of tannins, prolonged use or the consumption of large amounts of uva-ursi should be avoided.

Drug Interactions

No cases of interactions with conventional medications could be found. Theoretically, caution should be exercised with drugs known to interact with hydroquinone.

Selected Reference

Larsson B, Jonasson A, Fianu S. Prophylactic effect of UVA-E in women with recurrent cystitis — a preliminary report. Current Therapeutic Research — Clinical Experience 1993 Apr;53(4):441–43.

Dosage Regimens

* Dried leaves: 1.5–4 g three times daily.
* Fluid extract (1:1 in 25% alcohol): 1.5–4 mL three times daily.

Note: The ESCOP monograph recommends "cold water infusions of the crude drug equivalent to 400–800 mg arbutin per day in divided doses." The duration of treatment should be limited to 2 weeks and medical attention sought if there is a worsening of symptoms. Cold water infusions are preferable to hot ones because they contain fewer tannins. Uva-ursi is often given with an alkalinizing agent, such as sodium bicarbonate.

Valerian

Valeriana officinalis L.
and other species of *Valeriana*

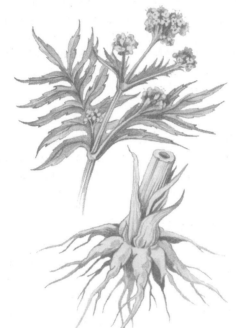

Introduction

Family
- Valerianaceae

Synonyms
- All-heal
- Amantilla
- Balderbrackenwurzel
- Baldrian
- Baldrianwurzel
- Capon's tail
- Cat's tail
- Fragrant valerian
- Garden heliotrope
- Katzenwurzel
- Racine de valeriane
- Setewale
- Setwall
- Valerian root
- *Valerianae radix*
- Valeriane

Medicinal Forms
- Dried root or rhizome
- Tincture

Description

There are more than 200 valerian species and variants found in Australia, China, Europe, India, Japan, and North America, including Mexico. This perennial plant grows up to 125 centimeters (4 feet) in height, with pairs of opposing, almond-shaped, serrated leaves arising from a grooved, hollow stem. Small, rose-colored flowers bloom from the top of the stem in the summer months. The root produces an odor variously described as offensive, distinctive, and penetrating.

Parts Used

The tuberous root and dried rhizome of three species — *V. officinalis* L., *V. jatamansi* Jones (Indian valerian), and *V. edulis* Nutt. ex. Torr. & Gray sp. *procera* F.G. Meyer (Mexican valerian) — are most often used for medicinal purposes.

Traditional Use

Although not specifically mentioned in classical Greek or Roman medical writings, the use of valerian has been attributed to Hippocrates as early as 425 BC. Valerian's medicinal use in Asia, Australia, Europe, the Middle East, and North America has been documented in Greek, Anglo-Saxon, Medieval, and Renaissance texts. It has been used as a sedative and an antinauseant, as well as for gastrointestinal and urinary symptoms.

Current Medicinal Use

While valerian is primarily used in the treatment of mild insomnia, it is increasingly being found in herbal products used to treat muscle spasms and pain.

Relevant Research

Preventative and Therapeutic Effects

Constituents
- Amino acids: gamma-aminobutyric acid (GABA).
- Alkaloids: actinidine, chatinine, skyanthine, valerianine, valerine.
- Iridoids (valepotriates): valerate(s), dihydrovalerate(s), valerosidate.
- Volatile oils: monoterpenes, sesquiterpenes (e.g. valerenic acid), valerenyl esters.
- Phenylpropanoids: caffeic acid, chlorogenic acid.
- Sesquiterpenoids: valerenolic acid, acetylvalerenolic acid.

Sedative and Hypnotic Effect

Valerian is most often used as a sedative and hypnotic agent. Because of the herb's historical use as a sedative, most basic science research has been directed at the interaction of valerian constituents with the GABA neurotransmitter receptor system. These studies remain inconclusive, and all require independent replication. The mechanism of action of valerian in general, and as a mild sedative in particular, remains unknown.

Valerian extracts appear to have some affinity for the GABAA (benzodiazepine) receptor, but this activity does not appear to be mediated by valerenic acid but rather by the relatively high content of GABA itself. The amount of GABA present in aqueous extracts of valerian is sufficient to account for the release of GABA from synaptosomes, and also may inhibit reuptake. However, GABA does not cross the blood-brain barrier efficiently at low concentrations, so these in vitro results cannot account for the clinical data. Catabolism of GABA may be inhibited by valerenolic acid and acetylvalerenolic acid.

Interactions with the serotonin neurotransmitter system have also been investigated, and hydroxypinoresinol was found to have high affinity for the 5-HT1A receptor. One paper reports an interaction with the adenosine receptor but not with the benzodiazepine receptor.

Insomnia

The most common use for valerian is the management of sleep disorders, including insomnia. However, the scientific evidence is both inconsistent and inconclusive. A 2006 meta-analysis of 16 clinical trials involving 1,093 patients concluded that valerian might improve sleep quality. However, the authors noted that there was a wide range of valerian preparations and doses, further complicated by the poor methodological quality of the studies and evidence of publication bias. They argue for more research before a definitive conclusion can be made.

In contrast, a 2007 systematic review identified 37 distinct studies (29 controlled trials that assessed safety and efficacy and 8 open-label trials that assessed safety alone). The authors reported that most studies found no significant differences between valerian or placebo treatments and that none of the most recent or most methodological rigorous studies reported positive effects. Overall, the authors concluded that the evidence indicates that valerian is not clinically efficacious as a sleep aid for insomnia.

> *The most common use for valerian is the management of sleep disorders, including insomnia. However, the scientific evidence is both inconsistent and inconclusive.*

Antianxiety

Several clinical trials provide some clinical evidence that valerian may be helpful in the management of anxiety-related symptoms; however, others produced negative results, and many of the trials have poor methodological quality, in that valerian was only one of several active compounds tested in combination with other products. Additional research is needed to confirm the preliminary findings to date.

One randomized, double-blind, controlled pilot study found no significant differences in total Hamilton Anxiety Scale (HAS or HAMA) scores between 36 individuals diagnosed with generalized anxiety disorder who took valerian (mean daily dose 81.3 mg valepotriates daily) compared with diazepam (mean daily dose 6.5 mg) and a placebo — all groups improved significantly from baseline scores. Given the small number of participants in this pilot study, the authors indicated that their results must be viewed as preliminary and recommended additional studies.

A second randomized, placebo-controlled trial enrolled 40 patients with mild anxiety. Participants took either valerian (100 mg) or a placebo three times daily for 21 days. The statistical analysis of the results was very poorly presented; however, the authors conclude that the valerian group had statistically significant reductions in anxiety compared to those taking a placebo.

Miscellaneous Effects
Benzodiazepine Withdrawal
A randomized, double-blind, placebo-controlled study assessing the use of valerian (100 mg Valmane three times daily) on benzodiazepine withdrawal reported subjective sleep quality improvement after 2 weeks of treatment of insomniacs who had withdrawn from benzodiazepines. The authors also reported an objective decrease in wake time after sleep onset in those treated with valerian, but those taking valerian took longer to get to sleep compared with the placebo control group. Overall, the authors concluded that valerian had a positive effect on withdrawal from benzodiazepine use.

Depression
One open-label study suggests that using valerian and St. John's wort in combination was better than St. John's wort alone for the treatment of depression that is combined with anxiety. A total of 500 patients diagnosed with mild to moderate depression and anxiety were given either 500 mg of valerian and 600 mg of St. John's wort daily (Group 1) or 1,000 mg of valerian and 600 mg of St. John's wort daily (Group 2) for 3 months. The study compared their results with those of a multi-center study of 2,166 patients using only St. John's wort and concluded that the combination treatment resulted in faster improvement (no statistics were reported). Additional research is needed to confirm this preliminary finding.

Other Effects
Valerian has been reported to decrease gastrointestinal motility. There is also some suggestion that valerian extracts have an antipyretic or anti-inflammatory effect.

Adverse Effects
Clinical trials report very few adverse effects associated with valerian. Gastrointestinal upset, headaches, and vivid dreams have been reported in a few patients in clinical trials. Tachycardia and high-output cardiac failure were reported following withdrawal (stopping valerian) in one case of a patient suffering from coronary artery disease who had been self-medicating with high doses of valerian (530 mg to 2 g per dose five times daily) for many years. Hepatotoxicity has been reported with herbal sleep remedies, but these contained other ingredients in combination with valerian, and thus it is not clear if this toxicity is related in any way to use of valerian.

Cautions/Contraindications
Valerian should be used with caution in children under 3 years of age. Individuals taking valerian should be cautious when operating a motor vehicle or hazardous machinery.

Valerian is not recommended for use in pregnant and breastfeeding women because in vitro studies have shown that the valepotriates and baldrinals appear to have cytotoxic and mutagenic properties. It is important to note that such substances are unstable and are generally not found in commercially available valerian products; however, until more research is available, caution is recommended. An open-label retrospective study of 860,215 women on the Swedish birth registry identified that less than 1% had ingested any herbal product during their pregnancy and that valerian was among the most common three herbs used by women who had taken an herb. No signs of unfavorable effects on pregnancy outcome were noted; however, since the number of exposures was so low, effects on rare outcomes could not be excluded.

Drug Interactions
The following valerian-drug interactions have been documented or identified as theoretically possible. In addition, valerian has been found to be a non-competitive inhibitor of CYP 2D6, and thus theoretically may interact with medications metabolized by this liver enzyme.

- **Anti-anxiety medications:** Clinical trials indicate that valerian may have an additive effect if taken together with conventional anti-anxiety medication. In animal studies, valerian has been found to increase the effects of central nervous system depressants and prolong barbiturate-induced sleeping time.

- **Sedatives:** Animal studies suggest that valerian may have an additive effect when taken with other sedatives, but clinical studies in humans have not documented increases in side effects from the combination. Caution is warranted until additional evidence is available.

- **Monoamine oxidase inhibitors (MOAIs):** Valerian may increase both the therapeutic and side effects (e.g., drowsiness) of antidepressants. However, this is an area that needs more research before definitive conclusions can be made.

- **Selective serotonin reuptake inhibitors (SSRIs):** Valerian may increase both the therapeutic and side effects (e.g., drowsiness) of antidepressants. However, this is an area that needs more research before definitive conclusions can be made. There is one case report of a patient taking fluoxetine (Prozac) who had reported that, 12 hours after taking valerian tablets, he experienced mental status changes and lost control of his left arm. The patient's symptoms resolved after another 12 hours, and whether valerian was ascosiated with the symptoms was not conclusively determined.

- **Loperamide:** There is one case of a patient suffering a brief episode of acute delirium while taking valerian with loperamide. It is important to note that this patient was also taking St. John's wort, so it was difficult to know whether valerian was the cause of this event.

- **Beta blockers:** In a randomized, double-blind, placebo-controlled trial, a combination of 100 mg valerian and 20 mg propranolol impaired subjects' performance on a written concentration test more than valerian alone. The effect of propranolol alone was not tested during the study, which made it difficult to know whether this effect was due to an interaction between valerian and propranolol or to propranolol alone.

- **Anticonvulsants:** Valerian products might interact with antiseizure agents, although there has been no evidence of such an interaction in clinical studies.

Dosage Regimens
- Dried root or rhizome (or equivalent dry extracts): 2–3 g three times daily or at bedtime.
- Tincture (20% concentration by volume in a 70% ethanol solution): 1–3 mL three times daily or at bedtime.
- Insomnia: Doses range widely, from 300–1,800 mg of aqueous or aqueous-ethanolic extracts (corresponding to 1.5–6 g of herb)
- Children: There is not enough evidence to recommend valerian for use in children.

Selected References

Andreatini R, Sartori V, Seabra M, Leite J. Effect of valepotriates (valerian extract) in generalized anxiety disorder: a randomized placebo-controlled pilot study. Phytotherapy Research 2002;16:650–54.

Bent S, Padula A, Moore D, Patterson M, Mehling W. Valerian for sleep: A systematic review and meta-analysis. American Journal of Medicine 2006;119(12):1005–12.

Taibi DM, Landis CA, Petry H, Vitiello MV. A systematic review of valerian as a sleep aid: Safe but not effective. Sleep Medicine Review 2007;11(3):209–30.

Wild Yam

Dioscorea villosa L.

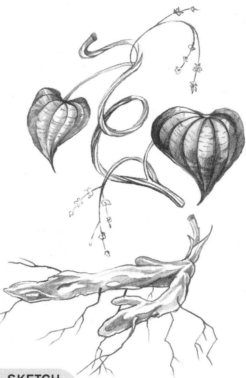

Common Uses
- Gynecological problems (dysmennorhoea and ovarian pains)

Active Constituents
- Steroidal glycosides (based on the sapogenin diosgenin)

Adverse Effects
- Gastrointestinal upset and headaches (rare)

Cautions/Contraindications
- Pregnancy
- Hormone-sensitive conditions (e.g., breast cancer)

Drug Interactions
- None could be found

Doses
- *Dried root:* 2–4 g daily in divided doses
- *Capsules:* 250 mg taken one to three times daily
- *Liquid extract (45% alcohol):* 2–4 mL daily in divided doses
- *Tincture:* 4–12 drops taken three to five times daily
- *Children:* Not recommended for consumption by children

Introduction

Family
- Dioscoreaceae

Synonyms
- Atlantic yam
- Barbasco
- Colic root
- China root
- Devil's bones
- Dioscoreae
- Mexican yam
- Rheumatism root
- Shan yao
- Wild yam root

Medicinal Forms
- Tincture
- Creams

Description

Many different species of the genus *Dioscorea* exist, but within the complementary medical model, *Dioscorea villosa* is the one most often used. Wild yam (*Dioscorea villosa*) is distinct from the vegetable often referred to as yam (*Ipomoea batatas* (L.) Lam., Convolvulaceae). *Dioscorea villosa* is a perennial vine, growing to 6 meters (20 feet), with small green flowers, heart-shaped leaves, and a large, fibrous root stock. The plant is native to the eastern United States and Central America. It has a characteristic taste often described as insipid.

Parts Used

The tuberous roots are the part used medicinally. The therapeutic actions disappear on storage, so it is best harvested annually.

Traditional Use

The Aztecs, Mayans, and other Native peoples of North and Central America used wild yam to treat painful menstruation and labor. The plant was also known as colic root and rheumatism root. This herb was used extensively by Eclectic physicians in the United States during the mid to latter part of the 19th century. Diosgenin, a steroid-like substance found in wild yam, was used in the development of modern contraceptives.

Current Medicinal Use

Unprocessed wild yam products are primarily used to treat digestive disorders, such as colic, diverticulitis, and irritable bowel syndrome. Semi-synthetic products containing hormones made from diosgenin are used in treating a number of gynecological conditions, although more research is needed to confirm this use.

Relevant Research

Preventative and Therapeutic Effects

Constituents
- Steroidal saponins (based on the sapogenin diosgenin), including dioscin and dioscorin.
- Dioscorein is not an actual constituent but refers to a dried solid extract.

Common Uses

Wild yam is reputed to have antispasmodic, anti-inflammatory, diuretic, hepatic, and anti-rheumatic properties. Oral consumption is considered useful in the treatment of digestive conditions, such as intestinal colic, diverticulitis, irritable bowel syndrome, and bilious indigestion. As a traditional anti-rheumatic, it is used in situations of arthritis and joint inflammation. It is also considered a "relaxing remedy" and is used to treat a number of gynecological problems, such as ovarian pain, painful menstruation, and pain in labor.

Hormone Effects

Diosgenin, isolated from Mexican yam, was originally considered of prime importance in the pharmaceutical manufacture of a number of steroidal substances, including early oral contraceptives. Confusion has arisen because of claims that diosgenin can be converted into a number of steroidal substances, including dehydroepiandrosterone (DHEA) and progesterone, following oral or topical administration. Some products have been marketed as "hormonal precursors." No evidence could be found to substantiate these claims.

One study demonstrated that oral administration of a compound containing 90% wild yam extract did not increase serum dehydroepiandrosterone sulfate (DHEA-S) levels in a group of 7 patients over 65 years of age. The results of this study were supported by a similar investigation in which saliva specimens were analyzed in a group of women taking products containing Mexican yam.

Concerns have been expressed about the use and marketing of wild yam extracts as "hormonal precursors." There appears to be no evidence to support this claim. This confusion seems to be particularly important in the use of natural progesterone products.

> *Diosgenin, isolated from Mexican yam, was originally considered of prime importance in the pharmaceutical manufacture of a number of steroidal substances, including early oral contraceptives.*

Menopausal Symptoms

A 2001 double-blind, placebo-controlled crossover study reported that the application of wild yam cream, known to contain steroidal saponins, to 23 healthy, menopausal woman over a 3-month period had no significant effects on their menopausal symptoms of flushing and nocturnal sweats. No changes in serum lipids and hormones or salivary progesterone were observed. The authors concluded that short-term treatment with topical wild yam extract in women suffering from menopausal symptoms is safe but does not appear to have any effect on menopausal symptoms. Additional studies are required to confirm these findings.

> *The authors concluded that short-term treatment with topical wild yam extract in women suffering from menopausal symptoms is safe but does not appear to have any effect on menopausal symptoms.*

Diosgenin, a steroidal component of wild yam, has been postulated to influence endogenous steroidogenesis in humans when applied topically to the skin. The exact pathway through which this is supposed to take place is not known. Wild yam has been reported to be a weak antagonist of estrogen but with no progestational activity. It has been postulated that the ingestion of wild yam can lead to an increase of serum dehyroepiandrosterone (DHEA); however, available human research suggests that humans lack the enzymes needed to convert orally ingested wild yam to DHEA.

Lipid-Reducing Effects

One randomized, controlled, open-label, human trial (N=7) reported that daily ingestion of a commercial preparation containing 90% Mexican wild yam extract (the remaining 10% was a composition of kola nut extract, country mallow, cellulose, atlantic kelp, cayenne pepper, silica, manapol, and stearic acid) for 8 weeks produced a significant decline in serum triglyceride and phospholipid levels compared to a placebo. No significant change was observed in plasma total cholesterol.

Many scientists investigating the effects of diosgenin, a compound found in wild yam, on the absorption and synthesis of cholesterol in animals, mainly rats, have reported that ingestion of diosgenin causes lower absorption of cholesterol in the body and a concurrent increase in the biosynthesis of cholesterol within the body, with no negative side effects reported. The results of animal studies are promising, and more human trials are recommended.

Miscellaneous Effects
Antioxidant
Two experiments suggest that dioscorin, which is one of the chemical constituents of wild yam, exhibits antioxidant activities.

Cancer Prevention
One in vitro experiment suggested that wild yam extract may be helpful as a cancer chemopreventive agent in the treatment of Epstein-Barr virus–induced B-cell lymphoma. The researcher reported significant inhibition of the activation of the virus by the wild yam root. Further experimentation is warranted to reproduce these findings.

Adverse Effects
Adverse effects appear to be rare but include gastrointestinal upset, nausea and vomiting, fever, headache, sleep disturbances, and dry mouth.

Cautions/Contraindications
Due to potential progestinic and uterine-contracting effects, avoid use during pregnancy. Avoid in patients with hormone-sensitive illnesses, such as cancer of the reproductive organs, due to potential hormonal effects.

Drug Interactions
There have been no reports of drug interactions in humans. However, based on animal and in vitro study data, a number of theoretical interactions with drugs are possible, including:

- Cholesterol-lowering agents: Wild yam may potentiate the effects of other lipid-lowering agents, warranting caution.

- Hormone replacement therapy (HRT) or oral contraceptives: A small study reported that wild yam suppressed progesterone synthesis in women, suggesting that wild yam may interfere with hormonal therapies. However, further clinical studies are warranted, as anecdotal reports suggest that wild yam products are sometimes contaminated with synthetic progesterone.

- Non-steroidal anti-inflammatory drugs (NSAIDs): An animal study reported that wild yam lowered serum indomethacin (an NSAID) levels in rats, attenuating intestinal inflammation. Caution is warranted when using NSAIDs in conjunction with wild yam.

Dosage Regimens
- Dried root: 2–4 g daily in divided doses (unconfirmed by scientific studies).
- Capsules: 250 mg taken one to three times daily (unconfirmed by scientific studies).
- Liquid extract (45% alcohol): 2–4 mL daily in divided doses (unconfirmed by scientific studies).
- Tincture: 4–12 drops taken three to five times daily (unconfirmed by scientific studies).
- Children: Not recommended for consumption by children.

Selected References
Araghiniknam M, Chung S, Nelson-White T, Eskelson C, Watson RR. Antioxidant activity of dioscorea and dehydroepiandrosterone (DHEA) in older humans. Life Science 1996; 59(11):147–57.

Komesaroff PA, Black CV, Cable V. Effects of wild yam extract on menopausal symptoms, lipids, and sex hormones in healthy menopausal women. Climacteric 2001; 4(2):144–50.

Willow

Salix spp.

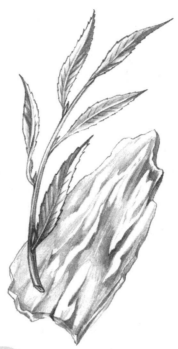

Common Uses
- Arthritic conditions
- Analgesic

Active Constituents
- Phenolic glycosides (including salicin and salicortin)

Adverse Effects
- Nausea, headache, digestive upset (rare)

Cautions/Contraindications
- Classic ones applicable to salicylates (e.g., aspirin)

Drug Interactions
- Classic ones applicable to salicylates (e.g., aspirin)

Doses
- *Raw herb:* 5–10 g three times daily
- *Willow preparations (dried, hydroalcoholic, or aqueous extracts, tinctures, or fluid extracts):* equivalent to 60–120 mg (up to 240 mg) of salicin daily
- *Salicin:* 20–40 mg three times daily (maximum of 240 mg of salicin daily)
- *Liquid extract (1:1 in 25% ethanol):* 1–2 mL three times daily
- *Hydroalcoholic tincture (1:5 in 25% ethanol):* 5–8 mL three times daily

Introduction

Family
- Salicaeae

Synonyms
Members of the Salix genus commonly used medicinally include:

- *S. fragilis* L. (crack willow)
- *S. nigra* Marsh (black willow)
- *S. alba* L. (white willow)
- *S. purpurea* L. (purple osier willow)
- *S. daphnoides* Villars (European daphne willow)
- *S. cinerea* L. (large gray willow)

Medicinal Form
- Raw herb
- Willow preparations (dried, extracts, tincture)
- Salicin

Description
Members of this genus of trees, native to Europe, Asia, and North America, range in height from 10 to 25 meters (30 to 70 feet), with soft green, "willowy" leaves and a soft bark that is easily separated or peeled from the young branches. While in North America white willow and black willow are most often used, pharmacologically these may not be the most active. Other members of the genus (e.g., *S. fragilis* L., *S. purpurea* L., and *S. daphnoides* Villars) are richer in the medicinally active phenolic glycosides.

Parts Used
The bark of young branches is the part most commonly used medicinally. However, it has been shown that the leaves of some species may contain as much and maybe more of the phenolic glycosides than the bark. Accordingly, it has been argued that there is no reason why these parts cannot be used therapeutically.

Traditional Use
Willow has a long history in many different healing traditions. It was especially popular in the treatment of rheumatism and ague (i.e, fever, chills).

Current Medicinal Use
Willow products are considered "natural painkillers" and are typically used in the treatment of joint pains, notably from arthritis, and in low back pain. Since willow does not contain aspirin (acetylsalicylic acid), it should not used as an aspirin substitute in thinning the blood.

Relevant Research

Preventative and Therapeutic Effects

Constituents
- Phenolic glycosides: include salicin, salicortin, tremulacin, salireposide.
- Miscellaneous: include condensed tannins, flavonoids, catechins.

Note: There is great variability among species of the *Salix* genus, and of particular importance are the phenolic glycoside components. While *Salix purpurea* can contain up to 8% salicin and *Salix fragilis* up to 10%, *S. alba* often has less than 1% salicin.

Common Uses
Preparations of white willow bark have been used in the treatment of feverish conditions and rheumatism and as a mild pain killer in such conditions as headaches. Given the rela-

tively low amount of phenolic glycosides, notably salicin, when compared to conventional salicylate medications, it has been argued that, in pharmacological terms, it is unlikely that any willow preparation will be effective in the management of these conditions.

The pharmacological action of willow appears to be determined not only by salicin content, however. The other phenolic glycosides also have therapeutic properties. It is hypothesized that the phenolic glycosides do not act directly but rather as pro-drugs. They are converted in multiple stages, primarily in the liver and intestines, to the active moieties, most notably salicylic acid. The action is therefore slower in onset than conventional salicylic acid but has a longer duration of action. It should be noted that salicin does not irreversibly inhibit platelet aggregation, as is the case with acetylsalicylic acid.

Limited in vivo studies demonstrate that a number of the phenolic glycosides have anti-inflammatory properties. Little research has been conducted on the salicylates and salicylic acid obtained from plant sources such as willow.

Low Back Pain

One review of herbal medicines for back pain cautiously concluded that extracts of willow appear to be effective for providing short-term improvements of low back pain. Three of the trials in the review specifically evaluated willow. The first trial was an open, randomized, post-marketing 4-week study. A total of 228 patients were assigned to receive a daily dose of an herbal extract containing 240 mg of salicin or 12.5 mg of the drug rofecoxib. At the end of the trial, there was no significant difference in low back pain symptoms between the treatments, with 60% of patients from both treatment groups reporting improvement.

The second randomized, double-blind, placebo-controlled trial involved 51 patients and reported that a daily dose of willow extract containing 240 mg salicin was more effective than the placebo at reducing platelet aggregation (a marker for inflammation) in patients suffering from low back pain exacerbations but was not as effective as acetylsalicylate (ASA).

The third randomized, double-blind, placebo-controlled 4-week trial included 210 patients and reported that willow bark extract (120 mg or 240 mg of salicin) was more effective (dose-dependent effects were noted) than the placebo in treating patients with exacerbations of chronic low pack pain. While promising, more research is necessary to confirm these findings.

> *One review of herbal medicines for back pain cautiously concluded that extracts of willow appear to be effective for providing short-term improvements of low back pain.*

Osteoarthritis

A randomized, placebo-controlled, double-blind 2-week trial (N=78) reported that willow extract containing 240 mg salicin given daily significantly decreased pain (as assessed by the WOMAC Osteoarthritis Index, patient diary, and visual analog scores) associated with osteoarthritis. As with the results for back pain, additional studies are needed to confirm these findings.

Anticancer Effect

One test tube study reported that willow extract was effective at stopping the growth of human colon and cancer cells. Clinical studies are needed to confirm these findings.

Adverse Effects

Adverse effects seem to be rare and mild, limited to nausea, digestive upset, skin allergies, and headache. A case of hemorrhage in a 64-year-old women with glucose-6-phosphate dehydrogenase (G6PD) deficiency has been documented following the consumption of an Ayurvedic product containing *Salix caprea* L. No information is given in the case report with regard to other ingredients present in the preparation.

A clinical trial (N=35) confirms that willow extract with 240 mg salicin in a daily dose reduces arachidonic acid–induced platelet aggregation compared to a placebo but does not reduce it as much as 100 mg of acetyl-salicylate (ASA). The authors suggest that further research is necessary to determine whether these effects are of clinical relevance for patients with impaired thrombocyte function.

One participant in a clinical trial who was randomized to the willow bark group experienced a severe allergic reaction (swollen eyes and pruritis). These symptoms resolved 2 days after discontinuing willow (containing 120 mg of salicin).

Cautions/Contraindications
The contraindications applicable to the use of conventional salicylate preparations are believed to be applicable to the consumption of willow products. Consequently, use should be avoided in individuals with such conditions as asthma, diabetes, gout, hemophilia, hyper-thrombinemia, hepatic or renal disease, active peptic ulcer disease, and glucose-6-phosphate dehydrogenase (G6PD) deficiency, and indi-viduals sensitive to aspirin. Until more detailed information is available, preparations con-taining willow should not be administered during pregnancy or lactation. No information could be found regarding the use of willow products in children, given that salicylate-containing products are normally restricted to individuals over 12 years of age.

Drug Interactions
One clinical study involving 171 people examined the risk of warfarin-related bleeding events and reported that patients taking warfarin along with willow and at least one other natural health product were nine times as likely to report an adverse bleeding event. The authors also noted that no indi-vidual natural health product by itself significantly increased the risk of excessive blood thinning.

No cases could be found in the literature, but prudence suggests that drug interactions common to conventional salicylates may be applicable to willow-containing products.

Dosage Regimens
- Raw herb: 5–10 g three times daily.
- Willow preparations (dried, hydro-alcoholic or aqueous extracts, tinctures, or fluid extracts): equiva-lent to 60–120 mg (up to 240 mg) of salicin daily.
- Salicin: 20–40 mg three times daily.
- Liquid extract (1:1 in 25% ethanol): 1–2 mL three times daily.
- Hydroalcoholic tincture (1:5 in 25% ethanol): 5–8 mL three times daily.

Selected References

Chrubasik S, Eisenberg E, Balan E, Weinberger T, Luzzati R, Conradt C. Treatment of low back pain exacerbations with willow bark extract: A randomized double-blind study. American Journal of Medicine 2000;109(1):9–14.

Chrubasik S, Kunzel O, Model A, Conradt C, Black A. Treatment of low back pain with a herbal or synthetic anti-rheumatic: A random-ized controlled study. Willow bark extract for low back pain. Rheumatology 2001;40(12):1388–93.

Krivoy N, Pavlotzky E, Chrubasik S, Eisenberg E, Brook G. Effect of salicis cortex extract on human platelet aggregation. Planta Medica 2001;67(3):209–12.

Canadian Cataloguing in Publication Data

Boon, Heather

55 most common medicinal herbs: the complete natural medicine guide / Heather Boon, Michael Smith. — 2nd ed.

Previously published under title: The complete natural medicine guide to the 50 most common medicinal herbs.

Includes bibliographical references and index.

ISBN 978-0-7788-0215-0

1. Herbals. 2. Naturopathy. 3. Herbs—Therapeutic use. I. Smith, Michael J., 1963–. II. Title. III. Title: Fifty-five most common medicinal herbs.

RS164.B66 2009   615'.321   C2008-907703-2

Index

More Great Books from Robert Rose

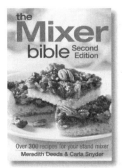
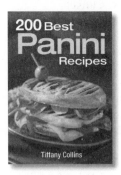
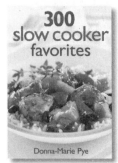
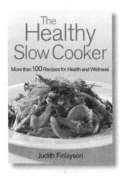

Appliance Cooking

- The Dehydrator Bible
  *by Jennifer MacKenzie,
  Jay Nutt & Don Mercer*
- The Mixer Bible
  Second Edition
  *by Meredith Deeds and
  Carla Snyder*
- The Juicing Bible
  Second Edition
  by Pat Crocker
- 200 Best Panini Recipes
  by Tiffany Collins
- 200 Best Pressure
  Cooker Recipes
  by Cinda Chavich
- 300 Slow Cooker
  Favorites
  by Donna-Marie Pye
- The 150 Best Slow
  Cooker Recipes
  by Judith Finlayson
- Delicious &
  Dependable Slow
  Cooker Recipes
  by Judith Finlayson
- 125 Best Vegetarian
  Slow Cooker Recipes
  by Judith Finlayson
- The Healthy Slow
  Cooker
  by Judith Finlayson
- The Best Convection
  Oven Cookbook
  by Linda Stephen
- 250 Best American
  Bread Machine
  Baking Recipes
  *by Donna Washburn
  and Heather Butt*
- 250 Best Canadian
  Bread Machine
  Baking Recipes
  *by Donna Washburn
  and Heather Butt*

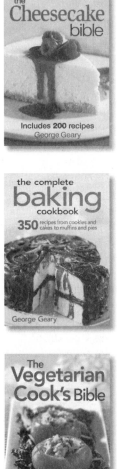
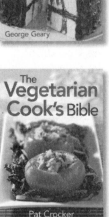
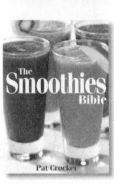

Baking

- The Cheesecake Bible
  by George Geary
- 1500 Best Bars, Cookies,
  Muffins, Cakes & More
  by Esther Brody
- The Complete Book
  of Baking
  by George Geary
- The Complete Book
  of Bars & Squares
  by Jill Snider
- The Complete Book
  of Pies
  by Julie Hasson
- 125 Best Chocolate
  Recipes
  by Julie Hasson
- 125 Best Cupcake
  Recipes
  by Julie Hasson
- Complete Cake
  Mix Magic
  by Jill Snider

Healthy Cooking

- The Vegetarian Cook's
  Bible
  by Pat Crocker
- The Vegan Cook's
  Bible
  by Pat Crocker
- 125 Best Vegetarian
  Recipes
  *by Byron Ayanoglu
  with contributions from
  Algis Kemezys*
- The Smoothies Bible
  by Pat Crocker
- 125 Best Vegan
  Recipes
  *by Maxine Effenson Chuck
  and Beth Gurney*

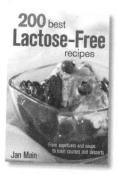

- 200 Best Lactose-Free Recipes
  by Jan Main
- 500 Best Healthy Recipes
  Edited by Lynn Roblin, RD
- Complete Gluten-Free Cookbook
  by Donna Washburn and Heather Butt

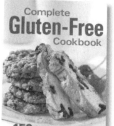

- 125 Best Gluten-Free Recipes
  by Donna Washburn and Heather Butt
- The Best Gluten-Free Family Cookbook
  by Donna Washburn and Heather Butt
- Diabetes Meals for Good Health
  Karen Graham, RD
- Canada's Diabetes Meals for Good Health
  Karen Graham, RD

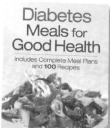

- America's Complete Diabetes Cookbook
  Edited by Katherine E. Younker, MBA, RD
- Canada's Complete Diabetes Cookbook
  Edited by Katherine E. Younker, MBA, RD

Recent Bestsellers

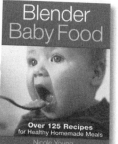

- 125 Best Soup Recipes
  by Marylin Crowley and Joan Mackie
- The Convenience Cook
  by Judith Finlayson
- 125 Best Ice Cream Recipes
  by Marilyn Linton and Tanya Linton

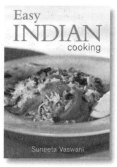

- Easy Indian Cooking
  by Suneeta Vaswani
- Baby Blender Food
  by Nicole Young
- Simply Thai Cooking
  by Wandee Young and Byron Ayanoglu

Health

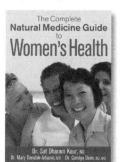

- The Complete Natural Medicine Guide to Women's Health
  by Dr. Sat Dharam Kaur, ND, Dr. Mary Danylak-Arhanic, MD and Dr. Carolyn Dean, ND, MD
- The Complete Natural Medicine Guide to Breast Cancer
  by Dr. Sat Dharam Kaur, ND

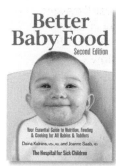

- Better Baby Food Second Edition
  by Daina Kalnins, MSc, RD, and Joanne Saab, RD
- Canada's Baby Care Book
  by Dr. Jeremy Friedman MBChB, FRCP(C), FAAP, and Dr. Norman Saunders MD, FRCP(C)
- The Baby Care Book
  by Dr. Jeremy Friedman MBChB, FRCP(C), FAAP, and Dr. Norman Saunders MD, FRCP(C)

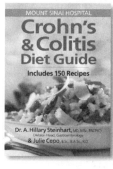

- Crohn's & Colitis
  by Dr. A. Hillary Steinhart, MD, MSc, FRCP(C)
- Crohn's & Colitis Diet Guide
  by Dr. A. Hillary Steinhart, MD, MSc, FRCP(C), and Julie Cepo, BSc, BASc, RD